Expert Pain Management

SPRINGHOUSE CORPORATION
Springhouse, Pennsylvania

Staff

Executive Director
Matthew Cahill

Editorial Director
June Norris

Art Director
John Hubbard

Managing Editor
David Moreau

Acquisitions Editors
Patricia Kardish Fischer, RN, BSN;
Louise Quinn

Copy Editors
Cynthia C. Breuninger (manager),
Christine Cunniffe, Brenna Mayer,
Christina P. Ponczek

Designers
Arlene Putterman (associate art
director), STELLARViSIONs (book
design and illustrations), Jacalyn
Facciolo (illustrations)

Manufacturing
Deborah Meiris (director), Pat Dorshaw
(manager), Anna Brindisi, T.A. Landis

Production Coordinator
Margaret A. Rastiello

Editorial Assistants
Beverly Lane, Mary Madden,
Jeanne Napier

Ⓡ A member of the Reed Elsevier plc group

Printed in the United States of America.

EPM-010796
ISBN 0-87434-777-7

Library of Congress Cataloging-in-Publication Data
Expert pain management
p. cm.
Includes bibliographical references and index.
1. Pain—Treatment. 2. Nursing. I. Springhouse Corporation.
[DNLM: 1. Pain—therapy—nurses' instruction. WL 704 E96 1997]
RB127.E97 1997
616'.0472—dc20
DNLM/DLC   96-3089
ISBN 0-87434-777-7 (alk. paper)   CIP

Expert Pain Management

Contents

Consultant, Contributors, and Reviewers

Springhouse Corporation wishes to acknowledge the assistance of the American Pain Society in identifying chapter authors. At the time of publication, the consultant, contributors, and reviewers held the positions listed.

Consultant

Paula Bakule
Editor
Doylestown, Pa.

Contributors

Mary F. Bezkor, MD
Assistant Professor of Clinical
    Rehabilitation Medicine
School of Medicine
New York University
New York

Raeford E. Brown, Jr., MD
Professor of Anesthesiology and
    Pediatrics
Executive Vice Chairman
Department of Anesthesiology
University of Arkansas for Medical
    Sciences
Little Rock

Michael G. Byas-Smith, MD
Assistant Professor
Department of Anesthesiology
School of Medicine
Emory University
Atlanta

Corey L. Cleland, PhD
Adjunct Assistant Professor
Department of Physiology and
    Biophysics
University of Iowa
Iowa City

Betty R. Ferrell, RN, PhD, FAAN
Associate Research Scientist
Nursing Education and Research
City of Hope National Medical
    Center
Duarte, Calif.

Bruce A. Ferrell, MD, FACP
Associate Professor of Medicine
    and Geriatrics
School of Medicine
University of California at Los
    Angeles
Sepulveda VA Medical Center
Sepulveda, Calif.

G. F. Gebhart, PhD
Professor and Head
Department of Pharmacology
College of Medicine
University of Iowa
Iowa City

Richard V. Gregg, MD
Director, Greater Cincinnati Pain
    Consortium
Associate Professor
Department of Anesthesiology
College of Medicine
University of Cincinnati

Rajat Gupta, MD
Pain Fellow, Instructor
Department of Neurosurgery
School of Medicine
Johns Hopkins University
Baltimore

Asteghik Hacobian, MD
Clinical Fellow of Anesthesia
Harvard Medical School
Boston
Chief of Staff
Northeast Pain Consultation and
    Management
Somersworth, N.H.

Julie Hammack, MD
Assistant Professor
Department of Neurology
Mayo Clinic
Rochester, Minn.

Suzanne L. Howell, RN, PhD
Assistant Research Professor
School of Nursing
University of Colorado
Denver

Sharon L. Jones, PhD
Associate Professor
Department of Pharmacology
College of Medicine
University of Oklahoma
Oklahoma City

Mathew H.M. Lee, MD, MPH, FACP
Medical Director and Professor
Rusk Institute of Rehabilitation
    Medicine
New York University Medical Center
New York

Peter S. Staats, MD
Chief, Division of Pain Medicine
Assistant Professor
Department of Anesthesiology and
    Critical Care Medicine
Department of Oncology
School of Medicine
Johns Hopkins University
Baltimore

Dennis C. Turk, PhD
Professor of Psychiatry and
    Anesthesiology
Director, Pain Evaluation and
    Treatment Institute
University of Pittsburgh Medical
    Center

Ann Tuttle, MD
Assistant Professor of Clinical
    Anesthesia
University of Cincinnati Medical
    Center
Director, Barrett Center
University of Cincinnati Pain
    Consortium

Carol A. Warfield, MD
Associate Professor of Anesthesia
Harvard Medical School
Director, Pain Management Center
Beth Israel Hospital
Boston

Reviewers

Gary J. Bennett, PhD
Chief, Neuropathic Pain and Pain
    Measurement Section
Neurobiology and Anesthesiology
    Branch
National Institute of Dental
    Research
National Institutes of Health
Bethesda, Md.

Rebecca D. Elon, MD, MPH
Medical Director, Johns Hopkins
   Geriatrics Center
Associate Professor of Medicine
School of Medicine
Johns Hopkins University
Baltimore

Brian L. Fellechner, DO
Medical Director, Pain
   Rehabilitation Program
Good Shepherd Rehabilitation
   Hospital
Allentown, Pa.

Noreen Frisch, RN, PhD
President, American Holistic
   Nurses' Association
Chair, Department of Nursing
Humboldt State University
Arcata, Calif.

Francis J. Keefe, PhD
Professor of Medical Psychology
Department of Psychiatry and
   Behavioral Sciences
Duke University School of
   Medicine
Durham, N.C.

Wilhelmina C. Korevaar, MD
Pain Relief and Rehabilitation
Bala Cynwyd, Pa.
Clinical Associate Professor of
   Anesthesiology
Hahnemann University School of
   Medicine
Philadelphia

Thomas H. Kramer, PharmD
Assistant Professor
Department of Anesthesia
University of Pennsylvania School
   of Medicine
Hospital of the University of
   Pennsylvania
Philadelphia

Elliot S. Krames, MD, FACPM
Medical Director
Pacific Pain Treatment Center
San Francisco

Eugenie A.M.T. Obbens, MD
Medical Director
Barrow Neurological Institute Pain
   Clinic
St. Joseph's Hospital and Medical
   Center
Phoenix

Barbara S. Shapiro, MD
Clinical Assistant Professor of
   Pediatrics
University of Pennsylvania School
   of Medicine
Children's Hospital of Philadelphia

Preface

Throughout the ages, the fear of suffering unrelieved pain has been a very real concern that crosses all socioeconomic, political, and cultural lines. Just as pain has existed since the beginning of time, so have attempts at treating it. Early humans often attributed pain to demons and therefore attempted to ward them off with charms, amulets, rattles, and incantations. Eventually, sorceresses and shamans, seen as pain exorcists, became an integral part of human culture. Shrines such as the pyramids were built to appease the gods, and priests used charms and sacrificial offerings as a treatment for pain.

References to pain and pain-relieving techniques abound throughout recorded history. Pain relief was depicted on Babylonian clay tables, Egyptian papyri, and the artifacts of ancient Persia and Troy. About 4,600 years ago, the Chinese first described Yin and Yang, two opposing yet unifying forces in the body, an imbalance of which was thought to be the source of pain. The Egyptians recorded the use of opium for pain relief as early as 1550 BC.

Opium and its active ingredient, morphine, were widely used for many years until eventually the pendulum swung toward the contemporary concern with addiction. Today the widespread fear of drug abuse and addiction has resulted in inadequate and inappropriate treatment of pain. Although recent medical research has provided tremendous technological advances in pain relief, the wealth of knowledge and techniques available are widely underutilized by the health care community.

Inadequate pain management was thought to be such a public health problem that a few years ago, the Agency for Health Care Policy and Research (a division of the U.S. Department of Health and Human Services) convened panels of scientists and health care specialists to compose guidelines for pain treatment. Despite the official recognition of untreated pain as a major public health issue, however, formal medical education and training in pain management lags far behind other topics.

Today pain medicine is a board-certifiable subspecialty. Important breakthroughs in our understanding of pain mechanisms have spurred the development of improved pain management techniques, including intraspinal and transdermal opioid delivery systems, patient-controlled analgesia, and implantable spinal cord stimulators. Using this new knowledge, researchers have also produced several new medications involving nerve transmission of pain.

Perhaps one of the most important advances in pain management has been the development of a multidisciplinary approach. Several years ago the pain therapy prescribed for a patient was primarily determined by a particular practitioner's specialty. For example, if a patient had back pain, an acupuncturist would recommend acupuncture, a physiatrist would recommend physical therapy, a chiropractor would recommend manipulation, an internist would recommend analgesics, an orthopedic surgeon would recommend surgery, a psychiatrist would recommend psychotherapy, and so on. The advent of the multidisciplinary pain clinic brought together the expertise of numerous specialties and drew attention to the importance of the pain management team.

Today this team is composed not only of physicians specializing in pain management, but also nurses, physical therapists, physician assistants, paramedics, pharmacists, psychologists, and other health care practitioners. Each has a unique role in managing pain. In fact, the pain management physician is seldom the first practitioner to assess the patient in pain. More commonly, paramedical personnel must make important assessments and decisions in the triage of such patients. Without this team approach, modern-day pain therapy would be ineffective.

One of the most important requirements of this team approach to pain management is that all of us as colleagues in various health care fields have a solid knowledge of the current pain treatment techniques as well as an understanding of their physiologic and pharmacologic bases. This shared foundation of basic knowledge encourages each of us to draw upon the expertise of our pain management colleagues and thus provide each patient the optimal course of treatment for pain.

Expert Pain Management provides the reader with crucial information about the pathophysiology and mechanisms of pain perception as well as an introduction to the gamut of pain therapies available and the indications for choosing each. It also provides an invaluable clinical guide to treatment of common pain problems. I hope that this text inspires not only implementation of improved pain management techniques, but also a reordering of patient-care priorities such that relief of the patient's pain becomes a primary measure of our effectiveness as health care professionals.

Carol A. Warfield, MD
Associate Professor of Anesthesia
Harvard Medical School
Director, Pain Management Center
Beth Israel Hospital
Boston

CHAPTER 1

Principles of nociception and pain

Corey L. Cleland, PhD
G.F. Gebhart, PhD

Pain is anything but a simple sensation. Classically, the principal senses include sight, sound, smell, taste, and touch. Pain, however, is a unique and complex experience that is influenced by a person's culture, by his or her anticipation and previous experience, by a variety of emotional and cognitive contributions, and by the context in which the pain occurs. Accordingly, reactions to stimuli that produce pain vary among individuals and even within the same individual at different times.

The stimuli that produce pain were termed *noxious* (nocuous) by the great physiologist Sir Charles Scott Sherrington. Noxious stimuli are those that damage or threaten to damage tissue, such as pinches, cuts, and burns. Thus, pain serves as a notice of injury and is a vital protective mechanism important to normal life. Individuals born congenitally insensitive to pain are often injured without being aware of it, which can lead to disfigurement and early death. Noxious stimuli set into motion a series of events that contributes to the experience of pain. Noxious stimuli activate a special category of sensory receptors called *nociceptors* (noxious *(noci)* + receptive). Nociceptors and the axons of neurons with which they are associated convey nociceptive information to the spinal cord where autonomic and nociceptive reflexes are activated; simultaneously the information is transmitted to the brain supraspinally.

The autonomic reflex responses typically produced by painful or noxious stimuli include increases in heart rate, blood pressure, and respiration and can be used, for example, to estimate whether the depth of anesthesia is sufficient during a surgical procedure. Nociceptive reflexes are protective withdrawal (motor) reflexes that are organized at the level of the spinal cord. For example, if a person touches an unexpectedly hot surface with his hand, the result will be reflex withdrawal followed by conscious appreciation that he has just burned himself. The conscious appreciation of a peripheral event as painful requires supraspinal integration of the information in several areas of the brain and, most importantly, interpretation of the event. This supraspinal integration and interpretation are what make pain the unique experience it is.

A subtle but important distinction exists between nociception and the experience of pain. Nociception and pain are not synonyms. The term *nociception* refers to the neural events and reflex responses produced by a noxious stimulus. The term *pain* refers to an unpleasant sensory and emotional experience associated with actual or potential tissue injury or described in terms of such injury. Pain is always subjective. Accordingly, nociception can occur in the absence of the perception of pain, and pain can arise in the absence of nociception. For example, among persons with spinal cord injury, such as paraplegics or quadriplegics, noxious stimuli applied below the level of spinal cord injury can evoke nociceptive withdrawal reflexes because the peripheral nociceptors and spinal reflex circuitry are intact. However, because the information cannot be transmitted above the spinal injury to the brain, such a patient does not perceive noxious stimuli as painful. An example of pain in the absence of peripheral nociceptive input is central poststroke pain syndrome, a condition in which typically deep, aching or burning pain develops in the area of sensory loss or neurologic disability contralateral to the side of the cerebral infarct. Also, a number of pain syndromes show no evident pathophysiology, yet the pain associated with these syndromes can be debilitating.

Pain sensory channel

Sensations arising from skin, joints, muscles, and viscera may be thought of in terms of sensory channels. The term *sensory channel* means the peripheral receptors and nerves, the neurons in the spinal cord upon which the peripheral nerves terminate and transfer their message, the ascending tracts in the spinal cord that carry the information supraspinally, and the sites in the brain where integration and interpretation of input occur. For example, the temperature sensory channel is associated with separate cold and heat peripheral receptors and central pathways. Activation of a sensory channel provides information about the location, onset, intensity, and duration of the stimulus. The sensory channel for pain is generally considered to be composed of two parts: a sensory-discriminative component and a motivational-affective component.

Sensory-discriminative component

The sensory-discriminative component of pain is directly linked to the noxious stimulus and generally refers to pain as a physical sensation. That is, a noxious stimulus activates nociceptors and initiates a series of neural events that ultimately reaches the cortex of the brain to allow a person to determine the location of the stimulus as well as its intensity and duration. Personal experience reveals the importance of the ability to determine easily the location and characteristics of pain; for example, a person does not normally wonder whether a pain is in the left or right hand or even, given a painful finger, which of two adjacent fingers is the correct location. This exquisite ability to characterize and locate the site of pain is best developed in the skin but relatively poorly developed in deeper tissues such as the viscera.

Motivational-affective component

The motivational-affective component of pain includes the nature and intensity of emotional responses that make pain personal and unique for each person. The sites in the brain that contribute to the motivational-affective component and the spinal pathways that convey nociceptive information to these brain sites are different from those associated with the sensory-discriminative component of pain. The motivational-affective component of pain is considered to be served by older, relatively indirect neural pathways that are conserved phylogenetically; that is, they are common to all vertebrates. Whereas the sensory-discriminative component of pain is organized to give information about the location, the time, and the duration of the nociceptive event, the motivational-affective component of pain emotionally colors a person's response to the nociceptive input.

Overlying the sensory-discriminative and motivational-affective components of pain are learned cultural and cognitive contributions to the interpretation of and concern about pain. The cognitive contributions include attention, anxiety, anticipation, and past experiences. For example, if past experience with a potentially painful procedure has been bad, then anxiety about the procedure and anticipation that it will be painful will influence a person's interpretation of and response to any nociception that arises during the procedure. Similarly, attention to or distraction from a potentially painful procedure can influence a person's response. Thus, cognitive contributions can significantly modulate the response and reaction to a painful stimulus.

Pain classifications

Pain can be conveniently classified according to its duration or source. Classification according to duration is important because pain associated with tissue injury sets into motion changes that contribute to altered sensations. Classification according to source is important because the mechanisms of pain associated with superficial structures are different from pain mechanisms associated with the viscera.

Classification according to duration

Pain is most commonly described in terms of its duration as acute, prolonged, or chronic and in terms of its source as somatic or visceral. Most of the above material relates to acute pain. Acute pain has a short duration, is protective, and is not associated with significant tissue injury. Acute pain often evokes a withdrawal reflex but fails to evoke or evokes modest autonomic reflexes and emotional reactions. Venipuncture and paper cuts are examples of acute pain. Both the sensory-discriminative and the motivational-affective components of pain are involved, but past experience instructs that the consequences of the event are not serious.

Chronic pain, in many ways the polar opposite of acute pain, can be of unlimited duration, is not protective, and is associated with significant tissue damage. Chronic pain is typically defined as pain lasting longer than six months. It usually arises from nerve damage, including brain damage, tumor growth, or inexplicable, abnormal responses by the central nervous system to tissue injury. Chronic pain often exists in the absence of obvious pathology long after the initial injury has apparently been repaired or surgery has corrected the damage. Obviously, the motivational-affective and cognitive contributions to chronic pain are very significant. In addition to the personal suffering and debilitation caused by chronic pain, tremendous economic and societal consequences are associated with the millions of chronic-pain sufferers in the U.S. Chronic pain serves no useful purpose and can, if severe and intractable, lead to depression and sometimes suicide. (See *Treatment of chronic pain* for additional comments on the difficulties of treating chronic pain.)

Perhaps the most common pain is described as prolonged, meaning that it lasts days to weeks. Prolonged pain is always associated with tissue injury and inflammation, such as sunburn, sprains, or surgery. One consequence of tissue injury and inflammation is the development of an exaggerated response to a normally painful stimulus, a phenomenon termed hyperalgesia. For example, a pinprick may cause the experience of severe pain in an inflamed finger. In hyperalgesia, chemicals released or synthesized at the site of injury

Treatment of chronic pain

Chronic pain is the most difficult type of pain to treat. Even ancient cultures resorted to surgical procedures such as drilling holes in the skull to let the evil spirits escape. Modern surgical procedures such as cutting the ascending spinothalamic tract (cordotomy) are sometimes used to treat chronic pain unresponsive to less invasive therapy. Unfortunately, although the pain disappears immediately following surgery, it often reappears over the following 6 to 12 months. Possible reasons for the reappearance of pain offer interesting insights into the mechanisms underlying nociception. One possible explanation for the reappearance of pain following cordotomy is that alternative, parallel nociceptive pain pathways are engaged following surgery. Alternatively, information in nonnociceptive pathways may be used to estimate noxious stimuli. These hypotheses underscore the robustness of the nociceptive system.

increase the sensitivity of nociceptors. Because of the increased activity of nociceptors, central neurons upon which nociceptors terminate also undergo a change and they become more easily excited. Thus, prolonged pain is characterized by a change in the function and behavior of almost all elements that comprise the sensory-discriminative component of pain. Importantly, these changes are normal and reversible. It follows then that the neural components of the sensory channel for pain are not static and immutable but exhibit remarkable flexibility and plasticity. Prolonged pain, like acute pain, serves an important protective function. The tenderness and increased sensitivity of tissue surrounding the site of an injury help to protect the site and prevent further damage.

Classification according to source

Sensory input from the body (soma) to the central nervous system has traditionally been referred to as somatosensory input. However, based on the current understanding of pain mechanisms as well as on the observation that the qualities of pain vary according to the site of pain origin, it is more appropriate to refer to pain as either somatic or visceral, depending on the origin of the pain. If somatic pain arises from skin, it is called superficial pain. If it arises from muscle, joints, or connective tissue, it is called deep pain. Visceral pain, which arises from internal organs, is different in significant ways from somatic pain and is considered a separate quality of pain.

Somatic pain

The skin is continuously exposed to the external environment and thus to a wide variety of stimuli. Consciousness of itch, touch, temperature, pain, and the like are distinguishable from one another and are generally easy to localize. The skin is densely innervated by a wide variety of specialized sensory receptors, including nociceptors, which give a person   the ability to distinguish light touch from noxious pinch and to localize the movement of even a single hair on the back of the hand. Superficial pain is thus best characterized by its ability to be easily and accurately localized. Because the skin is a protective barrier against the environment, noxious stimuli applied to skin typically evoke protective withdrawal reflexes.

In the case of deep somatic tissues (muscles, joints, connective tissues), the prominent sensation that reaches consciousness is pain. Most sensory nerve activity arising from muscles and joints does not reach consciousness, but joint sprains and deep muscle bruises can be very painful. Damage to a joint or muscle does not generally evoke the same type of withdrawal reflex associated with noxious stimulation of the skin, but pain from joints and muscles serves a similar protective function. Joints and muscles are innervated by nociceptors, and just as is true for skin, pain from these deeper structures is generally well localized. A person rarely attributes the source of muscle or joint pain to the wrong muscle or joint. Because pain from joints and muscles is commonly associated with tissue injury and inflammation, the sensitivity of nociceptors innervating the injured tissue increases, and the sensory channel for pain undergoes a reversible plastic change. One consequence of such plasticity is referral of pain to the overlying skin. Careful sensory examination of the overlying skin will reveal that its sensitivity to stimulation has increased and it has become hyperalgesic. In this example of an injured joint or muscle, referred pain and hyperalgesia help to protect the deeper structures from further damage.

Visceral pain

Visceral pain is a separate quality of pain that is in most ways unlike pain in skin, muscles, or joints. Visceral pain is diffuse and difficult to localize and is typically referred to other deep visceral or nonvisceral structures and to the skin. The complexity of visceral pain is illustrated by the pain associated with insufficient oxygen supply to the heart, angina pectoris. Anginal pain is typically referred to the skin and muscles of the upper left chest, shoulder, and arm. A similar pattern of referred pain is produced by obstruction of the gall bladder or by pain arising from the esophagus. Esophageal or gallbladder pain is typically confused with anginal pain. Thus, visceral pain is often not correctly localized to the site of its cause.

Whether the viscera are innervated by nociceptors has long been argued and remains uncertain at present, but it is apparent that the sensory-discriminative component of visceral pain is poorly developed with respect to localization of the source. Because a person usually has little or no previous experience with visceral pain and cannot easily assess the significance of the pain, the motivational-affective component of pain arising from internal organs is significant. Many people experience acute visceral pain on occasion that passes without concern. The common response to repetitive or aching visceral pain, on the other hand, is fear of a serious disorder or disease. Indeed, among the most intense chronic pains are those associated with tumor growth that distends and distorts a viscus.

Not easily placed in the categories described above is the pain arising from veins and the pain referred to as migraine headache. Veins, but not arteries, appear to be innervated by sensory nerve endings that function like nociceptors when a vein is distended or exposed to a cold infusion or a solution with low pH. Accordingly, intravenous drug administration or infusions can be unintentionally painful. Migraine headache has long been considered to be a disorder of the brain and meningeal vasculature. Recently, however, it has been established that many headaches are neurogenic in that the neural innervation of the meningeal vasculature and sinuses initiates the events that produce headache. Indeed, headache resembles visceral pain in many ways in that it is diffuse in character, difficult to localize, and referred to other structures, such as the eyes, teeth, or head and neck muscles.

Four neural stages of nociception

Functionally, nociception can be divided into four stages:

- transduction—the conversion of stimulus energy into neural activity
- central processing and abstraction—the processing of nociceptive neural signals by the central nervous system to extract relevant information
- modulation—the adaptation of nociceptive activity to changes in the environment and needs of the individual
- development and plasticity—long-lasting or permanent changes in the neural mechanisms that mediate nociception in response to development, experience, and injury.

Each of these stages will be considered in detail below.

Transduction

The first stage in nociception is the reception of a nociceptive stimulus by a primary afferent neuron, which consists of a specialized receptor that transduces somatic or visceral stimuli, an axon that conveys the electrical information toward the spinal cord or cranial nuclei, and the cell body located in a dorsal root ganglion or ganglion of a cranial nerve (see *Transduction: The first stage of nociception and pain*).

Transduction, which occurs in all sensory systems, is the conversion of stimulus energy into changes in nerve membrane electrical potentials. Somatovisceral receptors, specialized sensory nerve endings in skin, deep tissue, and viscera convert mechanical, thermal, and chemical energy into action potentials. An individual primary sensory afferent fiber innervates several receptors distributed over a localized region of tissue. The sensory receptors can be excited only by stimuli applied in the innervated region, known as the receptive field. Receptive fields of different primary afferent fibers vary greatly in size and can be continuous or discontinuous; adjacent receptive fields overlap extensively.

Mechanism of transduction

Although the transduction mechanisms differ for thermal, mechanical, and chemical stimuli, they share the common principle that the stimulus interacts with highly specialized transducer molecules embedded in the receptor membrane. The transducer molecule subsequently undergoes a transformation that directly or indirectly causes sodium channels in the receptor membrane to open. Sodium influx from the extracellular fluid then causes the receptor to depolarize, an event that initiates an action potential. Transduction occurs rapidly, requiring but a few milliseconds for mechanical stimuli. Transducer molecules vary according to the type of stimulus they transduce. Chemosensitive transducer molecules have binding sites that will accept only one type of chemical. Mechanosensitive ionic channels are opened by mechanical distortion of the cell membrane. Thermosensitive transducers have molecular gates that open when heated or cooled. Whether individual transducer molecules can respond to more than one type of stimulus is yet to be determined.

Different receptors exhibit varying degrees of specificity for different types of stimuli. Receptors that respond to only one type of stimulus energy, heat for example, are termed *unimodal receptors*. *Polymodal receptors* respond to two or more types of stimuli. Receptors also differ in their sensitivity, which is the number of action potentials evoked by a given stimulus. Somatovisceral receptors vary greatly in their selectivity and sensitivity.

Somatovisceral receptors can be divided into two groups: *nonnociceptive*, or innocuous, *receptors*, which can be activated by stimuli that do not cause damage or produce pain, such as touch and hair movement, and *nociceptive-specific receptors*, or nociceptors, which respond only to stimuli that potentially or actually damage tissue. Consequently, nociceptors are viewed as specialized sensory receptors for sensing pain.

Transduction: The first stage of nociception and pain

In transduction, noxious stimuli (mechanical, thermal, or chemical) cause the membrane of a nociceptor to become permeable to sodium ions. The influx of sodium gives rise to an action potential, which travels along the nerve cell axon to the dorsal horn of the spinal cord.

Nociceptors are present throughout the body as unencapsulated free nerve endings. The two classes of superficial somatic nociceptors (A-δ and C fibers) differ in their conduction velocities and receptive fields.

Enlargement of free nerve ending receptor

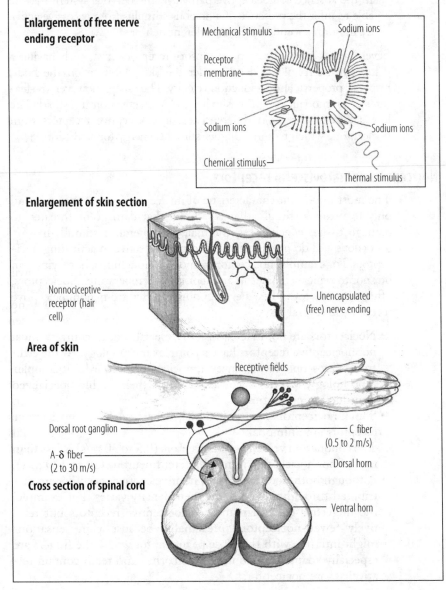

Mechanical stimulus — Sodium ions

Receptor membrane

Sodium ions — Sodium ions

Chemical stimulus

Thermal stimulus

Enlargement of skin section

Nonnociceptive receptor (hair cell)

Unencapsulated (free) nerve ending

Area of skin

Receptive fields

Dorsal root ganglion — C fiber (0.5 to 2 m/s)

A-δ fiber (2 to 30 m/s) — Dorsal horn

Cross section of spinal cord

Ventral horn

Nonnociceptive somatovisceral receptors

Although they do not usually signal pain directly, nonnociceptive somatovisceral receptors contribute to pain perception in several ways:

- Innocuous sensory input can modulate the perception of pain (see "Modulation," page 20).
- In some pathological conditions, innocuous stimuli can become painful (see "Hyperalgesia and plasticity," page 25).
- In the absence of nociceptive pathways, the nervous system may be able to infer the presence of a noxious stimulus from excessive activity in nonnociceptive primary afferent neurons.

Several types of nonnociceptive sensory receptors exist, each having a distinctive morphology, depth under the skin, location on the body, response property, and conduction velocity. They share, however, the features of unimodality, high sensitivity, and low activation threshold. The low activation threshold differentiates nonnociceptive receptors from nociceptors, which require a higher stimulus energy for activation.

Nociceptive somatovisceral receptors

The most important characteristic of nociceptors is that they respond only to noxious stimuli, that is, stimuli that damage or threaten to damage tissue. Mechanical, thermal, and chemical stimuli that are innocuous and do not damage tissue are ineffective in activating nociceptors. For example, nociceptors respond to touching a hot frying pan but not to typical changes in ambient room temperature. Nociceptors, often referred to as free nerve endings, differ from nonnociceptive receptors in several ways:

- Nociceptors are not macroscopically specialized. In contrast, most nonnociceptive receptors have a complex morphology. At the electron microscopic level, however, nociceptors also exhibit complex morphology, which is consistent with their highly specialized transduction properties.
- Some nociceptors are polymodal, whereas all nonnociceptive receptors are unimodal.
- The conduction velocity of nociceptors (0.5 to 30 m/s) is less than that of nonnociceptive primary afferent neurons (30 to 120 m/s).
- Although both nociceptors and nonnociceptive receptors are distributed throughout the body, their density varies. For example, the fingertips contain many nonnociceptive receptors but relatively fewer nociceptors, presumably because pain sensations might interfere with the sense of touch, for which the fingers are especially adapted. In contrast, the cornea and teeth contain relatively more nociceptors.

Capsaicin: Culinary ingredient, experimental probe, and clinical treatment

Pharmacological probes (specialized molecules used in pharmacological research) often have complex names, such as N-methyl-D-asparate and obscure origins like tetrodotoxin, a puffer fish toxin that only scientists remember. Capsaicin, however, is not only one of the most important pharmacological tools and a recently developed clinical drug, but it is also the subject of an ages-old international culinary legacy; capsaicin is the ingredient that makes hot peppers hot.

Capsaicin's fame rests on its ability to selectively and potently excite C fiber afferents, thereby inducing the long-lasting, burning sensation associated with hot peppers. Capsaicin's lack of effect on A-δ and non-nociceptive mechanoreceptors have made it a useful research probe for distinguishing the relative contributions of the two types of nociceptors. Repeated capsaicin application to C fibers eventually kills them, making capsaicin preparations useful for topical treatment of some painful skin conditions such as postherpetic neuralgia. The demise of C fibers frequently exposed to capsaicin also explains why people who repeatedly eat hot food become more tolerant of the hotness.

• Nociceptors, but not nonnociceptive receptors, can be activated by chemicals, such as endogenous inflammatory mediators or exogenous compounds, including hot chili peppers (see *Capsaicin: Culinary ingredient, experimental probe, and clinical treatment*). Furthermore, these same chemicals can sensitize nociceptors and contribute to hyperalgesia (see "Hyperalgesia and plasticity," page 25).

Superficial somatic nociceptors

Nociceptors occur throughout the skin, deep tissue, and viscera. Although broadly similar, they differ somewhat in nomenclature and response properties (see *Somatovisceral nociceptors*, page 12). Somatic superficial, or cutaneous, nociceptors are currently the best understood.

The stimulation threshold for evoking a single action potential in a nociceptor is lower than the stimulation threshold for the perception of pain. For example, the heat threshold for a single action potential in heat nociceptors is 43° to 44° C (109.4° to 111.2° F), but the threshold for human perception of pain is 45° to 47° C (113° to 116.6° F). Similarly, mechanical nociceptor thresholds to pressure are lower and cold nociceptor thresholds are at a higher temperature than are their perceptual counterparts. The explanation for these disparities is that a threshold stimulus that evokes one action potential in one nociceptor is not sufficient to be perceived as painful; either spatial summation (one action potential occuring simultaneously in many nociceptors) or temporal summation (many action potentials occurring closely in time in a single nociceptor) is required. Consequently, suprathreshold stimuli are necessary to produce the temporal and spatial summation required for perception of pain.

Somatovisceral nociceptors

Location (m/s)	Fiber Type	Specificity	Myelinated	Conduction Velocity (m/sec)
skin	A-δ	unimodal	yes	2 to 30
	C	polymodal	no	0.5 to 30
viscera	A-δ	unimodal	yes	2 to 30
	C	polymodal	no	0.5 to 2
muscle and joints	III (II)	unimodal	yes	2 to 30 (30 to 72)
	IV	polymodal	no	0.5 to 2

Two types of somatic superficial nociceptors exist: unimodal and polymodal. Unimodal receptors give rise to myelinated, afferent nerve fibers with conduction velocities in the A-δ fiber range (2 to 30 m/s) and consequently are usually referred to as A-δ fibers. The receptive field of a typical A-δ fiber ranges from 1 to 8 cm^2. Activation of A-δ fibers evokes sharp, well-localized pain sensations. (See *Fast vs. slow pain*.) The two types of A-δ fiber receptors are those that respond only to mechanical stimuli and those that respond primarily to thermal stimuli.

Polymodal nociceptors give rise to unmyelinated, slowly conducting afferent fibers with conduction velocities in the C fiber range (0.5 to 2 m/s) and consequently are usually referred to as C fibers. Polymodal nociceptors are more plentiful than unimodal nociceptors, constituting over 75% of all nociceptors. The typical C fiber receptive field consists of 3 to 20 small (<1 mm^2), noncontiguous, punctuate receptive fields. Polymodal receptors respond to mechanical and thermal as well as chemical stimuli. They are particularly responsive to chemicals released during inflammation, exercise, or disease, as well as to capsaicin, the hot ingredient in chili peppers. Their absolute firing rates are typically lower than unimodal nociceptors, and they rarely are active in the absence of stimulation. Activation of polymodal nociceptors typically evokes long-lasting, burning pain.

Deep somatic nociceptors

Deep somatic nociceptors occur in muscle, fascia, connective tissue, and joints. Although similar to cutaneous nociceptors, deep nociceptors differ in both nomenclature and response properties. Historically, afferent fibers in muscle nerves were classified as belonging to group I, II, III, or IV rather than to the A-α, A-β, A-δ, or C categories used for skin nerves, with groups III and IV being similar in myelination, conduction velocity, and response properties to A-δ and C fibers in skin. Some group II afferents (30 to 72 m/s) also terminate in unen-

Fast vs. slow pain

In most sensory systems, perception occurs instantaneously following a sensory stimulus because of the rapid conduction velocity of most afferent fibers, including A-δ nociceptor afferents (up to 30 m/s). Consequently, the sensory-discriminative component of pain activated by a noxious stimulus applied to the foot will occur with a latency of only about 67 milliseconds in a person 6 feet tall (2 meters/30m/s). In contrast, C fiber nociceptor afferents have a conduction velocity of 0.5 to 2 m/s, resulting in a latency of 1 sec (2 meters/2 m/s).

The difference is readily perceived as a first pain that is sharp, brief, and easily localized, followed by a second pain that is long-lasting and burning . Thus, as expected based on differences in their response properties and conduction velocities, activation of A-δ and C fibers produce dramatically different pain sensations.

capsulated nerve endings and respond like nociceptors. Deep nociceptors are well matched to stimuli that evoke deep pain. For example, excessive force that can occur in traumatic injury and chemicals, such as lactate and potassium, that can cause muscle pain all effectively excite deep nociceptors.

Visceral nociceptors

Viscera were once considered to lack nociceptors because direct manipulation, a pinch for example, and surgical incisions failed to produce pain when surgical anesthesia was allowed to become light. Commonly experienced pain, such as appendicitis and angina, however, instructs that pain does arise from internal organs or viscera. Current knowledge indicates that slowly conducting A-δ and C fiber unencapsulated nerve endings occur throughout viscera as well as somatic structures. The stimuli that produce pain when applied to the viscera, however, are different from those that produce pain when applied to skin. Moreover, the appropriate noxious visceral stimulus differs among the organs. For example, in hollow organs, like the colon and stomach, nociceptors are excited by distension, whereas in solid organs like the testes, compression is the most effective noxious stimulus.

Central processing and abstraction

The incoming information provided by nociceptors can be thought of as a "picture" of noxious stimulation. The brain, however, does not simply "print" that picture within the nervous system. Instead, the nervous system abstracts the features of the picture that are important. This is similar to visual processing and abstraction, where instead of seeing a color photograph as a matrix of colored dots, a person perceives features of the photograph, such as who is in the picture, what type of camera lens was used, or where the picture was taken. Processing and extraction of relevant features of sensory input is referred to as abstraction. (See *Abstraction: The second stage of nociception.*)

Anatomy of the sensory channel for pain

Pain sensations consist of two components. The sensory-discriminative component includes perception of the intensity, location, and type of stimulus. The motivational-affective component is the subjective, emotional response, which lacks any detailed parametric sense of the stimulus.

The distinction between the sensory-discriminative and motivational-affective components of the sensory channel for pain begins at the spinal cord, where information from A-δ and C fiber nociceptors, nonnociceptive receptors, and descending modulatory pathways is integrated to give rise to three ascending pathways: neospinothalamic, paleospinothalamic, and spinobulbar (spino–brain stem). The neospinothalamic pathway principally conveys information important to the sensory-discriminative component of pain. The paleospinothalamic pathway largely mediates the motivational-affective component of pain, and the spinobulbar pathway contributes primarily to activation of descending modulation of nociception. (See "Three ascending tracts," page 16).

The cell bodies of nociceptors are found in the dorsal root ganglia located next to the spinal cord. The dorsal root ganglion neuron gives rise to two axons; one travels peripherally to become the nociceptor, and the other projects centrally through the dorsal roots to terminate in the spinal cord and synapse onto higher-order spinal neurons.

The spinal cord gray matter can be divided anatomically and functionally into three regions: the dorsal horn, the intermediate region, and the ventral horn. Generally, the dorsal horn processes sensory information, the intermediate region integrates sensorimotor information, and the ventral horn generates motor commands for spinal reflexes. The spinal cord can be further divided into ten laminae, or layers, with laminae I through VI corresponding to the dorsal horn gray matter, laminae VII and X corresponding to the intermediate region, and lamina VIII and IX corresponding to the ventral horn gray matter.

The central terminations of nociceptive and nonnociceptive afferent fibers initially synapse in different laminae; nociceptive afferent fibers synapse in laminae I, II, V, and VI, whereas nonnociceptive afferent fibers synapse in laminae III and IV. The spatial segregation of nociceptive and nonnociceptive information in the spinal cord disappears with subsequently converging higher-order projections.

Abstraction: The second stage of nociception

During abstraction, nociceptive and nonnociceptive information travels via afferent fibers that project to distinct laminae of the dorsal horn gray matter. After extensive convergence, nociceptive information is conveyed to ventral horn neurons that initiate motor and autonomic reflexes and to ascending tract cells in the dorsal horn and intermediate regions. The ascending tract cells give rise to long axons that cross the spinal midline and then project to the brain contralaterally via three different ascending tracts.

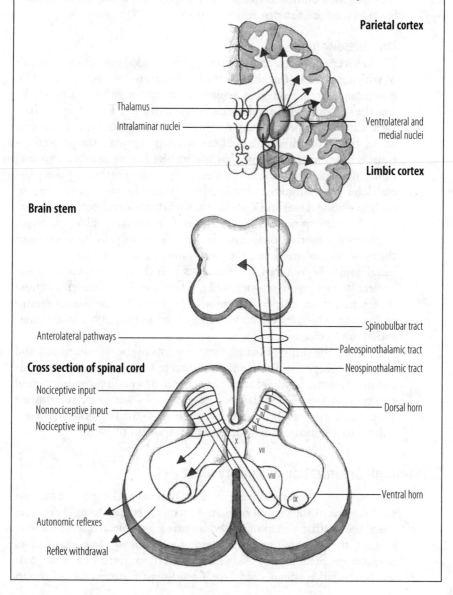

Parietal cortex

Thalamus

Intralaminar nuclei

Ventrolateral and medial nuclei

Limbic cortex

Brain stem

Anterolateral pathways

Spinobulbar tract

Paleospinothalamic tract

Neospinothalamic tract

Cross section of spinal cord

Nociceptive input

Nonnociceptive input

Nociceptive input

Dorsal horn

Ventral horn

Autonomic reflexes

Reflex withdrawal

Following processing in the spinal cord, nociceptive information is conveyed to motor/autonomic output neurons in the ventral horn and spinal autonomic nuclei and to ascending tract cells in the dorsal horn and intermediate regions. The somatic motor neurons and preganglionic autonomic neurons mediate spinal motor and autonomic reflexes such as the protective flexion withdrawal reflex. The ascending tract cells give rise to long axons that cross the spinal midline over several segments and then project contralaterally through the spinal funiculi (the bundles of tracts that compose the white matter) to the brain to mediate the perception of pain.

Three ascending tracts

The nociceptive ascending neurons can be divided into three tracts, all of which ascend in the anterolateral quadrant of the spinal cord. The neospinothalamic tract is an evolutionarily newer pathway that mediates the sensory-discriminative component of pain. The neospinothalamic pathway projects to the ventrolateral and ventromedial portions of the thalamus adjacent to but not overlapping with the projections from other sensory systems that are involved in sensory discrimination. Subsequently, the thalamus projects to the portions of the parietal lobe cerebral cortex that mediate perception and processing of both nonnociceptive and nociceptive somatosensory information.

The paleospinothalamic tract, an evolutionarily older pathway, mediates the motivational-affective component of pain. In contrast to the neospinothalamic tract, the paleospinothalamic tract projects to the intralaminar portions of the thalamus, which are involved with the subjective aspects of sensory input rather than with discrimination. The intralaminar nuclei then project primarily to the limbic system and cortex, which mediate motivational, subjective, and affective sensations and behavior.

Lastly, the spinobulbar pathway consists of the spinoreticular and spinomesencephalic tracts, which ascend to the medulla and the midbrain, respectively, where they can activate descending modulation of nociception (see "Modulation," page 20). In addition, subsequent projections from the brainstem or midbrain to the thalamus may contribute to the motivational-affective component of pain.

Somatotopic organization of sensory input

Somatosensory receptors from adjacent regions of skin project to adjacent regions of the central nervous system. This somatotopic arrangement means that a map of the body surface is projected onto the surface of the central nervous system. Dermatomes, one example of somatotopy, are regions of skin innervated by axons from a single dorsal root of the spinal cord (see *Somatotopic organization of sensory*

Somatotopic organization of sensory input

Sensory input is organized somatotopically in the central nervous system. Skin dermatomes, an example of somatotopic organization, are regions of skin whose sensory neurons project to specific spinal cord segments. The viscerotomes demonstrate the somatosensory locations of referred visceral pain.

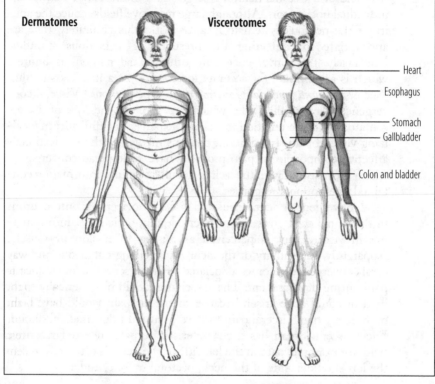

Dermatomes   **Viscerotomes**

Heart
Esophagus
Stomach
Gallbladder
Colon and bladder

input). A similar organization is found in the thalamus and the cortex in the sensory-discrimination pathway. Presumably, the accurate mapping aids in the spatial perception of somatic stimuli. Both nonnociceptive and nociceptive processing are somatotopically organized. In contrast, the viscera do not appear to be somatotopically represented in the thalamus or cortex; this observation is consistant with the difficulty in localizing visceral stimuli.

Spatial and temporal processing

Nociceptive information undergoes spatial and temporal processing in the spinal cord and in supraspinal structures. Processing is closely matched to the needs of the sensory-discriminative and motivational-affective components of pain.

Spatial processing

Spatially, some spinal cord neurons receive extensive convergence from many individual nociceptors. Consequently, the resulting receptive field of the spinal neuron is larger than the receptive field of the individual nociceptors. Although large receptive fields reduce the ability of the nervous system to localize a stimulus accurately, they are appropriate for detecting the presence of a noxious stimulus. Conversely, the convergence onto other spinal neurons is limited, which is appropriate for accurate localization of a noxious stimulus. (See *Spatial and temporal processing of nociceptive input*.) Visceral convergence is especially wide, which may explain the lack of a clear somatotopic representation as well as the perceptual difficulty in localizing visceral pain. In addition, neurons mediating the motivational-affective component of pain probably have widespread convergence, which is consistent with the lack of detailed stimulus information contained in emotional responses.

Convergence of cutaneous and visceral nociceptors onto neurons in the spinal cord gives rise to referred pain, which is pain originating in viscera that is perceived as arising from skin or muscle. Apparently, the activity of the neurons receiving cutaneous and visceral convergence becomes associated with the sensation of cutaneous pain during development. The association could be genetically specified or could have arisen because cutaneous pain would have been more likely than visceral pain to have occurred in normal childhood. Each visceral organ has a characteristic somatic referred receptive field; for example, pain in the left side of the heart is often referred to the left shoulder, side of the neck, pectoral muscle, and arm.

Temporal processing

Nociceptive signals are transformed through time, too. For example, conventional postsynaptic potentials, which arise when neurotransmitters bind to receptors that are directly coupled to ion channels, are 5 to 20 milliseconds in duration. In contrast, postsynaptic potentials evoked by activation of C fibers can persist for 1 to 60 seconds.

The prolongation of depolarization occurs because the postsynaptic receptor is not directly coupled to an ion channel. Instead, the postsynaptic receptor initiates a complex intracellular second messenger cascade, utilizing G-proteins for example, that ultimately opens ion channels. The intracellular cascade then takes longer to recover than do simple ligand-linked ion channels.

These prolonged postsynaptic potentials partially underlie the prolonged second pain evoked by C fiber afferents. The long-lasting post-

Spatial and temporal processing of nociceptive input

Some spinal cord neurons receive input from many individual nociceptors (A.). Others receive input from a limited number of receptors. Conventional fast, short-duration neurotransmission in the spinal dorsal horn results from the binding of neurotransmitters to receptor-linked ion channels (B.). C fibers produce slow, long-lasting post-synaptic potentials that depend on intracellular second messengers to open ion channels (C.).

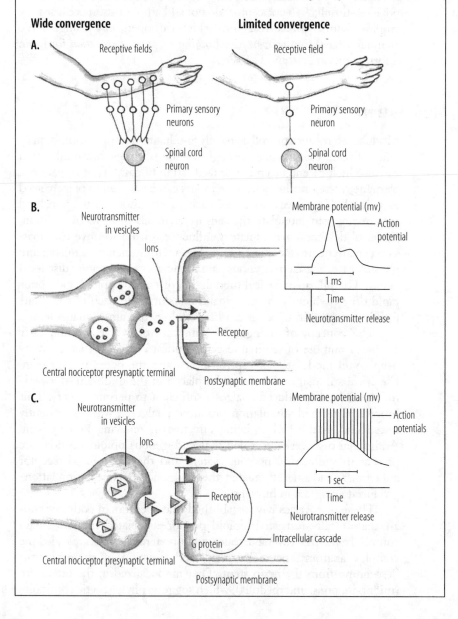

Wide convergence

A.
Receptive fields
Primary sensory neurons
Spinal cord neuron

Limited convergence

Receptive field
Primary sensory neuron
Spinal cord neuron

B.
Neurotransmitter in vesicles
Ions
Receptor
Central nociceptor presynaptic terminal
Postsynaptic membrane

Membrane potential (mv)
Action potential
1 ms
Time
Neurotransmitter release

C.
Neurotransmitter in vesicles
Ions
Receptor
G protein
Intracellular cascade
Central nociceptor presynaptic terminal
Postsynaptic membrane

Membrane potential (mv)
Action potentials
1 sec
Time
Neurotransmitter release

synaptic potentials are also necessary if temporal summation is to occur because the firing frequencies of C fiber nociceptors is so low. Intracellular cascades can also provide amplification of the original nociceptive signal because a single receptor molecule can open many ionic channels, whereas a conventional channel-linked receptor can open only a single ionic channel. In contrast to the prolonged postsynaptic potentials seen in C fiber activity, A-δ nociceptors evoke brief postsynaptic potentials, which can enhance temporal discrimination of noxious stimuli; A-δ nociceptors do not add amplification because they employ channel-linked receptors, which can open only a single ionic channel. (See *Microneurography: Linking receptors to sensation* for more information on A-δ and C fibers.)

Modulation

Modulation means control. Typically, modulation implies inhibition or relief of pain, for example, through the use of drugs, but modulation can also include enhancement or facilitation of pain. That is, pain can be made worse or nonnociceptive inputs can be altered to be perceived as painful. Cognitive influences such as attention, distraction, and anticipation can modulate the sensory channels of pain. In addition, powerful descending modulatory influences on nociceptive transmission can attenuate or enhance pain. The anatomy, neurochemistry, and physiology of these endogenous pain modulatory systems are discussed below. The pharmacological modulation of pain by opioid and nonopioid drugs, which is the principal therapeutic approach to pain control, is discussed in Chapter 2, Pharmacology of Pain Management.

The concept of endogenous pain control evolved in the early 1970s. A number of seminal research findings revealed that the body itself could modulate nociceptive inputs and the perception of pain. Electrical stimulation by electrodes placed in the midbrain of experimental animals produced analgesia sufficient to permit surgery. This procedure, termed stimulation-produced analgesia, was subsequently tested and established as being effective in relieving human pain. Additional discoveries revealed that endogenous opioid peptides are present in the central nervous system and that the opioid receptor antagonist naloxone attenuated the analgesic effects of stimulation-produced analgesia in humans.

These discoveries have established that the human body contains an anatomically restricted, opioid peptide–associated means of pain control. In the past several decades, additional research has revealed the complex anatomy, neurochemistry, and function of these systems descending from the brain stem. They are localized in the brainstem (midbrain, pons, and medulla), which suggests phylogenetic continuity

Microneurography: Linking receptors to sensation

What sensations do A-δ or C fiber nociceptors produce? Answering this question became possible only through a technique called microneurography developed by Vallbo and Hagbarth in Sweden. Slender metal microelectrodes are inserted by hand through the skin into a peripheral nerve of a human volunteer. The microelectrode is so small that it can record the activity of individual afferent fibers while thermal, mechanical, chemical, or other stimuli are applied to the subject's arm, thus allowing classification and characterization of the afferent fiber. Subsequently, small amounts of current are injected through the microelectrode to excite only the fiber that had been recorded. The subject can then describe the sensation felt by activation of the nociceptive afferent fiber. Microneurography thus makes it possible to associate specific pain perceptions with the activity of individual, identified nociceptor afferents. These studies were instrumental in determining the roles of A-δ and C fibers in nociception.

among vertebrates. Indeed, pain modulatory influences descending from the brain stem have been found in all vertebrate species studied.

Anatomy and neurochemistry of pain modulation

The midbrain periaqueductal and periventricular gray matter is the nodal point of the endogenous pain modulatory system. At this anatomical site both exogenously administered opioids like morphine and endogenously released opioid peptides activate inhibitory influences that descend to the spinal cord. (The principal anatomical features of this modulatory system are illustrated in *Endogenous systems that modulate pain,* page 22.) There is a critical synapse between the midbrain and spinal cord in the rostral part of the ventral medulla. Thus, descending influences on spinal nociceptive transmission activated in the midbrain are indirect in that there exists a relay between the midbrain and spinal cord. From the medulla, descending influences are direct. Axons of neurons in the medulla descend in the spinal cord to terminate on spinal neurons where the nociceptive message from the periphery is received.

An important aspect of descending inhibitory modulation is that the system is tonically active. That is, a moderate brake was applied to spinal neurons by the descending inhibitory system even under normal circumstances. Thus, increases or decreases in spinal nociceptive transmission could be produced by alterations in the activity of this tonic descending system.

The neurotransmitter chemicals that mediate descending inhibition are principally serotonin and norepinephrine. Serotonin is contained in the terminals of neurons descending from the ventral medulla, and norepinephrine is contained in the terminals of neurons

Endogenous systems that modulate pain

Pain modulation includes both inhibition (indicated by - sign) and facilitation (indicated by + sign). Although descending inhibition and facilitation employ different spinal tracts and neurotransmitters, both types of modulation arise from the brainstem. Both endogenous and exogenous descending inhibitions are mediated by neural activity at the periaqueductal gray (PAG) area of the midbrain.

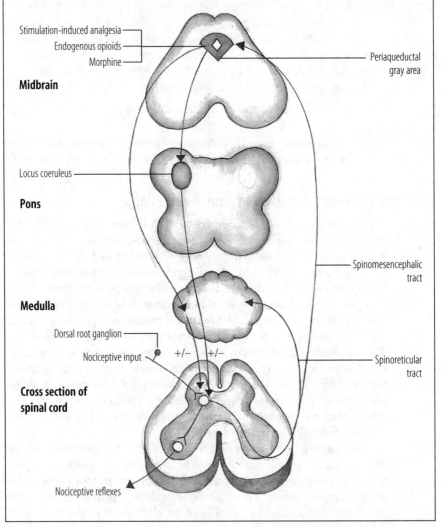

descending from the dorsolateral pons such as the locus coeruleus. Accordingly, drugs that mimic the actions of serotonin and norepinephrine are analgesic when given directly into the spinal epidural or intrathecal space. For example, clonidine is analgesic in humans and has been used to treat cancer pain because it acts in the spinal cord like norepinephrine at the α_2-adrenergic receptor. Opioids given exogenously or released endogenously are analgesic because of action at opioid receptors, but at least part of their action is effected in the spinal cord by the monoamine transmitters serotonin and norepinephrine. This means that pain control by opioids should be enhanced by drugs that mimic or facilitate the actions of serotonin or norepinephrine such as certain antidepressants. Indeed, this has been documented in clinical trials; consequently, these drugs can be an important adjunct to pain control with the added benefit of reducing the opioid dose requirements and thus slowing the rate of tolerance development.

Facilitation of nociception

The principal focus of investigation has been on inhibitory modulation of nociceptive transmission, but it is now appreciated that descending systems can also facilitate nociceptive transmission in the spinal cord. Since facilitatory modulation of nociceptive transmission is a relatively recent subject of investigation, it is less well understood than is inhibitory modulation. The anatomical components of facilitatory modulation in the brainstem are similar to, if not overlapping, those of inhibitory modulation. That is, either inhibition or facilitation can be produced from the same sites in the brainstem, depending upon input. Full understanding of how the inputs may differ has not yet been attained. It is clear, however, that axons mediating facilitatory influences descend from the brainstem in different spinal tracts and contain neurotransmitters different from those described above for inhibitory modulation. These neurotransmitters act at cholinergic, cholecystokinin, and kappa opioid receptors and can contribute to the facilitation of nociceptive transmission.

Activation of endogenous pain modulation

A wide variety of influences can activate endogenous pain modulation, both inhibitory and facilitatory. Stress, fear, and pain itself can activate descending systems that inhibit pain. An injured animal's escape from a predator, even in the presence of pain, has been cited as an example of the survival role of pain-activated endogenous modulation. In less life-threatening circumstances, pain can inhibit pain by activation of the same endogenous mechanisms, a phenomenon referred to as counterirritation. Pathophysiology such as hypertension can also contribute to activation of descending inhibitory systems and attenuation of pain. Documentation shows that both experimental increases in blood pressure and preexisting hypertension lessen sensitivity to noxious stimuli.

Anxiety and apprehension can lead to enhancement of pain; however, descending facilitation of pain may play a particularly large role in unusual chronic pain states. It is possible but not yet proven that the pain facilitating system can be activated and subsequently not turned off by normal mechanisms, thus contributing to tonic facilitation, rather than tonic inhibition, of spinal neuron activity. Obviously, there are circumstances in which facilitation of nociceptive information is protective, such as during tissue repair, yet if such a system remains inappropriately activated after tissue repair is complete, normal, nonnociceptive inputs could conceivably acquire nociceptive character. Because the mechanisms of chronic pain are poorly understood, there is considerable interest and potential importance in better understanding endogenous systems that can enhance pain.

Modulation via spinal gate control

Some pain modulation techniques do not involve descending systems. A number of therapeutic pain management approaches are independent of descending endogenous systems or involve descending systems only minimally, such as acupuncture, dorsal column stimulation, transcutaneous electrical nerve stimulation (TENS), and so on. A popular and heuristically important concept that explains the success of some of these therapeutic approaches was introduced in the mid-1960s with the publication of a new theory of spinal modulation of pain (Melzack and Wall 1965). The theory holds that the cells in the spinal cord that transmit nociceptive information to supraspinal sites function as a spinal gate; hence, the gate control theory of pain control. According to this model the gate opens and nociception is facilitated by activity in the small-diameter afferent fibers, the A-δ and C fibers. The gate is then closed by activity in the large-diameter, myelinated nonnociceptive afferent fibers, the A-α and A-β fibers. It is hypothesized that the balance in activities between nociceptive and nonnociceptive afferent fiber inputs to the spinal cord affects the position of the gate: a relatively open gate means more pain; a relatively closed gate means less pain. The intensity of pain is thereby modulated. Subsequent modifications of the gate control theory have included the addition of influences descending from the brainstem that modulate the gate. Sensory-discriminative, motivational-affective, and cognitive components are currently believed to contribute to central nervous system integration and interpretation of and reaction to noxious inputs.

The mechanisms of dorsal column stimulation and TENS are not entirely understood but are generally explained by application of the gate control theory of pain control. For example, electrical stimulation of large-diameter, myelinated fibers in the dorsal column of the spinal cord or in peripheral nerves through the application of TENS is considered to close the spinal gate and thus reduce pain. Similarly, some forms of acupuncture that activate large-diameter peripheral myelinated axons may close the spinal gate. Different forms of acupuncture probably employ varying mechanisms of pain control, such as counterirritation, which are not all explicable by the gate control theory. The application of these and other methods of pain modulation is discussed in greater detail in Chapter 6, Noninvasive Techniques for Managing Pain.

Development and plasticity

Human perception of sensory stimuli is not constant; it changes in response to development, environmental experience, and disease and injury. These changes are collectively referred to as plasticity. Plasticity can be brief, defined as lasting minutes to hours, prolonged, defined as lasting hours to weeks, or relatively permanent. Learning and memory are forms of plasticity that are familiar. The response of the nervous system to nociceptive stimuli also exhibits plasticity. A person's perception of pain depends on childhood experiences, psychological attitudes toward pain, and how recently long-lasting traumatic or inflammatory tissue damage has occurred.

Development

A long-held but mistaken concept is that newborns have an incomplete, immature nociceptive system and thus do not perceive pain as do adults. While it is obvious that newborns and children lack the experiences that shape adult behaviors when confronted with a noxious stimulus, the peripheral and central anatomy and chemistry that comprise the sensory-discriminative component of pain are intact and functional at birth. Accordingly, nociceptors and nociceptive and autonomic reflexes are present, and supraspinal integration of the nociceptive information occurs just as it does in adults. The motivational-affective component of pain is intact anatomically, but emotional experiences and cognitive features of responses to noxious stimuli remain to be developed.

Hyperalgesia and plasticity

In adults as well as in children, certain types of injury or disease can lead to hyperalgesia, which is an enhanced pain perception in response to a normally painful stimulus, for example, the perception that a pinprick is extremely painful. Allodynia is the perception of pain in response to a normally nonpainful stimulus such as perceiving that a bedsheet touching a wounded limb causes pain. Hyperalgesia and allodynia can arise from inflammatory tissue damage, injury to peripheral nerves, or damage to portions of the central nervous system that mediate pain sensations. The tissue damage that leads to this heightened sensitivity can arise from many sources, including trauma and medical procedures.

Hyperalgesia is divided into primary and secondary forms. Primary hyperalgesia occurs when the site of injury corresponds to the site of hyperalgesia. Secondary hyperalgesia occurs when the site of hyperalgesia differs from the site of injury, such as when the ankle shows enhanced sensitivity following injury to the foot. Typically, primary hyperalgesia always occurs following injury, while secondary hyperalgesia is sometimes present and is usually weaker than the primary hyperalgesia.

Inflammatory hyperalgesia

Pain commonly arises from damage to tissue, such as sunburn, the abrasion of skin in a fall, or the occlusion of a ureter by a kidney stone. In addition to directly and briefly exciting nociceptors, damage to tissue initiates a repair process known as inflammation. During inflammation, chemical mediators, such as bradykinin, serotonin, histamine, cytokines, peptides, and prostaglandins, are released from local and circulating cells. These chemical mediators then cause vasodilation, swelling, and the eventual removal and replacement of damaged tissue. Importantly, chemical mediators can directly activate nociceptors and sensitize nociceptors to subsequent stimuli. Nociceptor sensitization caused by inflammation contributes significantly to primary hyperalgesia.

Although both A-δ and C fiber nociceptors can be activated and sensitized by chemical mediators, C fiber nociceptors appear to be particularly responsive to chemical stimuli. A subset of primarily C-fiber nociceptors are called silent nociceptors because they are usually unresponsive to typical noxious stimuli. Following chemical sensitization, they become spontaneously active and responsive to normal thermal and mechanical stimuli.

C fiber nociceptors also contribute to inflammation and hyperalgesia via neurogenic inflammation. Unlike most sensory neurons, C fiber nociceptors release neurotransmitters both centrally in the spinal cord and peripherally at receptor endings in tissue. Furthermore, the peptide neurotransmitters released—substance P and perhaps others—enhance the inflammatory process as do other inflammatory mediators, thus resulting in further activation of the C fiber nociceptor and further release of substance P. The resulting positive feedback significantly enhances the inflammation and resulting hyperalgesia. (See *Two mechanisms for development of hyperalgesia*).

Neurogenic inflammation is also responsible for the spread of reddening and soreness following a localized injury. As a single C fiber approaches the skin, it branches several times to innervate separate small patches of skin. Consequently, if a localized injury activates only one branch of the C fiber, the evoked orthodromic (traveling in the normal direction) action potential will induce antidromic (traveling in the opposite direction) action potentials in other branches. The

Two mechanisms for development of hyperalgesia

Hyperalgesia associated with peripheral sensitization is caused by a positive feedback loop that develops when peripheral C fiber terminals release neurotransmitters such as substance P. These chemical messengers then cause inflammatory cells to release chemical mediators that in turn reactivate C fiber release of substance P. Hyperalgesia associated with central sensitization can arise from the death of inhibitory spinal interneurons (1.), sprouting of new synapses between nonnociceptive afferent fibers and nociceptive neurons (2.), or sensitization of spinal dorsal horn neurons that receive C fiber input (3.).

Hyperalgesia associated with peripheral sensitization

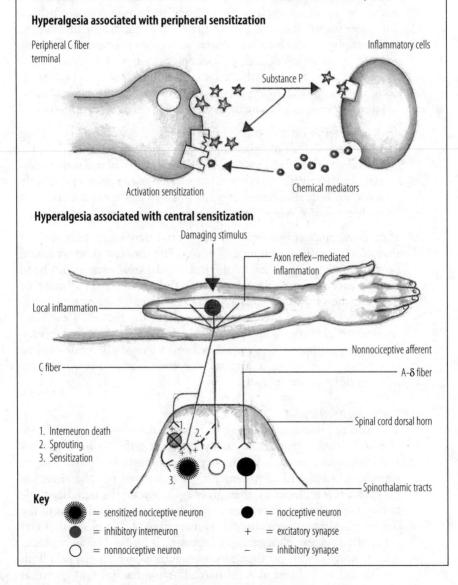

Peripheral C fiber terminal

Inflammatory cells

Substance P

Activation sensitization

Chemical mediators

Hyperalgesia associated with central sensitization

Damaging stimulus

Axon reflex–mediated inflammation

Local inflammation

Nonnociceptive afferent

C fiber

A-δ fiber

Spinal cord dorsal horn

1. Interneuron death
2. Sprouting
3. Sensitization

Spinothalamic tracts

Key

= sensitized nociceptive neuron

= nociceptive neuron

= inhibitory interneuron

+ = excitatory synapse

= nonnociceptive neuron

− = inhibitory synapse

antidromic action potentials will then travel to the nociceptor ending, causing release of substance P, inflammation, and nociceptor sensitization. This process is sometimes known as the axon reflex or axonal flare.

Sensitization of peripheral nociceptors readily accounts for primary hyperalgesia, the hyperalgesia that occurs at an injury site. But this explanation does not work as well for secondary hyperalgesia in which pain sensitivity is distant from the injury. Recent research has shown that changes in spinal cord neurons associated with enhanced pain perception, or central sensitization, occur in both secondary and primary hyperalgesia. Apparently, strong nociceptive input to the spinal cord causes higher-order nociceptive neurons to become more sensitive. The more painful the stimulus, the greater the central sensitization. As with peripheral sensitization, central sensitization is more effectively induced by activation of C fiber nociceptors than of A-δ nociceptors.

Structural changes, which may underlie chronic hyperalgesia, occur in inflammatory and particularly in nerve damage–evoked (neurogenic) hyperalgesia. Some of the structural changes identified are:

- death of inhibitory spinal interneurons due to toxicity arising from a powerful excitatory input
- rearrangement of afferent fiber terminals such as when nonnociceptive afferent fibers synapse into spinal cord regions previously receiving only nociceptor input, a possible cause of allodynia
- proliferation of sympathetic efferent fibers into sensory ganglia.

If excessive nociceptive input to the central nervous system, such as that occurring during surgery, is responsible for central sensitization or structural changes, then the logical clinical treatment would be to employ preemptive analgesia to block the nociceptive pathways or decrease the central nervous system's response. These types of preemptive analgesia, if maintained throughout the period of excessive nociceptor activity, keep central sensitization from developing. Recently, preemptive analgesia has been successfully accomplished using a centrally acting analgesic, morphine, and in some instances using peripheral nerve blocks.

Neurogenic hyperalgesia

Traumatic or infectious damage to peripheral nerves is a special case of tissue damage that results in hyperalgesia differing in symptoms and mechanisms from inflammatory hyperalgesia (see *Sympathetically maintained pain*). Initially, damaged or transected peripheral nerves die back a few millimeters, then grow again toward the periphery, following the pathway left by the injury debris and myelin sheaths of the old nerve. Although growth and reinnervation of skin or another target is often successful, sometimes regrowth is blocked by an obstacle. The growing nerve end then forms a neuroma, which acquires both mechanical and chemical sensitivity. The mechanical and chemical

Sympathetically maintained pain

A number of unusual, poorly understood, and difficult-to-treat pain syndromes involve the sympathetic nervous system. Causalgia, reflex-sympathetic dystrophy, and sympathetically maintained pain are clinical pain syndromes characterized by abnormal pain sensations, including spontaneous pain, burning pain, and pain evoked by gentle touch and warm or cool breezes across the skin. These pain syndromes result from damage to peripheral nerves or dorsal roots following a case of the shingles (herpes zoster), traumatic nerve damage, or even soft tissue injury.

The abnormal pains seem to depend on activity in the sympathetic nervous system. The sympathetic nervous system normally functions to control blood vessel diameter and blood flow in skin, which are important to temperature regulation. Accordingly, the affected tissue (typically a limb) is edematous, undergoes swings in temperature and, because it is so sensitive, often has long, overgrown nails that the patient finds painful to trim.

It is believed that the neurotransmitter of the postganglionic sympathetic nerves, norepinephrine, acts on α-adrenergic receptors that have become more sensitive to norepinephrine as a consequence of the injury.

Treatment is injection of local anesthesia at the appropriate sympathetic ganglia or infusion of an α-adrenergic receptor blocker like phentolamine into the affected limb. If treatment is initiated early enough, one or two treatments sometimes will produce complete and permanent reversal of the pain syndrome. Many times, however, surgical sympathectomy is required.

sensitivity results in the generation of ectopic (generated from an abnormal point) action potentials at the neuroma. Consequently, pain can be produced by even gentle pressure or by release of norepineph-rine from nearby sympathetic nerve endings. In other instances, even with largely successful nerve regrowth and no apparent pathology, chronic pain occurs for as yet unknown reasons.

Amputation, an extreme form of nerve damage, can lead to a unique pain sensation known as phantom pain. Although the pain is very real to the patient, it is labeled phantom because the patient describes it as arising from the missing tissue. Phantom limb pain is most common, but phantom breast and phantom anus pain syndromes have also been described following mastectomy and surgery for colorectal cancer. Phantom pain is typically present within the first week after amputation and in most cases gradually diminishes and vanishes. Phantom pain has been reported to persist in as few as 3% of amputees and in as many as 50% of amputees. Although not well studied, phantom pain is believed to arise at least partially from the ectopic activity of neuromas formed by the surgically transected nerves. Another component of phantom pain apparently arises from the central nervous system; preemptive treatments to block nociceptor discharges during the amputation surgery have been reported to prevent or significantly reduce the incidence of phantom pain. In either case, the pain is localized to the absent body part because afferent pathways are labeled according to the region innervated early in development. Consequently, activity in that pathway will be localized according to the original mapping, regardless of the origin of the activity.

Central pain states

Trauma, ischemia, or degeneration of the brain can also lead to hyperalgesia or hypoalgesia when the neural tissue involved is part of the central nervous system's pain processing system. Damage to the spinothalamic pathway at any level can lead to diminished pain perception. On the other hand, damage to some parts of the thalamus can lead to thalamic pain syndrome, a disorder characterized by hyperalgesia and allodynia. Presumably, the damaged neurons are part of a local nociceptive inhibitory system and are similar to those that descend to the spinal cord from the brainstem. Central pain that originates from damage to higher structures can be difficult to treat because many therapies such as TENS interrupt nociceptive transmission peripheral to the central lesion. An incorrect diagnosis of true central pain as psychogenic has in some instances deprived patients of traditional physiologically based treatments.

REFERENCES

Bonica, J.J. *The Management of Pain*, 2nd ed. Baltimore: William & Wilkins, 1990.

Casey, K.L. *Pain and Central Nervous System Disease: The Central Pain Syndromes.* Philadelphia: Lippincott-Raven Press, 1991.

Fields, H.L. *Pain: Mechanisms and Management.* New York: McGraw Hill, 1992.

Gebhart, G.F. *Visceral Pain.* Seattle: IASP Press, 1995.

Gebhart, G.F. "Somatovisceral Sensation" in *Neuroscience in Medicine.* Edited by Conn, P.M. Philadelphia: Lippincott-Raven, 1995.

Kandel, E.R., et al. *Principles of Neural Science.* 3rd ed. Norwalk, CT: Appleton & Lange, 1991.

Melzack, R., and Wall, P.D. "Pain Mechanisms: A New Theory," *Science* 150(699):971-979, 1965.

Melzack, R., and Wall, P.D. *The Challenge of Pain.* New York: Penguin, 1989.

Mense, S. "Nociception from Skeletal Muscle in Relation to Clinical Muscle Pain," *Pain* 54(3):241-289, 1993.

Ness, T.J., and Gebhart, G.F. "Visceral Pain: A Review of Experimental Studies," *Pain* 41(2):167-234, 1990.

Price, D.D. *Psychological and Neural Mechanisms of Pain.* Philadelphia: Lippincott-Raven, 1988.

Schmidt, R.F. *Fundamentals of Sensory Physiology,* 3rd ed. Berlin: Springer-Verlag, 1981.

Wall, P.D., and Melzack, R. *Textbook of Pain.,* 3rd ed. New York: Churchill Livingston, 1994.

Willis, W.D. *Hyperalgesia and Allodynia.* Philadelphia: Lippincott-Raven Press, 1992.

Willis, W.D. *Sensory Mechanisms of the Spinal Cord,* 2nd ed. New York: Plenum, 1991.

CHAPTER 2

Pharmacology of pain management

Sharon L. Jones, PhD

Pain is a complex sensory phenomenon that can be caused by many stimuli and can assume many qualitative properties. Pain also is a dynamic phenomenon that can cause both transient and long-lasting changes to occur in the periphery and in the central nervous system.

Recent studies indicate that untreated or inadequately treated pain can have profound negative physiologic effects on the body, including the release of stress hormones, impaired immune responses, altered respiratory patterns, and cough suppression. These physiologic responses can, in turn, produce secondary effects that can delay patient recovery, such as pneumonia, delayed ambulation, and inability to participate effectively in physical therapy. In contrast, the aggressive prevention and treatment of pain has been shown to have significant positive health benefits for patients, as evidenced by more rapid recovery rates and shorter hospital stays.

And yet, surprisingly, a review of the literature (Marks and Sachar 1973; Perry 1984) reveals that in addition to the poor management of chronic pain, the routine management of acute post-operative pain is often inadequate, even in modern institutions. A poor understanding of the basic pharmacology of pain medications by physicians, nurses, and other health professionals is frequently cited as a cause of inadequate pain treatment and management. (See *How ignorance of pharmacology leads to ineffective pain management*, page 32.)

This chapter reviews the pharmacology of the major classes of analgesics, including:

- the nonsteroidal anti-inflammatory agents (NSAIDs)
- the opioid analgesics
- the local anesthetics.

How ignorance of pharmacology leads to ineffective pain management

One startling example of the way in which a poor understanding of the pharmacology of pain medications can contribute to the inadequate treatment of pain was described by Loper et al. (1989). One hundred twelve medical/surgical house staff personnel and 258 nurses in an intensive care unit were questioned about the analgesic and anxiolytic effects of pancuronium (a neuromuscular junction blocking agent) and diazepam (a benzodiazepine anxiolytic agent).

- Of the responding physicians and nurses, 5% and 8%, respectively, endorsed the use of the neuromuscular junction blocking agent, pancuronium, for analgesia.

- Of the responding physicians and nurses, 50% and 75%, respectively, endorsed the use of pancuronium for anxiety relief.
- When asked about their impressions concerning the analgesic efficacy of diazepam, 78% and 44% of the responding physicians and nurses, respectively, endorsed the use of diazepam for analgesia.

Pancuronium is a drug used to induce paralysis and diazepam is a drug used to relieve anxiety. Neither drug has any significant analgesic properties. Clearly, the lack of understanding of the pharmacology of particular drugs can have a direct and profound negative impact on patient care.

Alternative pharmacologic agents recently found to be useful in pain management will also be discussed.

Nonsteroidal anti-inflammatory drugs

Agents having a variety of chemical structures make up the class of NSAIDs. (See *Chemical structures of common NSAIDs* for examples.) Although varied in structure, these agents are weak organic acids that have similar mechanisms of action and share clinically important antipyretic (fever-reducing), anti-inflammatory, and analgesic properties. NSAIDs are used to treat mild to moderate pain and are particularly useful for the management of painful conditions that have an inflammatory component. These agents are widely used because:

- they can be taken orally
- unlike the opioid analgesics, they do not cause central nervous system or respiratory depression at therapeutic doses
- several are available without a prescription.

Aspirin is the prototypical NSAID.

Chemical structures of common NSAIDs

Although the chemical structures of NSAIDs vary (as shown below), all the agents that make up this class are weak organic acids that bring about similar analgesic effects.

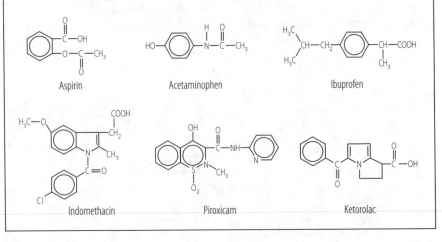

Aspirin

Acetaminophen

Ibuprofen

Indomethacin

Piroxicam

Ketorolac

Pain and inflammation

Although pharmacologic interventions are designed to inhibit them, pain and inflammation are protective mechanisms that are essential for human survival. Pain alerts humans as well as other species to the presence of potentially harmful stimuli, and the inflammatory process functions to remove noxious agents from the site of injury, repair physical damage, and return tissue function to normal. In most cases, pain and inflammation are triggered by stimuli that produce tissue injury; tissue injury can be caused by disease processes, surgical interventions, physical traumas, or antigens that are viral, fungal, bacterial, and so on. The resultant pain and inflammation develop along common pathways regardless of how the injury was initiated. *Biochemical steps to the development of inflammation,* page 34, shows the biochemical events initiated by tissue injury. *Sequence of events of the inflammatory process,* page 35, describes the basic physiologic events in tissue injury and repair. Except in cases of massive injuries, tissue function eventually will return to normal. However, if pain and inflammation continue unchecked and become chronic processes, progressive tissue destruction rather than repair can result.

Biochemical steps to the development of inflammation

Tissue injury results in the release of phospholipids from cell membranes and their subsequent conversion to arachidonic acid. Arachidonic acid is the most important precursor of prostaglandins, leukotrienes, prostacyclins, and thromboxanes, hormonelike compounds that mediate the inflammatory response as well as the production of pain and fever.

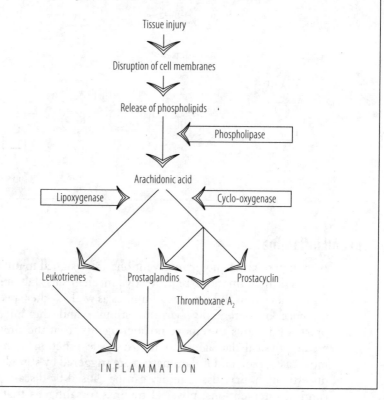

Many different substances play a role in the generation of pain and inflammation. The importance of these substances has been determined experimentally by using enzyme inhibitors to prevent their synthesis and by using selective antagonists to prevent their pharmacologic effects. Although it is clear that no single substance is responsible for the inflammatory process, prostaglandins (PGs) have been demonstrated to play a significant role in the development of pain and inflammation. Experimental evidence linking prostaglandins with inflammation includes the presence of PGs in inflammatory fluids and the capacity of PGs to induce vasodilation, increased capillary permeability, and increased sensitivity to pain. In addition, PGs have been shown

---

Sequence of events of the inflammatory process

1. Tissue injury.
2. Vasodilation of the vessels of microcirculation leads to increased blood flow to the injured area.
3. Mediators of inflammation produce increased vascular permeability.
4. Fluid moves from the vasculature into the tissue to produce edema.

5. White blood cells exit from the blood vessels into the tissue to phagocytize and destroy microbes and debris.
6. Tissue repair.

---

to induce fever when injected into cerebral ventricles and to induce severe disabling arthritis when injected into the knee joint. (For more information, see *Mediators of pain and inflammation*, page 36.)

Mechanism of NSAIDs' action

The antipyretic, anti-inflammatory, and analgesic properties of NSAIDs are attributed to their ability to inhibit prostaglandin synthesis by inhibiting the enzyme cyclo-oxygenase. Classically, this has been thought to occur in the periphery at the site of tissue injury. NSAIDs inhibit pain by preventing the activation of primary afferents that convey pain-producing information from the periphery to the central nervous system, so NSAIDs traditionally have been referred to as "peripheral" analgesics. However, recent evidence suggests that this term may no longer be accurate and that NSAIDs may also produce analgesia by influencing enzymes and neurotransmitter systems in the brain and spinal cord (McCormack 1994). Further research is required to determine the extent to which central nervous system effects contribute to the analgesic efficacy of NSAIDs.

Adverse effects of NSAIDs

The widespread use of NSAIDs makes them responsible for approximately 20% of all adverse drug effects reported to the Food and Drug Administration (Gardner and Simkin 1991). Some adverse effects are unique to specific NSAIDs, but adverse gastrointestinal, hematologic, and renal effects are shared to some degree by most NSAIDs. Less common adverse effects include agranulocytosis, alopecia, aplastic anemia, asymptomatic hepatitis, peripheral edema, photosensitivity, rash, central nervous system effects (headache, memory loss, tinnitus), and breathing problems in asthmatics.

Mediators of pain and inflammation

The complex events of inflammation and pain take place through the action of a number of different substances. These substances have varying chemical structures and other possible roles besides mediating inflammation. For example, serotonin, an amine synthesized in many different tissues, affects brain cell metabolism and smooth muscle contraction as well as affecting the vasodilation that accompanies inflammation.

Bradykinin

The polypeptide bradykinin exists in the plasma as an inactive precursor (kininogen). Following tissue injury, bradykinin is activated by factors in the cascade of reactions involved in the blood clotting process. Bradykinin sensitizes free nerve endings to painful stimuli and produces vasodilation and edema. Bradykinin is metabolized rapidly and as a result plays a role in the early phases of inflammation and pain.

Histamine

The cyclic amine histamine is found in many tissues in the body and exists in an inactive form bound to granules in mast cells or basophils. Mechanical and chemical injury and antigen-antibody reactions can trigger the release of free histamine from mast cells. Histamine sensitizes free nerve endings to painful stimuli, produces vasodilation, and increases capillary permeability. Like bradykinin, free histamine is metabolized rapidly, so the role of histamine in inflammation is early, transient, and nonessential for subsequent events in the inflammatory process. Thus, antihistamines have little use as general anti-inflammatory or analgesic agents.

Interleukin

The polypeptide interleukin is produced by activated macrophages. Interleukin mimics the symptoms of chronic inflammation and stimulates the activation of lymphocytes and the production of fever.

Leukotrienes

Leukotrienes are a number of fatty acids that result from the metabolism of arachidonic acid via lipoxygenase. Leukotrienes cause changes in capillary permeability. NSAIDs do not inhibit the lipoxygenase enzyme and as a result, do not inhibit leukotriene synthesis.

Prostaglandins

Prostaglandins, a group of fatty acids, are the cyclooxygenase products of arachidonic acid metabolism. They are produced in response to tissue injury. A large body of evidence suggests that prostaglandins are potent mediators of inflammation and pain.

Serotonin

The exact role of the amine serotonin in the inflammatory process is not clear; however, the subcutaneous injection of serotonin produces vasodilation and increased capillary permeability.

Gastrointestinal side effects

Gastric irritation and ulceration are the most common adverse effects produced by NSAIDs. Although the gastric irritation can be minimized by taking NSAIDs with food, milk, or antacids, it can limit their use, particularly by people who require high doses. Because NSAIDs are weak acids, local irritation of the gastric mucosa can occur following oral administration. However, because gastric irritation and ulceration can also occur following parenteral administration

(administration other than via the GI tract such as intravenous injection), local irritation is not considered to be the primary mechanism. Prostaglandins produced by the gastric mucosa serve a protective function in the gastrointestinal system. They inhibit gastric acid secretion, increase mucosal blood flow, and stimulate the secretion of gastric mucus. Because NSAIDs inhibit prostaglandin synthesis, these protective mechanisms are lost, and the gastric mucosa is left susceptible to irritation and damage.

Estimates state that 1% to 2% of all patients taking NSAIDs for longer than three months experience some degree of ulceration, bleeding, or perforation (Gardner and Simkin 1991). The high incidence of gastric ulceration following chronic NSAID use has caused research to be focused on developing agents to minimize this adverse effect. Misoprostol, a methyl analogue of prostaglandin E_1, has recently been approved by the Food and Drug Administration for the prevention of ulcers induced by the chronic administration of NSAIDs. Misoprostol inhibits gastric acid secretion by inhibiting histamine-stimulated cyclic adenosine monophosphate (cAMP) production. However, misoprostol has adverse effects of its own including dose-dependent diarrhea. As a result, it is reserved primarily for use in patients who have a history of ulcers and in whom NSAID therapy cannot be terminated.

Hematologic side effects

Disruption of normal platelet function occurs because NSAIDs inhibit the formation of thromboxane A_2, a potent aggregating agent that is synthesized by platelets. Normal bleeding time can be doubled by as little as one 325-mg aspirin tablet. This side effect is of particular concern in patients who have bleeding disorders and who concurrently are on anticoagulant therapy. Additionally, patients undergoing operative procedures may be advised to discontinue NSAID use prior to surgery to minimize blood loss.

Although the effect of NSAIDs on platelet aggregation generally is considered to be an adverse effect, it also has been used to advantage. Aspirin has been proven to be an effective prophylactic agent for the prevention of transient ischemic attacks and unstable angina in men and may reduce the incidence of thrombosis following coronary artery bypass grafts.

Renal side effects

NSAIDs have no significant effects on renal function in normal, healthy individuals. However, when renal function is compromised by conditions such as congestive heart failure and chronic renal disease, renal prostaglandins play a much more significant role in maintaining renal function. Renal prostaglandins promote renal blood flow, increase sodium and water excretion, and stimulate the secretion of renin, a kidney enzyme that helps to maintain normal blood pressure. Because NSAIDs inhibit prostaglandin synthesis, they may precipitate renal failure in compromised patients. In addition, hypertension may be more difficult to control in the presence of NSAIDs in renally compromised people.

Contraindications of NSAID use

The adverse effects associated with NSAIDs can limit their use in some populations. They should be used with caution by people who have active ulcers or a history of ulcers, because the gastrointestinal irritation produced by NSAIDs can precipitate internal bleeding or hemorrhage. Asthmatics also should be advised that aspirin and other NSAIDs can precipitate an asthmatic attack. This hypersensitivity reaction affects about 10% of adults with asthma, but is rare in asthmatic children. Additionally, diabetics should be advised of possible alterations in blood sugar levels when taking NSAIDs, because low and high doses of some NSAIDs can cause hyperglycemia and hypoglycemia, respectively. Plasma uric acid concentrations also may be affected by some NSAIDs. Low doses of salicylates can increase plasma urate concentrations and high doses can lower plasma urate concentrations, so patients who have gout should be cautioned about using NSAIDs. An increased incidence of Reye's syndrome, a fatal degenerative neurological condition, also has been identified in children who take aspirin in the presence of flu or chickenpox viruses. Additionally, for the reasons discussed previously, patients on anticoagulant therapy and patients with compromised renal function should use NSAIDs with caution.

Note that although acetaminophen is often classified as a nonsteroidal anti-inflammatory drug, it is different from other NSAIDs in terms of the side effects associated with its use. Gout patients, children with viral infections, and patients on anticoagulant therapy can take acetaminophen without risking the complications mentioned above. However, acetaminophen lacks anti-inflammatory properties and when used alone will not relieve pain associated with inflammation.

Selected NSAIDs

A large number of NSAIDs are currently available. Several are discussed below in detail. Most importantly, no agent has been proved clearly superior to aspirin with regard to efficacy or toxicity, but newer NSAIDs do offer some advantages:

• Many of the newer NSAIDs are associated with fewer side effects than are associated with aspirin.

- Some of the newer NSAIDS have very long durations of action, which allows them to be administered as a single daily dose. This is important for patients who are taking NSAIDS on a long-term basis and often results in better compliance.
- Patients often have difficulty accepting that a drug as easily obtained and as inexpensive as aspirin can be as effective as newer, more expensive NSAIDs that require a prescription. As a result, newer NSAIDS may be more readily accepted.

Aspirin

Aspirin was first synthesized in 1853 and used clinically in 1899, when it was found to be an effective treatment for arthritis. Aspirin's long history of use, relative safety, low cost, and availability without a prescription make it the standard against which the efficacy of all other NSAIDs are measured. Aspirin is an effective antipyretic, anti-inflammatory, and analgesic agent. A single 650-mg dose of aspirin is sufficient to achieve maximal analgesic and antipyretic effects. In contrast, daily doses of up to 5 grams are required to achieve maximal anti-inflammatory effects.

Aspirin is effective when taken orally and is rapidly absorbed from the stomach and small intestine. It is a weak acid and, because the majority of a dose remains in the nonionized form in the stomach, absorption is favored from the stomach. However, as with most drugs, the large surface area of the small intestine provides for maximal absorption. The half-life (the time required for a drug to fall to one-half its original plasma concentration) of aspirin is 15 to 20 minutes, as it is quickly metabolized by plasma esterases to salicylic acid and acetic acid.

Toxicity and poisoning can be caused by aspirin because it is so readily available and used so frequently. Chronic aspirin toxicity, also known as salicylism, can occur when large doses of aspirin are taken on a chronic basis. For example, daily doses of up to 5 g of aspirin are required for the treatment of chronic inflammatory conditions such as rheumatoid arthritis. Salicylism is not usually life-threatening, and toxic symptoms are mild (see *Symptoms of aspirin toxicity*, page 40). Tinnitus, or ringing in the ears, frequently is a warning sign that toxic plasma levels of aspirin have been reached and that the dosage of aspirin should be decreased.

In contrast, the metabolic changes that occur following acute aspirin toxicity are life-threatening. Aspirin frequently is the cause of accidental poisoning in children because it is so commonly found in the home. The metabolic changes associated with acute aspirin toxicity include hyperventilation and respiratory alkalosis, followed by respiratory and metabolic acidosis. The treatment for acute aspirin toxicity is supportive therapy.

Symptoms of aspirin toxicity

Mild	Moderate	Severe
Vertigo	Acneform eruption	Hallucinations
Tinnitus	Diarrhea	Convulsions
Nausea and vomiting	Drowsiness	Coma
	Confusion	Cardiovascular collapse
	Hyperventilation	
	Hyperthermia	
	Electrolyte imbalances	

Phenylpropionic acid derivatives

The gastric irritation produced by aspirin has led to the search for alternative compounds. Phenylpropionic acid derivatives constitute the largest group of aspirin alternatives. Agents in this group include ibuprofen, naproxen, fenoprofen, flurbiprofen, ketoprofen, and oxaprozin. Oxaprozin is the newest agent in this group; the major advantage this agent offers is its very long half-life of 58 hours, which allows for single daily dosing. This pharmacokinetic property is an important consideration with regard to patient compliance.

The phenylpropionic derivatives generally cause fewer gastrointestinal disturbances than aspirin, and these effects can be further minimized by taking the agents with food, milk, or antacids. Some studies also suggest that the phenylpropionic derivatives may be more efficacious analgesics than aspirin. As a result, these agents are being used in place of aspirin with increasing frequency. Several agents in this class, such as ibuprofen and naproxen, have recently become available as nonprescription drugs.

Other adverse effects associated with the phenylpropionic derivatives include nausea, skin rashes, pruritus, tinnitus, dizziness, headache, peripheral edema, nephrotoxicity, jaundice, and blood dyscrasias, such as agranulocytosis and aplastic anemia. People who experience hypersensitivity reactions to aspirin should be advised that similar hypersensitivity reactions may be encountered with the phenylpropionic derivatives.

Acetaminophen

Acetaminophen is often included with NSAIDs because it is a weak inhibitor of prostaglandin synthesis, but it is important to note that acetaminophen is unlike other NSAIDs in several ways. Acetaminophen has no significant anti-inflammatory properties, does not interfere with platelet aggregation, and does not affect uric acid levels. The reasons for these differences are unclear, because acetaminophen does weakly inhibit the enzyme cyclo-oxygenase. It has been hypothesized that acetaminophen may inhibit central nervous system cyclo-oxygenase more effectively than it inhibits peripheral cyclo-oxygenase.

Acetaminophen is an effective analgesic and antipyretic agent that has efficacy comparable to that of aspirin. It is the drug of choice when a mild analgesic or antipyretic agent is needed for people in whom aspirin is contraindicated. Acetaminophen is preferred over aspirin in the following cases:

• patients who demonstrate aspirin hypersensitivity reaction
• patients with a history of ulcers
• patients with gout
• children with viral infections.

Acetaminophen is a weak base that is well absorbed from the small intestine following oral administration. The half-life of acetaminophen is 2 to 4 hours. It is metabolized in the liver where it is conjugated with glucuronide and sulfate.

Adverse effects of acetaminophen are limited to situations of acute overdose. Acetaminophen has a high therapeutic index, and it is estimated that 6 g or more must be ingested for toxicity to occur. The most serious toxic effect of acetaminophen overdose is hepatotoxicity. The degree of liver damage is related directly to the amount ingested, and patients with preexisting liver disease are particularly susceptible. Hepatotoxicity occurs when the metabolic systems in the liver are overwhelmed, and a highly active, toxic metabolite accumulates. Clinical manifestations of acetaminophen overdose may not become apparent for several days after ingestion, making diagnosis and treatment difficult. Signs of acetaminophen toxicity include nausea, vomiting, diarrhea, and abdominal pain, all of which are indications of hepatic damage. Death is associated with central lobular necrosis of the liver (death of cells associated with liver lobules), with renal necrosis sometimes occurring. Treatment of acetaminophen overdose is primarily supportive. Acetylcysteine can be given to neutralize the toxic metabolite, but it is effective only if administered within 8 to 10 hours of the overdose.

Indomethacin

Indomethacin is a derivative of indoleacetic acid, which was synthesized in 1963 for the treatment of rheumatoid arthritis. It inhibits cyclo-oxygenase and prostaglandin synthesis and has potent antipyretic, anti-inflammatory, and analgesic properties. However, the adverse effects associated with indomethacin have limited its use, and it is not recommended for general use as an analgesic or anti-inflammatory agent. Indomethacin is indicated for several specific conditions, including acute gouty arthritis, ankylosing spondylitis, and extra-articular inflammatory conditions, such as carditis and pleurisy. Indomethacin also is used to accelerate closure of the ductus arteriosus in premature infants.

Indomethacin has a high incidence of dose-dependent adverse effects. Gastrointestinal effects associated with indomethacin use include abdominal pain, diarrhea, ulcerations, and hemorrhage. Acute pancreatitis also has been reported. Central nervous system effects are reported in 20 to 25% of people who take indomethacin for long periods of time and include severe frontal headaches, dizziness, and mental confusion. Hematologic effects, including neutropenia, thrombocytopenia, and aplastic anemia, and hypersensitivity reactions, such as rashes, pruritus, urticaria, and acute attacks of asthma have also been reported. These adverse effects cause approximately 20% of patients to discontinue treatment with indomethacin.

Piroxicam

Piroxicam is equal in potency to indomethacin as an inhibitor of prostaglandin synthesis and is an effective antipyretic, anti-inflammatory, and analgesic agent. A relatively new NSAID whose primary advantage is pharmacokinetic in nature, piroxicam is well absorbed orally, and peak plasma concentrations occur 3 to 5 hours after administration. The average half-life of 50 hours allows a single daily dose to be effective, an important factor for any drug taken on a chronic basis.

The reported incidence of adverse effects with piroxicam is 20%, but only about 5% of those taking the drug discontinue it because of adverse effects. As with other NSAIDs, piroxicam causes gastrointestinal irritation, inhibits platelet aggregation, and can cause hypersensitivity reactions in people who are sensitive to aspirin.

Ketorolac

Ketorolac is unique in that it is the first injectable NSAID available for clinical use. It has antipyretic, anti-inflammatory, and analgesic properties and was approved in 1989 primarily for short-term pain management.

The availability of an injectable NSAID is particularly important in the emergency room setting, where an analgesic agent may be required in situations in which the depressive effects of opioids on the central nervous system and respiration are undesirable. Ketorolac also is available in oral and ophthalmic preparations.

Opioid analgesics

For centuries opium has been an important drug. Ancient Egyptian, Greek, Roman, and Chinese cultures documented its use, recognizing even then that opium relieves not only severe pain but also diarrhea, cough, anxiety, and insomnia. Prior to the development of antibiotics, antipsychotics, and barbiturates, opium was used liberally and played an important role in medical treatment. In the 19th century, following the widespread use of parenteral morphine during the U.S. Civil War, the addictive liabilities of opium became apparent and began to cause concern.

Opium, sometimes referred to as "poppy juice" because it is obtained from the exudate of the poppy seed pod, contains about 20 alkaloids, including morphine, codeine, papaverine, and thebaine. Morphine, first isolated from opium in 1803 and present in concentrations of about 10%, and codeine, present in concentrations of less than 0.5%, are both potent analgesic agents.

Opioid chemistry

Examples of opioid compounds that have agonist, mixed agonist/antagonist, and antagonist properties are shown in *Chemical structures of common opioids,* page 44. A review of the chemical structures reveals that compounds that have agonist properties share common structural features, as do those that have antagonist properties.

Note that relatively small molecular alterations can dramatically change the action of these compounds; agonists can be converted into antagonists and vice versa. In general, antagonist properties are associated with the replacement of the methyl substituent on the nitrogen atom of an agonist with larger groups, such as in naloxone and naltrexone. Molecular alterations also can change the pharmacokinetic properties of compounds. For example, morphine undergoes significant first pass metabolism in the liver following oral administration and, as a result, has a low oral potency. A methyl substitution at the hydroxyl group at the C_3 position converts morphine into codeine, an opioid agonist that has a high oral potency.

Opioid receptors

Structural similarities that exist between opioid agonists and antagonists suggest that they produce their effects by acting at specific receptors. Three different opioid receptors have been identified and demonstrated to be the effectors of opioid actions (see *Opioid receptors and their effects,* page 45). Opioid receptors occur throughout the

Chemical structures of common opioids

In opioid chemistry, relatively small changes in molecular structure often profoundly affect drug function in the body. For example, substitution of a methyl group at the C$_3$ hydroxyl of morphine, an opioid that is not an effective oral analgesic, produces codeine, which is effective in oral form. Substitution of an N-propylene group for an N-methyl group converts the agonist morphine into the antagonist naloxone.

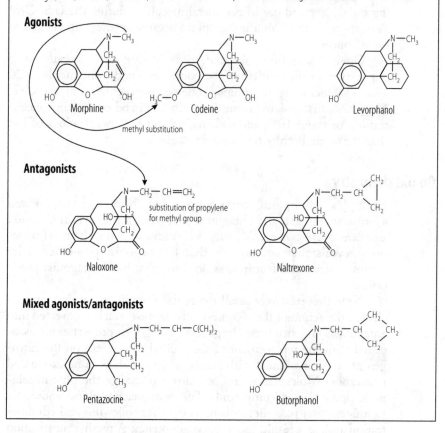

Agonists

Morphine

methyl substitution

Codeine

Levorphanol

Antagonists

substitution of propylene for methyl group

Naloxone

Naltrexone

Mixed agonists/antagonists

Pentazocine

Butorphanol

brain and spinal cord, and opioids produce their primary effects within the central nervous system. In contrast to NSAIDs, which often are referred to as "peripheral" analgesics, opioids are referred to as "central" analgesics.

The knowledge that different receptors have been shown experimentally to be responsible for different effects has allowed pharmaceutical manufacturers to develop opioid compounds that have high affinities for the receptors that mediate the desired effects. Although

Opioid receptors and their effects

Opioid receptors occur in the central nervous system and in other tissues such as the nerves of the gastrointestinal tract. Opioids relieve pain by binding at receptor sites in the central nervous system. A drug that binds at two or more receptor sites may have better properties than a drug that binds at only one type of receptor. For example, a drug that acts as an agonist at kappa sites and an antagonist at mu sites may provide analgesia without the risk of respiratory depression.

Receptor	Effect
Mu (μ)	analgesia, sedation, miosis, euphoria, constipation, respiratory depression, physical dependence
Kappa (κ)	analgesia, sedation, miosis, dysphoria
Delta (δ)	affective behavior

drugs may exhibit higher affinities for certain receptors than others, none is selective for only one receptor type.

Opioid effects at the spinal cord

In the spinal cord, primary afferents (A-δ and C fibers) that convey painful information from the periphery to the central nervous system synapse onto neurons in the substantia gelatinosa, a region of the dorsal horn of the spinal gray matter. These neurons, in turn, relay information to projection neurons located in deep laminae of the dorsal horn. Projection neurons have axons that cross the midline of the spinal cord and ascend contralaterally to supraspinal sites. The classic example of an ascending pathway that conveys painful information to supraspinal sites is the spinothalamic tract (see *Pathways of nociceptive input and inhibition,* page 46). In the spinal cord, opioids modulate the information about pain that is relayed supraspinally by presynaptically inhibiting neurotransmitter release from A-δ and C fibers and by postsynaptically inhibiting dorsal horn neuronal activity.

Opioid effects at the brainstem

Opioids also inhibit the transmission of painful information in the spinal cord by activating descending inhibitory systems in the brainstem (see *Pathways of nociceptive input and inhibition,* page 46). Multiple, distinct descending inhibitory systems have been identified that, when activated, inhibit noxious-evoked dorsal horn neuronal activity in the spinal cord. Opioid receptors have been localized in regions of the brainstem that support descending inhibition. At the spinal level, neurotransmitters, such as norepinephrine and serotonin, mediate the inhibition that originates in the brainstem.

Pathways of nociceptive input and inhibition

Almost all somatosensory information, including pain, enters the spinal cord through the dorsal roots of spinal nerves. Pain is transmitted via primary afferents (A-δ and C fibers) to the substantia gelatinosa, a region in the dorsal horn of the gray matter. In the dorsal horn, projection neurons cross the midline of the spinal cord and ascend contralaterally. They relay the information to brain sites such as the thalamus and the cortex.

Cross section of spinal cord

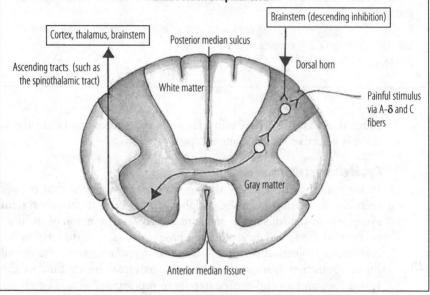

Opioid effects at the thalamus

The central perception of pain occurs in the thalamus and cortex. Opioids modulate pain perception by inhibiting neurons in these regions. Patients report that the "reaction" to a painful stimulus is very much affected by opioids (see discussion below).

Functional classification of opioids

Opioids often are classified according to function as agonists, antagonists or mixed agonist/antagonists (see *Opioid classifications*). Opioid agonists are morphine-like in that they act as agonists at mu, kappa, and delta receptors. The prototypical opioid agonist is morphine. Other opioid agonists are codeine, oxycodone, methadone, meperidine, fentanyl, and levorphanol.

Opioid antagonists lack agonist activity at any of the opioid receptors. They are used clinically to reverse the respiratory depres-

Opioid classifications

Agonists are compounds that bind to receptors (particular proteins necessary for cell function) to produce a biological effect. Morphine, the prototypical opioid agonist, has a high affinity to bind to mu receptors. Opioid agonists produce analgesia and other effects.

Antagonists are compounds that bind to receptors but do *not* produce a biological effect. Naloxone is the prototypical opioid antagonist. Naloxone is a compet-

itive antagonist, which means that it can "compete" with opioid agonists for binding to opioid receptors.

Mixed agonist/antagonists are compounds that may have agonist properties at one receptor type and antagonist properties at another receptor type. Pentazocine is the prototypical opioid mixed agonist/antagonist. It acts as an agonist at kappa receptors and as an antagonist at mu receptors.

sant effects produced by opioids (see discussion below). Opioid antagonists include naloxone, naltrexone, and nalorphine.

Opioids that have mixed agonist/antagonist properties have agonist properties at some receptors and antagonist or very weak agonist properties at others. Opioids with mixed agonist/antagonist properties function as agonists in opioid-naive patients, whereas in opioid-tolerant patients they can precipitate withdrawal symptoms. The prototypical mixed agonist/antagonist is pentazocine. Other mixed agonist/antagonists are butorphanol, nalbuphine, and buprenorphine.

Central nervous system effects of opioids

The predominant general effect of opioids in the central nervous system is inhibition; many of the specific effects reflect that depressant action. Tolerance, a decreased responsiveness to a pharmacologic effect of a drug as a consequence of prior administration of that drug, does develop to all of the central nervous system effects produced by opioids, with the exception of miosis (see *Development of tolerance to opioid effects,* page 48).

Analgesia

Opioids are effective analgesic agents and produce significant analgesia without the loss of other sensory modalities, such as vision, audition, and touch. Opioids suppress both the perception of and the reaction to pain. In the presence of opioids, patients report that although an awareness of the pain is maintained, it is no longer a source of discomfort.

Respiratory depression and sedation

All opioid agonists produce a dose-dependent respiratory depression that is mediated by brainstem mechanisms; high concentrations of

Development of tolerance to opioid effects

Tolerance to many of the central nervous system effects of opioids develops with repeated exposure. Constipation occurs as a result of a high density of opi-oid receptors in the gastrointestinal tract causing in opioid-induced inhibition of local enteric nerves.

Tolerance develops	No tolerance develops
Analgesia	Miosis
Respiratory depression	Constipation
Sedation	
Euphoria and dysphoria	
Cough suppression	
Nausea and vomiting	

opioid receptors have been localized in brainstem respiratory centers. In the presence of opioids, chemoreceptors in the brainstem exhibit a decreased responsiveness to CO_2. The respiratory depression produced by opioids is the major disadvantage of opioid use, and opioids should be used with caution by people with preexisting respiratory conditions such as asthma, chronic obstructive pulmonary disease, or emphysema. In opioid overdose, respiratory arrest is the usual cause of death. Tolerance does develop to the respiratory depressant effects produced by opioids, but even in opioid-tolerant patients, lethal respiratory depression can be produced by very high doses.

Sedation and mental clouding are common side effects produced by opioid agonists. Significant central nervous system depression can occur if opioids are combined with other depressant drugs, such as barbiturates or antipsychotics. The sedative effects produced by opioids can limit their use by some people, but tolerance does develop to the sedation. Note that it is not appropriate to use opioids as sedative-hypnotic agents unless the insomnia is due to pain.

Other central nervous system effects

Euphoria, a sense of well-being, is the affective response experienced by most people who are taking opioids for pain relief. In contrast, 25% of people who take opioids but are not in pain experience dysphoria, a sense of restlessness and malaise.

Opioids have long been recognized to be effective cough suppressants, an effect that is the result of suppression of the cough reflex center in the brainstem.

Miosis, or constriction of the pupils, is a central nervous system effect produced by all opioid agonists. Because no tolerance develops to this effect, the presence of miosis can be used as an indicator of opioid use or abuse, although it should be recognized that other drugs and pathophysiologic conditions may also alter pupillary diameter.

Initial doses of opioids can stimulate the chemoreceptor trigger zone in the medulla and cause nausea and vomiting in some individuals. A higher incidence exists in ambulatory patients compared to recumbent patients, suggesting a secondary effect on the vestibular apparatus. This effect of opioids is transient, and larger or subsequent doses suppress the chemoreceptor trigger zone.

Increased tone of the large trunk muscles, or truncal rigidity, occurs in some individuals following rapid administration of large doses of opioids for anesthesia. This effect is thought to be mediated both at the supraspinal and spinal levels. It can interfere with respiratory function, particularly in compromised patients.

Peripheral effects of opioids

Although the majority of opioid receptors are in the brain or spinal cord, there is also evidence that there are opioid receptor sites in the periphery. The effects of opioids on peripheral systems vary.

Gastrointestinal effects

Constipation is a recognized peripheral side effect of opioid agonists, and opioid receptors have been identified in the gastrointestinal tract. Stimulation of these receptors increases the resting tone and decreases the propulsive activity of the gastrointestinal tract, resulting in constipation. Minimal tolerance develops to this effect of opioids, and constipation can be a significant and limiting effect, particularly in people who are required to take opioids on a chronic basis for pain management.

Cardiovascular effects

Most opioid agonists have no significant direct effects on the cardiovascular system at doses required for analgesia. However, intravenous administration of opioids can cause histamine release that, in turn, can cause hypotension and flushing and itching at the site of injection. Opioid agonists also can worsen hypovolemic shock and should be used with caution in patients who have decreased blood volume.

Other peripheral effects

Opioid agonists can increase urethral sphincter tone and precipitate urinary retention, which can be a particular problem in postoperative patients. Therapeutic doses of opioid agonists also may prolong labor and affect the degree to which the mother is able to cooperate in the delivery. Opioid agonists constrict the smooth muscles of the biliary tract and the sphincter of Oddi and can produce symptoms of biliary colic and epigastric distress. They can also precipitate biliary colic in patients with bile duct or gallbladder disease.

Therapeutic uses of opioids

Clinically, opioids are used as analgesic agents, antitussive agents, antidiarrheal agents, and as adjunct medications for anesthesia. Opioids should not be used as sedative-hypnotic agents unless the insomnia is due to pain. Opioids provide symptomatic treatment only, and in all cases the underlying cause of the symptoms should be sought.

Analgesics

Opioids continue to be the most efficacious analgesic agents available for the treatment of moderate to severe pain. Opioids are particularly effective for the treatment of visceral pain, and severe, dull, constant pain is better relieved by opioids than is sharp, stabbing pain. Patients vary greatly in their analgesic dose requirements, so opioid dosing schedules should be individualized and titrated for each patient to maximize the analgesic effects and minimize the adverse effects produced by opioids. For example, since opioid metabolism and elimination decrease with age, pain relief provided by opioids increases with age. Thus, opioid doses that provide effective analgesia for older patients may not be appropriate for younger patients.

Unfortunately, despite their effectiveness as analgesics, the fear of addiction to opioids by health care professionals and patients often limits their appropriate use. Physicians tend to prescribe inadequate doses of opioids, health care providers do not administer them as frequently as required to provide adequate pain relief, and patients often are reluctant to request adequate pain relief medications. Tolerance and physical dependence, which is defined as an abnormal physiologic state produced by repeated drug administration and characterized by the necessity of continued drug use to prevent a withdrawal syndrome, do develop with repeated opioid use, but they should not inhibit the use of opioids to treat pain. Following chronic administration, withdrawal symptoms can be minimized by gradually terminating the opioid. The development of psychological dependence, which is defined as drug-seeking behavior contrary to the rational best interest of the individual, and opioid abuse as a consequence of the use of opioids for medical reasons is unsubstantiated. It is essential that health care professionals and patients be educated about the addiction liabilities that are associated with opioid use. Additionally, the positive health benefits that result from effective pain control, particularly in the postoperative patient must be acknowledged.

Adjunct medications for anesthesia

An ideal general anesthetic is one that produces unconsciousness, analgesia, and muscle relaxation. Most general anesthetics used today are not ideal. Ideal anesthesia is achieved by administering preoperative medications in combination with a primary anesthetic. Opioids are frequently used as preoperative drugs prior to anesthesia and surgery because of their sedative, anxiolytic, and analgesic properties.

Because opioids have few significant effects on the cardiovascular system, high doses of certain opioids like fentanyl, alfentanil, and sufentanil can be used as primary anesthetics in situations in which it is desirable to minimize cardiovascular depression such as in cardiac surgery. Muscle relaxants and nitrous oxide or small doses of other inhalation anesthetics are usually administered in combination with the opioid.

Other therapeutic uses

Opioids such as codeine are very effective antitussive agents, and cough suppression can be obtained at doses lower than those needed for analgesia. Synthetic agents like dextromethorphan and noscapine that are neither addictive nor analgesic are now replacing the use of codeine for cough control.

Opioids increase the resting tone and decrease the propulsive activity of the gastrointestinal tract, so they can be used effectively to control diarrhea. Many antidiarrheal medications contain paregoric, an opium-containing tincture. Diphenoxylate and loperamide also are opioid derivatives that are used to control diarrhea. It should be emphasized that opioids provide symptomatic treatment only. If the diarrhea is associated with an infection, opioids should not be used as substitutes for appropriate antibiotic therapy.

Selected opioid agonists

Numerous opioids are available for the treatment of moderate to severe pain (see *Selected opioid agents*, page 52). Most opioid agonists exhibit pharmacologic properties that are qualitatively similar to morphine. As the prototypical opioid agonist, morphine remains the standard against which new analgesics are measured. To date, no other opioid has been demonstrated to be clearly superior to morphine as an analgesic agent.

Morphine and related compounds

Morphine, the prototypical mu receptor agonist, is available for oral use and for injection. However, oral administration results in significant first-pass metabolism and has been shown to be only one-sixth as effective as parenteral administration. Codeine, hydromorphone,

Selected opioid agents

Both agonists and mixed agonist/antagonists are used for analgesia. The agonist/antagonist drugs have a reduced potential for causing respiratory depression.

Pure antagonists (naloxone, naltrexone) are used clinically to reverse opioid-related respiratory depression.

Agonists	Mixed agonist/ antagonists	Antagonists	Antitussives	Antidiarrheals
Morphine	Pentazocine	Naloxone	Dextromethorphan	Diphenoxylate
Codeine	Nalbuphine	Naltrexone	Noscapine	Loperamide
Hydromorphone	Butorphanol			
Oxymorphone	Buprenorphine			
Oxycodone				
Heroin				
Meperidine				
Fentanyl				
Sufentanil				
Alfentanil				
Methadone				

oxymorphone, and oxycodone are compounds that are structurally related to morphine and can be used in place of morphine. Heroin also is a morphine-related compound that has significant analgesic properties. Although the use of heroin is prohibited in the United States because of the potential for its abuse, it is used to treat cancer pain in some countries. Recently, there has been a movement in the United States to legalize the therapeutic use of heroin even though it offers no significant clinical advantages over morphine for the treatment of severe chronic pain.

Meperidine and related compounds

Meperidine (Demerol) is a synthetic mu agonist that has effects similar to those of morphine. Meperidine is available for oral use and for injection and, like morphine, it is less effective when administered orally. Meperidine has a significantly shorter half-life than morphine, and frequent dosing is required to maintain pain relief. As a result, meperidine is infrequently used. Additionally, meperidine is unique because it can cause central nervous system excitation, such as seizures, tremors, and muscle twitches, an effect that is due to the accumulation of the metabolite normeperidine.

Fentanyl, sufentanil, and alfentanil are synthetic opioids that structurally are related to meperidine. They are mu agonists and are estimated to be 80 times more potent than morphine. Currently, no oral formulations are available for these drugs. High doses of these drugs can be used as primary anesthetics when it is desirable to minimize cardiovascular effects, and they can be used intrathecally and epidurally for postoperative analgesia. Fentanyl is also used in a transdermal formulation for the treatment of chronic intractable pain.

Methadone

Methadone also has pharmacologic properties that are qualitatively similar to morphine, but methadone offers several advantages over morphine including:

- reliable effects following oral administration
- the ability to suppress withdrawal symptoms in opioid-dependent individuals for an extended duration of action
- a slower development of tolerance and physical dependence
- milder withdrawal symptoms after abrupt termination of the drug.

Methadone is used for pain relief, for the treatment of opioid abstinence syndromes, and for the treatment of heroin addiction.

Mixed agonist/antagonists

Pharmaceutical companies have pursued the development of opioids with mixed agonist/antagonist properties in an effort to develop effective analgesics that lack respiratory depressant effects and abuse potential. This endeavor has yielded new compounds with limited abuse potential. Opioids that have mixed agonist/antagonist properties are effective analgesic agents for mild to moderate pain, but they should not be used by people previously treated with opioid agonists because they can precipitate withdrawal symptoms. Pentazocine is the prototype mixed agonist/antagonist.

Pentazocine

Pentazocine is an agonist at kappa receptors and a weak antagonist at mu receptors. It has a pharmacologic profile similar to morphine, including the respiratory depressant effects and the development of tolerance and physical dependence. Currently, pentazocine is the only mixed agonist/antagonist that is available for oral administration.

Nalbuphine

Nalbuphine, a kappa agonist and mu antagonist, was released in 1979. Structurally, it is related to both naloxone and oxymorphone, and it has a spectrum of effects similar to those of pentazocine. In contrast to morphine, the respiratory depressant effects produced by nalbuphine exhibit a ceiling effect; increasing doses beyond 30 mg produces no further respiratory depression. Nalbuphine is not classified as a controlled substance, and few cases of abuse have been reported since its release. Nalbuphine is available as an injectable for parenteral administration.

Butorphanol
Butorphanol, thought to be a kappa agonist, was introduced in 1978. It has a pharmacologic profile similar to that of pentazocine. Butorphanol is not classified as a controlled substance, and addicts actually express a dislike for it. It is available as an injectable for parenteral administration and as an intranasal formulation.

Buprenorphine
Buprenorphine is a semisynthetic opioid that is derived from thebaine, an alkaloid found in opium. It is a partial agonist at mu receptors and is 25 to 50 times more potent than morphine. The analgesic effects produced by buprenorphine are qualitatively similar to morphine, but the respiratory depressant and sedative effects are much less significant. Recent clinical trials indicate that, like methadone, buprenorphine may be useful in the treatment of heroin addiction (Bowersox 1995). Buprenorphine is currently available only for parenteral administration in the United States.

Opioid antagonists

In normal individuals, opioid antagonists, such as naloxone and naltrexone, produce few effects when administered in the absence of an opioid agonist. Clinically, they are used as diagnostic agents for opioid abuse, to reverse opioid-induced respiratory depression, and as pharmacologic deterrents in opioid addicts. When endogenous opioid systems are activated as in hypovolemic shock, endotoxic shock, or spinal cord injury, for example, opioid antagonists can produce effects and may be useful in the treatment of shock, stroke, and brain and spinal cord injuries.

Naloxone
Naloxone is absorbed readily from the gastrointestinal tract, but it is metabolized rapidly by the liver and, as a result, must be administered parenterally. Naloxone has a half-life that is significantly shorter than morphine, so 1 to 4 hours and multiple doses may be required to reverse the depressant effects of opioids. Naloxone has a high affinity for mu receptors and is a competitive antagonist.

Naltrexone

In contrast to naloxone, naltrexone is efficacious with oral administration, and its half-life is considerably longer at 10 hours. Naltrexone also has a high affinity for mu receptors and is a competitive antagonist. It has been used in drug treatment programs to deter addicts from future opioid abuse and has recently been approved as an adjunct medication for the treatment of alcoholism.

Novel routes of opioid administration

Opioids are the most effective analgesic agents available; they continue to be the cornerstone of pain management. The pharmacokinetic properties of many opioids make them most effective when administered by the parenteral route. This route of administration is painful to the patient, expensive, and requires additional physician and nursing time and expertise. As a result, alternative routes of opioid administration are being investigated.

Sublingual administration

Buprenorphine, mentioned above as an effective synthetic opioid with reduced sedation and respiratory depressant effects, has been proven effective following sublingual administration. It is a lipophilic compound and is easily absorbed through the oral mucosa. A sublingual preparation of buprenorphine is not now available in the United States but is being used in other countries.

An oral transmucosal formulation of fentanyl was recently approved for human use by the Food and Drug Administration as a preoperative sedative, anxiolytic, and analgesic (Streisand 1994). Fentanyl does not produce effective analgesia following a single bolus sublingual dose, but it has been shown to be effective when incorporated into a candy base that can be kept in the mouth and sucked by the patient until adequate analgesia is achieved. This route of administration is noninvasive and has been shown to be particularly effective for pediatric patients.

Transdermal administration

Fentanyl is currently available in transdermal form and has been approved for the management of chronic pain requiring opioid therapy. The principal advantage offered by the transdermal system is conversion of a short-acting drug into one that produces up to 72 hours of effective analgesia once steady-state plasma levels have been achieved. Because a subcutaneous depot of the drug must develop after initial application of the product, several days must pass before steady-state plasma levels are reached and effective analgesia is produced. Thus, alternative means of analgesia are required during the initial period of the transdermal application. Obviously, transdermal routes of administration are not appropriate for acute pain management because of the slow onset of analgesia.

Patient-controlled analgesia

Patient-controlled analgesia has recently become a popular method of controlling acute postoperative pain. The patient is equipped with an indwelling intravenous catheter that is attached to an electronic injection device. The setup allows the patient to self-administer opioids as needed for adequate pain relief. This method of pain management provides patients with a greater sense of personal control over their situations, which may reduce anxiety and further improve analgesia. It also is a particularly useful method of pain management for people who are reluctant to request additional pain medications.

Other routes

Evidence suggests that rectal administration may provide an alternative route of administration for opioids, and it is a route that is common in hospice settings. Variable absorption rates represent the main disadvantage associated with rectal administration. Absorption rates are dependent on the placement site, rectal contents, and individual differences in venous drainage from the rectum.

Intranasal administration of opioids is another alternative route of administration that is noninvasive and that is being investigated further. Butorphanol has been demonstrated to provide effective analgesia for acute pain following intranasal administration (Cool et al. 1990).

Local anesthetics

Local anesthetics block the sensation of pain by interfering with the propagation of peripheral nerve impulses along nerve axons. When applied to a localized area, they can produce analgesia and muscle relaxation without hypnosis or sedation. As a class of agents, local anesthetics can be identified by the suffix, "caine," for example, procaine, lidocaine, benzocaine.

Cocaine, an alkaloid found in high concentrations in the leaves of the *Erythroxylum coca* plant, was the first local anesthetic agent to be discovered. The natives of Peru, recognizing the effects on the central nervous system of cocaine, chewed or sucked coca leaves to prevent hunger and fatigue and to provide a sense of well-being. In 1884 cocaine was introduced into medicine simultaneously by two physicians, Sigmund Freud and Karl Koller. Cocaine was used by Freud to treat morphine addiction and by Koller as an ophthalmologic anesthetic (Ritchie and Greene 1990). The use of cocaine rapidly increased to include dental and surgical procedures, but the potential for abuse of cocaine soon became apparent and the search for new local anesthetic agents was initiated. Since the introduction of cocaine, nonaddictive synthetic substitutes have been developed

Local anesthetic chemistry

Three structural characteristics are required for a compound to have local anesthetic activity:

- a lipophilic group
- a hydrophilic group
- an intermediate chain (see *Chemical structures of two local anesthetics,* page 58).

The lipophilic group, usually an aromatic group, confers lipid solubility on the compound and is required for the penetration by the agent through the nerve membrane to its site of action (see "Local anesthetic mechanisms"). The hydrophilic group, usually a secondary or tertiary amino group, confers water solubility on the compound and ensures that once injected, the drug will not precipitate in the interstitial fluid. The intermediate chain provides the necessary spatial separation between the lipophilic and hydrophilic ends of the compound. The chemical linkage between the intermediate chain and the aromatic group is used to classify local anesthetics as either esters or amides.

Local anesthetics are weak bases. Usually they are formulated as hydrochloric salts to increase their solubility and stability. In the body, local anesthetics exist as a nonionized base or as a cationic acid. Only the nonionized base can cross nerve cell membranes, but once inside the axon, the cationic acid acts as the anesthetic. Tissue acidity (low pH) fosters a balance in which a greater proportion of the anesthetic exists as the cationic acid, which does not readily diffuse into the nerve cell. This explains why local anesthetics are less effective in inflamed tissue, as inflamed tissues are acidic (have a low extracellular pH) and thus promote existence of a greater proportion of the anesthetic as the cationic acid.

Local anesthetic mechanisms

Local anesthetics block the conduction of action potentials along nerve axons by blocking the influence of stimulation on Na^+ channels (see *Changes in cell membrane potential associated with nerve conduction,* page 59). Local anesthetics must cross the cell membrane in order to be effective because they produce their effects by binding at specific

Chemical structures of two local anesthetics

Molecules of local anesthetics reversibly bind to the sodium channels in nerve cell membranes, an event that leads to cessation of the sodium current and loss of the cell's ability to generate an action potential. The lipophilic end of the molecule aids in its penetration through the lipid portion of the cell membrane. The hydrophilic end of the molecule ensures its solubility in interstitial fluid.

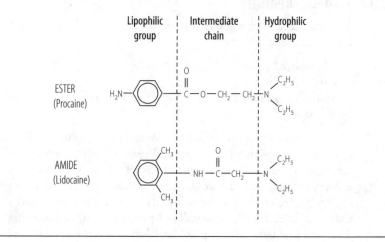

sites near the intracellular end of sodium channels. As the local anesthetic block develops, the threshold for excitation increases, the conduction rate of action potentials slows and, if sodium conductance is blocked along a critical length of axon, the ability to conduct action potentials fails (see "Fiber size and critical length" below).

Local anesthetics affect different types of nerve fibers to varying degrees. Large-diameter, myelinated A fibers, which convey information regarding motor function, pressure, proprioception, and touch, are relatively insensitive to local anesthetic blockade. In contrast, small-diameter sensory fibers, which convey information regarding temperature and pain, are very sensitive to local anesthetics. Modalities, listed in increasing order of resistance to conduction block, include pain, cold, warmth, touch, and deep pressure.

Several factors account for the selectivity of nerve blockade observed in local anesthetics, including fiber size, the critical length, and the firing frequency.

Fiber size and critical length

The critical length of a nerve fiber is defined as the length of nerve that must be blocked by the local anesthetic for nerve conduc-

Changes in cell membrane potential associated with nerve conduction

The conduction of action potentials along axons reflects changes in cell membrane permeability to sodium and potassium. In the resting state (A) the nerve membrane is impermeable to sodium ions, Na^+ channels are closed, and the membrane potential is negative (-80 mV). In the presence of a stimulus, Na^+ channels open, the Na^+ conductance increases (B), and the inside of the neuron becomes less electronegative (depolarized). If the transmembrane potential becomes sufficiently positive, an action potential occurs. This change in membrane potential and membrane permeability to Na^+ is transient and can occur at any given segment of the membrane. Following the generation of an action potential, Na^+ channels close, K^+ (potassium ion) channels open (C), and the nerve becomes refractory to stimulation. As the membrane potential returns to its resting state (D), the nerve regains the ability to conduct action potentials.

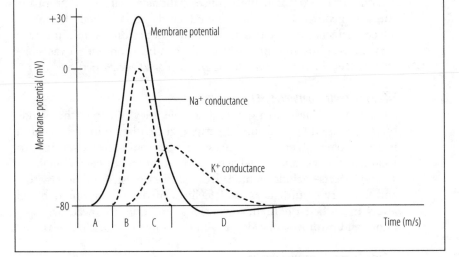

tion to fail. Myelinated nerve fibers conduct action potentials in a saltatory fashion between nodes of Ranvier. It is estimated that three successive nodes of Ranvier must be blocked to prevent nerve conduction. Larger nerve fibers are more resistant to blockade by local anesthetics because of larger distances between nodes of Ranvier and larger critical lengths.

Firing frequency

Local anesthetics have been demonstrated to have a higher affinity for Na^+ channels in the open, activated state than in the closed, resting state, and they more effectively inhibit nerve axons that exhibit high-frequency trains of action potentials than nerve axons that exhibit single action potentials. This phenomenon is known as use-dependent block. Because local anesthetics bind more effectively to open Na⁺ channels, neurons that are firing at high frequencies have greater exposure of their Na⁺ channel receptor sites to the anesthetic. Generally, pain fibers fire action potentials at a higher frequency than do motor fibers. As a result, they are more sensitive to local anesthetic blockade.

Adverse effects of local anesthetics

Local anesthetics can provide reversible analgesia within well-defined, localized regions of the body, but they do not selectively depress peripheral nerve conduction, and they can interfere with nerve conduction in any excitable tissue, particularly central nervous system tissue and cardiac tissue. Systemic effects produced by local anesthetics can occur if high concentrations are absorbed from the site of injection and if high blood levels are reached. However, adverse effects associated with local anesthetics can be minimized if they are administered properly and in combination with a vasoconstrictor (see *How to avoid adverse effects of local anesthetics*).

Effects on central nervous system
Because local anesthetics are lipid-soluble, they can cross the blood-brain barrier and pass from the peripheral circulation into the central nervous system. Central nervous system neurons are very sensitive to local anesthetics, and initial signs and symptoms of central nervous system effects include lightheadedness, dizziness, numbness, visual and auditory disturbances, and feelings of disorientation. If blood levels are sufficiently high, convulsions can occur, followed by respiratory and cardiovascular depression and a loss of consciousness.

Effects on cardiovascular system
Local anesthetics also can have direct effects on cardiac tissue. Some of these effects can be beneficial and have been used to clinical advantage. For example, local anesthetics are used to treat cardiac arrhythmias. In nontoxic doses, local anesthetics increase the effective refractory period of cardiac tissue and decrease cardiac automaticity. In toxic doses, membrane excitability and conduction velocity are depressed throughout the heart, which leads to decreased cardiac output, hypoxia and, ultimately, circulatory collapse.

Other adverse effects
Fainting as a result of the injection procedure is a frequently seen adverse effect of local anesthetic administration. Typically, fainting is a psychological response to the fear or pain of the injection and is not a pharmacologic effect of the local anesthetic.

How to avoid adverse effects of local anesthetics

1. Take a careful history.
2. Use the smallest dose possible that will provide effective anesthesia.
3. Use a vasoconstrictor with the local anesthetic to retard drug absorption.
4. Use proper injection techniques and aspirate before administering the local anesthetic to avoid intravascular injection.
5. Inject SLOWLY.
6. Avoid repeated injections into the same site over a prolonged period of time.

Allergic reactions, such as contact dermatitis, asthmatic attacks, and anaphylactic reactions, can occur with local anesthetic administration, although the incidence is infrequent. Health care personnel sometimes experience contact dermatitis if they frequently handle local anesthetics. Allergic reactions occur more commonly with the ester type of local anesthetic.

Addition of vasoconstrictors
Many local anesthetics inhibit myogenic activity and autonomic tone and produce vasodilation at the site of administration. To counteract this effect, vasoconstrictors are routinely added to local anesthetic solutions to localize the anesthetic, decrease systemic absorption, and prolong the duration of action. The most commonly used vasoconstrictors are sympathomimetic (adrenergic) drugs, including epinephrine, levonordefrin, norepinephrine, and phenylephrine. Clinically, epinephrine is considered to be the most effective vasoconstrictor when administered with local anesthetics. Local anesthetics combined with vasoconstrictors should not be used in fingers, toes, ears, or the penis because vasoconstriction in those locations could result in tissue necrosis.

Routes of administration
Local anesthetics are used widely for the relief of pain. They inhibit pain by anesthetizing the nerves that transmit information indicating pain. They are useful because they can produce analgesia and muscle relaxation without loss of consciousness. Depending on the extent and duration of anesthesia required, local anesthetics can be administered by several different routes. (See *Commonly used local anesthetics,* page 62.)

Commonly used local anesthetics

Local anesthetics are classified according to type of chemical linkage between opposing lipophilic and hydrophilic ends of the compound. The choice of anesthetic is usually determined by the desired duration of anesthesia. The effects of short- or moderate-duration anesthetics can be prolonged by adding a vasoconstrictive agent to the drug.

Drug	Anesthetic type	Duration of action
Procaine	ester	short
Prilocaine	amide	moderate
Mepivacaine	amide	moderate
Lidocaine	amide	moderate
Bupivacaine	amide	long
Tetracaine	ester	long
Etidocaine	amide	long

Topical application

Anesthesia of mucous membranes, such as the nose, mouth, throat, and trachea, and of injured skin can be achieved by directly applying local anesthetics to surface membranes. Aqueous solutions are used when coverage of large surfaces is required. Ointments or viscous gels are used when anesthesia of restricted areas is required. Benzocaine is an example of a local anesthetic that is effective when applied topically, but ineffective when administered parenterally.

Peripheral infiltration

Administration of local anesthetics by using infiltration and nerve block techniques allows anesthesia to be produced within restricted regions of the peripheral nervous system. Infiltration anesthesia is accomplished by the injection of local anesthetic into the subcutaneous or submucosal tissues that are to be anesthetized. Nerve endings in the anesthetized region rapidly become unresponsive. Nerve block anesthesia is accomplished by the injection of local anesthetic close to a nerve trunk, but proximal to the intended area of anesthesia. Following diffusion of the local anesthetic, tissues that are innervated by the distal portion of the affected nerve are anesthetized.

Spinal routes

Administration of a local anesthetic solution in the spinal cord subarachnoid space can be used to produce central nervous system anesthesia in all structures of the body below the diaphragm. The local anesthetic is usually administered in the lumbar subarachnoid space to avoid damage to the spinal cord, and circulating cerebrospinal fluid distributes the anesthetic to the spinal cord. The dose and volume of anesthetic administered determine the extent of distribution.

An alternative to subarachnoid anesthesia is epidural anesthesia. The local anesthetic is administered in the epidural space, which is between the dura mater (the outermost membrane of the spinal cord) and the walls of the vertebral canal. Epidural anesthesia generally is slower in onset, often requires more drug, and may be more difficult to control than spinal anesthesia.

Other pharmacologic agents

The human pain response is a complex phenomenon with both physiologic and affective components. The affective component can be influenced by many factors, including past experiences with pain, both personal and cultural, the reactions of others to pain, and the emotional context in which pain is experienced. So perhaps it is not surprising that drugs primarily used to treat psychiatric disorders also have been found effective in the treatment of chronic pain (Monks and Merskey 1989).

Psychotropic agents influence multiple neurotransmitter systems in the brain, and these changes in central nervous system neurotransmission could account for their analgesic efficacy. The changes in neurotransmission produced by these agents are not always comparable, however, and additional studies will be required to understand the specific mechanisms that account for the analgesic effects produced.

Antidepressants

Tricyclic antidepressants and monoamine oxidase inhibitors have been demonstrated to be effective treatment for certain chronic pain states, such as diabetic neuropathy, rheumatoid arthritis, and migraine headaches. The mechanisms of action that account for their analgesic efficacy are unclear. Many chronic-pain patients also experience reactive depression; thus, the initial hypothesis was that the analgesic effects of these agents were due to their antidepressant actions and to nonspecific physiologic effects, such as sedation, muscle relaxation, and decreased anxiety.

Evidence suggests, however, that the analgesic efficacy of antidepressants is not mediated entirely by their antidepressant and nonspecific actions. For example, time course studies reveal that the onset of analgesia produced by antidepressants is more rapid than the onset of antidepressant effects. Also, relief of chronic pain has been reported in patients who do not demonstrate symptoms of clinical depression, and not all antidepressants are effective analgesics. It has been suggested that the analgesic efficacy of these agents is due to their actions on central nervous system catecholamine and indolamine systems. Tricyclic antidepressants and monoamine oxidase inhibitors increase synaptic levels of dopamine, norepinephrine, and serotonin.

Other psychotropic agents

Antipsychotic agents that have been found to be useful in the treatment of chronic pain include phenothiazines, thioxanthenes, and butyrophenones. Because most chronic-pain patients do not experience delusional psychiatric disorders, the analgesic effects produced by these agents are probably distinct from their antipsychotic effects. Antipsychotic agents influence multiple neurotransmitter systems in the central nervous system. In contrast to the antidepressant agents, antipsychotic agents inhibit dopamine, norepinephrine, serotonin, and histamine neurotransmission.

In general, benzodiazepines, the most important class of anxiolytics, do not produce significant analgesic effects. They can be given to chronic-pain patients to relieve the anxiety, excessive muscle tension, and insomnia that can accompany chronic pain states; however, the dependence liability of benzodiazepines and their lack of long-term efficacy limits their usefulness. Benzodiazepines affect norepinephrine, serotonin, dopamine, and gamma-aminobutyric acid (GABA) neurotransmission.

REFERENCES

Bowersox, J.A. "Buprenorphine May Soon Be Heroin Treatment Option." *NIDA Notes* 10:8-9, 1995.

Cool, W.M., et al. "Transnasal delivery of systemic drugs," in *Advances in Pain Research and Therapy Series; Opioid Analgesia: Recent Advances in Systemic Administration*, Vol. 14. Edited by Benedetti, C., et al. Philadelphia: Lippincott-Raven, 1990.

Gardner, G.C., and Simkin, P.A. "Adverse Effects of NSAIDs," *Pharmacy and Therapeutics* 16:750-754, 1991.

Loper, K.A., et al. "Paralyzed with pain: the need for education," *Pain* 37(3):315-316, 1989.

Marks, R.M., and Sachar, E.J. "Undertreatment of medical inpatients with narcotic analgesics," *Annals of Internal Medicine* 78(2):173-181, 1973.

McCormack, K. "Non-steroidal anti-inflammatory drugs and spinal nociceptive processing," *Pain* 59(1):9-43, 1994.

Monks, R., and Merskey, H. "Psychotropic drugs," in *Textbook of Pain*, 3rd ed. Edited by Wall, P.D., and Melzack, R. New York: Churchill Livingstone, 1994.

Perry, S.W. "The undermedication for pain," *Psychiatric Annals* 14(11):808-811, 1984.

Ritchie, J.M., and Greene, N.M. "Local anesthetics," in *Goodman & Gilman's The Pharmacologic Basis of Therapeutics*, 9th ed. Edited by Gilman, A.G., et al. New York: McGraw-Hill, 1996.

Streisand, J.B. "OTFC: A new opioid delivery system," *American Pain Society Bulletin*, 4:1-3, 1994.

CHAPTER 3

Diagnostic tools in the management of pain

Rajat Gupta, MD

Peter S. Staats, MD

Pain is one of the most common reasons patients visit a doctor's office. It is the principal complaint in approximately half of all visits to a physician in the United States. Several years ago, estimates suggested that approximately one-third of the adult population in the United States suffered a chronic painful condition. Moreover, the annual health care costs, costs resulting from disability, and other indirect costs of chronic painful conditions totaled approximately $79 billion. That estimate did not include the enormous emotional stress of chronic pain (Bonica 1990, 180-81).

As the portion of elderly people in the population continues to increase, a trend that has been well established, chronic disorders, including those that produce chronic pain, will probably become more prevalent. Chronic pain is likely to become an even bigger problem than it already is and to result in increasingly numerous presentations to doctors' offices. Therefore, it is very important for those care providers who may encounter such patients to be well-versed in the workup, diagnosis, and management of chronic pain conditions.

Unfortunately, a pain complaint cannot be confirmed by a simple laboratory test, an X-ray, or any other objective modality. Pain can only be subjective, experienced uniquely by the patient in a complex interaction of biological, psychological, behavioral, and emotional factors. (Staats et al., *Pain Forum*, in press; Chapman and Turner 1990). Simply put, pain is what a person says it is; however, pain usually has a biological basis. A wide variety of tests are available to help the physician determine the etiology. Understanding the principles of pain management, the modalities available for pain assessment, including their strengths and weaknesses, and the indications for referral to a pain specialist is paramount to ensure the best possible outcome.

A comprehensive treatment program for a person with chronic pain cannot be implemented or even adequately formulated until a thorough evaluation of the problem has abeen completed. Many pain centers use a coordinated, multidisciplinary team effort in their approach to such a person. The main goal for the physician on the team is to formulate a differential diagnosis of the etiology of the pain. Determining a specific diagnosis is the first step in the evaluation of the person with pain, as it dictates the formulation of a specific treatment plan.

This chapter describes some of the tools utilized in the evaluation of people with chronic pain. Included in the physician's arsenal for establishing a diagnosis are a thorough history and physical examination; a variety of imaging modalities, such as conventional radiography, myelography, computed tomography (CT), and magnetic resonance imaging (MRI); laboratory studies; electrodiagnostic studies, such as electromyography (EMG) and nerve conduction studies (NCSs); and diagnostic nerve blocks.

History and physical examination

A thorough history and a physical exam are the most important diagnostic tools a health care practitioner has at his or her disposal. The history is obtained primarily by talking with the person and his or her family, but also through questionnaires that may be sent to the patient prior to the initial evaluation. Obtaining a history serves several functions:

- It allows the physician to gather the information required to make a differential diagnosis.
- It facilitates a directed physical examination.
- It assures the patient that the physician is listening and is interested in providing care.
- It allows the patient to develop self-understanding as well as the potential for self-help in managing the pain.
- It allows the physician and patient to develop a therapeutic relationship in which the patient can trust and confide in the health care practitioner and so will provide all of the information necessary for determining the source of the pain.
- It allows the patient and the physician to define their goals and design a plan for therapy.

Taking the history

The secret to taking a good history is to be a good listener while simultaneously leading the patient by means of directed questions that will provide vital information. It is important to understand the patient's functional status prior to the onset of the pain. This establishes a baseline treatment goal. The history should reveal to the evaluator a clear picture of the onset, course, and progression of the problem as well as how the pain is affecting the patient's life.

Because pain is often the result of a complex interaction of biological, psychological, behavioral, and emotional events, associated psychosocial and behavioral factors affecting the pain should be elicited during the initial evaluation. For example, if pain develops while the patient is at a job he dislikes but he is receiving worker's compensation because of the pain, it may be more difficult to return the patient to work. Likewise, pending litigation or other sources of secondary gain should also be noted and goals should be modified accordingly.

History of present illness

The history should include a clear chronological narrative indicating why the patient is seeking a consultation. A description of the pain problem should include when it developed, how it has progressed, and how it affects the patient's life. Various subassessments should be included:

- the location of the pain
- the quality of the pain
- the intensity of the pain as described on a visual analog scale or on a 0 to10 numeric scale
- the time course of the pain; that is, whether it is always present or it waxes and wanes throughout the day, week, or month
- aggravating factors, including things that the patient can do to exacerbate the pain
- alleviating factors, including things that the patient can do to help relieve the pain
- changes in functional status caused by the pain
- a complete review of results of all previous diagnostic modalities applied to the pain problem
- a complete review of the effectiveness of any previous therapeutic measures applied to the pain, such as transcutaneous electrical nerve stimulation (TENS), dorsal column stimulation, medication, nerve blocks, surgeries, biofeedback, rehabilitation programs, and the like.

Past medical history

Past medical history should include a review of the patient's general state of health, childhood illnesses as they relate to the current pain problem, adult illnesses, psychiatric disease, surgeries, major injuries, hospitalizations, allergies, and current medications, information that is important to the management of other diseases as well as to the management of the pain problem. Review of the patient's sleep patterns can provide insight into ongoing depression. Medical history should also include a discussion of the patient's habits, including a quantified review of the use of tobacco, alcohol, intravenous drugs, and nonprescription drugs to self-medicate.

In particular, the examiner should ask about the efficacy of the various pain medications the patient has tried. Data should include the dosage and frequency of each medication as well as how the patient's pain responds to a particular dosage paradigm. Determining which drugs have been tried, the dosages at which they were tried, the side effects noted, and the degree of pain relief achieved gives clues to the origin of the pain as well as to the most appropriate therapy.

As with all medical history-taking, an assessment of known allergies is critical. When an individual reports a true allergic reaction to a drug, such as throat-swelling, hives, or rashes, that drug and chemically related drugs should be avoided. Examiners should bear in mind that patients frequently report an allergy to a drug when what they really experience are drug side effects. Many drug side effects, for example, the nausea and sedation associated with opioids, are transient and will resolve with time.

Physical examination

After obtaining a clear description of the patient's pain problem, the examiner should perform a directed physical exam. If the patient has a unilateral limb pain syndrome, contralateral limbs should be assessed first. This provides an indication of what is normal in that individual and allows for a comparison to the affected side. The painful site should be inspected for erythema, discoloration, changes in skin color, nail growth, masses, induration, scars, or any other abnormalities when compared to the normal limb. The area should be palpated first with light touch to determine whether or not touch-evoked pain, or hyperalgesia, is present. In cases where neuropathic pain is suggested, a cold stimulus should be applied to the area in question to determine whether or not the patient has cold hyperalgesia.

Palpation along the site of a lesion will indicate whether or not masses are present or whether or not pain can be reproduced with palpation. A careful neurological examination can assess sensory and motor function as well as deep tendon reflexes, thereby evaluating peripheral nerve or nerve root involvement in the pain condition. Examination of the spine, including range of motion, is important in those patients with neck or low back pain and may also be used to gauge efficacy of treatment. In addition, certain procedures and maneuvers during the physical examination can help to localize the specific structures from which the pain may be originating, for example, hip joint, sacroiliac joint, or lumbar spine. During the examination it is also important to note the patient's mood, affect, and degree of "pain behavior."

Imaging studies

Technological advances in the past few decades have contributed greatly to the clinician's ability to assess and successfully treat painful conditions. Modern imaging techniques such as CT and MRI are among the most widely used by the medical community. These advanced modalities offer detailed images of internal structures with little or no risk to the patient by way of radiation exposure, invasiveness, or discomfort. Certain conditions that might have been difficult to diagnose or evaluate in the past can now be more easily identified. Additionally, diseases can now be discovered at earlier stages in their progression, which has lead to earlier treatment and improved outcomes.

Conventional radiography

Even though highly advanced imaging modalities are available, conventional radiographs, or plain X-rays, are still highly valued and frequently utilized. They are particularly helpful in diagnosing problems that involve musculoskeletal pain, for example back or neck pain or pains in limbs or joints. Radiographs are readily available in nearly all medical facilities, they may be obtained and interpreted quickly, and their cost is substantially less than that of other imaging techniques. Their noninvasive nature and short exposure times make plain radiographs acceptable to most people with chronic pain.

Uses of radiography
Most fractures are easily detected with conventional radiography, but those with little bone disruption might be missed. If a fracture is strongly suspected but not visible by means of plain radiography, several options for further evaluation exist, including tomography, which uses conventional X-ray technology to "home in" on a particular area. This technique improves the delineation of the area in focus but obscures the surrounding tissues. Radionuclide bone scanning, another option available for detection of subtle bone lesions, will be discussed later in this chapter.

Following skeletal trauma, radiographs are also used in the follow-up period to ensure that the bone is undergoing proper healing and alignment. Other conditions such as osteomyelitis (infection of the bone) and osteoporosis (thinning of the bone) may be easily detected. Pathological fractures, those that occur due to an underlying disorder such as metastatic cancer or osteoporosis, for example, can be diagnosed radiographically by demonstrating a fracture superimposed on a destructive bone lesion.

Radiographs are a primary means of detecting and assessing primary bone tumors. Tumor characteristics, such as size and shape, can be studied. Correlation of this information with other data, such as the specific site of the tumor, can lead the physician to formulate a list of possible diagnoses. Note, however, that bone metastases are usually more easily detected by radionuclide bone scanning than by a radiographical skeletal survey. A significant percentage of metastatic lesions may not be visible on plain X-rays yet may be easily seen on a bone scan.

Radiography is highly precise in the differential diagnosis of arthritic disorders. The radiographic appearance of the articular lesions together with the clinical presentation play a primary part in the diagnosis. As an example, when rheumatoid arthritis affects the hands, it usually involves the metacarpophalangeal joints, which may show narrowing of the joint space and erosions on the articular surface. Other arthritic abnormalities, such as osteophytes (bony outgrowths) and sclerosis (scarring), can also be detected easily.

Conventional radiography also aids in the evaluation of neck and low back pain. Radiographic findings that can be associated with spinal pain include spondylolisthesis (slippage of one vertebral body over another), disk space narrowing, abnormal kyphosis or scoliosis (exaggerated or abnormal curvatures of the spine), osteoporosis, hypertrophic spurring ("bone spurs"), as well as failure of prior spinal fusions (pseudoarthrosis), and so forth. Additionally, plain X-rays can detect the presence of spondylosis (degenerative change in one or more vertebrae) or pars interarticularis defects (a break in the posterior elements of the spine), abnormalities of the apophyseal joints (spinal facet joints). X-rays can also help to evaluate and visualize the neural foramina through which spinal nerve roots exit.

Conventional radiography is limited in its ability to visualize and detect abnormalities in soft tissue structures. For example, in cases in which a herniated disk is suspected, conventional radiographs would offer very little to support or refute that diagnosis. Better visualization of such soft tissue structures is offered by CT and MRI or by myelography.

Myelography

Myelography is performed by introducing a radiopaque fluid, the contrast medium, into the cerebrospinal fluid in the subarachnoid space of the spinal column and then exposing the area to X-rays. Because the contrast medium renders the cerebrospinal fluid opaque to X-rays, a relatively smooth column of white along with bilateral tent-like outpouchings corresponding to the neural foramina should appear on the developed film. In early myelography, air was used as a contrast medium because it appears as black on X-rays. Later technology used oily contrast mediums. Currently, water-soluble contrast mediums are used most often as they are easily absorbed and do not require removal after the procedure is complete.

Myelography is often used to demonstrate or exclude the presence of a surgically correctable lesion in the course of evaluating degenerative changes in the vertebrae and intervertebral disks. Prior to surgery, it is used to confirm the exact location of a lesion. Herniated disks are a common indication for the use of myelography. Significant herniated disks as well as other abnormal masses in the spinal column appear on a myelogram as focal-filling defects, circumscribed interruptions of the otherwise smooth and continuous column of white on the developed X-ray film. Large lesions may actually obstruct the free flow of the contrast medium in the subarachnoid space and appear on film as abrupt discontinuations of the white column. The absence of a tent-like outpouching at a particular level indicates compression of the neural foramen on that side, which is usually due to a herniated disk and can lead to symptoms and signs of a radiculopathy.

Risks involved with myelography should be considered prior to having a patient undergo the procedure. It involves lumbar puncture, an invasive procedure that can occasionally result in complications such as infection, bleeding, or spinal headaches. The contrast agent can induce inflammation, allergic reaction, or the development of arachnoiditis (inflammation of the arachnoid membrane). Irritation of the meninges, exiting nerve roots, and brain tissues can occur. Newer, nonionic agents have decreased the incidence of arachnoiditis and some of the other side effects.

Computed tomography scanning

CT scanning (also called computed axial tomography, or CAT scanning) is a method of X-ray evaluation that examines a thin slice, or single cross section, of tissue. A single, thin-volume X-ray beam is applied successively around the patient's body from many different directions but always on the same plane. This technique decreases superimposition of the surrounding tissue images over the area to be visualized and limits the scatter effects of conventional radiography. As the X-ray beam is applied at multiple angles around the patient, a series of detectors measure the amount of X-ray transmission passing through the area of interest. A computer collects the data gathered by the detectors and constructs the final radiographic image of a single plane of the body. The X-ray source completes one revolution around the patient's body, moves a short distance along an axis, and repeats the process. Through computer analysis of successive planes of exposure, a three-dimensional image can be constructed.

CT scanning may be performed with intravenous contrast enhancement in order to highlight certain abnormalities, such as areas of blood-brain barrier breakdown or areas of increased vascularity, such as tumors or abscess that might not be seen without the infusion of a contrast agent.

Uses of computed tomography

CT is often used as a noninvasive means of evaluating the bony structures and soft tissues of the spine. For example, a cross-sectional image of the axial plane (a plane perpendicular to the spinal cord) may reveal laterally placed herniated disk fragments that might not be visible on a myelogram.

CT scanning may follow a myelographic study to better evaluate and diagnose radicular pain (pain originating at a nerve root), which often results from a herniated disk compressing an exiting nerve root as it passes through its neural foramen. Facet joints can be imaged to reveal degenerative/hypertrophic changes, which are a common contributor to chronic spinal pain. Other spinal structures, such as ligaments and disks, can also be visualized in the CT axial images.

CT can provide images of the soft tissues of the thoracic and abdominal cavities as well as of the brain. Abnormalities such as hematomas, neoplasms, and abscesses can be examined. CT is often used in cases of suspected aortic aneurysm in the chest or abdomen and is the imaging modality of choice in the urgent evaluation of suspected stroke or brain hemorrhage. The introduction of a contrast agent enhances the examination of vascular structures, the urinary tract, or the gastrointestinal tract.

The advantages of CT are that it is more widely available than MRI and produces images in a shorter period of time. For these reasons, it will probably continue to be used frequently, especially for urgent evaluations, despite growing acceptance of MRI as a superior tool for many applications.

The risks inherent in CT are exactly those of conventional radiography, that is, exposure to X-ray radiation and its long-term effects on reproductive structures, skin, thyroid, and so forth. Another risk, though relatively rare in occurrence, is an allergic reaction to the intravenous contrast agent.

Magnetic resonance imaging

MRI differs significantly from other imaging methods, for it depends on the physical phenomenon of spinning protons, the particles that, along with neutrons, compose atomic nuclei. Each proton has a characteristic spin that will always be parallel or antiparallel to an applied external magnetic field. Nuclei with an even atomic number do not exhibit significant properties associated with spin, because the spin effects of an even number of protons tend to cancel each other out.

Atomic nuclei with an odd atomic number such as hydrogen assume a characteristic orientation to an applied magnetic field that is caused by the spin of the odd proton. The alignment of the nuclei to a magetic field is similar to the alignment of a compass needle with the Earth's magnetic field. When such an atomic nucleus is aligned within an applied magnetic field, it will absorb radio frequency energy in discrete amounts and then emit a discrete amount of radio frequency energy when the applied radio pulse ends. The actual frequency of the radio wave absorbed and released depends upon the element being examined. In medical applications, hydrogen is the most frequently detected element in MRI. Hydrogen gives off a strong radio frequency signal and is naturally abundant in biological tissues.

MRI is conducted by placing the patient within a strong magnetic field and then applying radio frequency energy in pulses. The radio frequency energy is absorbed by the hydrogen atoms in the body area to be examined. At the end of the pulse, the hydrogen atoms release a radio wave with a characteristic frequency that is detected by the MRI computer and used to construct an image.

Unlike routine CT, the images acquired in MRI can be presented in many different orientations, including axial, coronal, sagittal, and oblique planes. Other advantages of MRI are that it requires no ionizing radiation (radio waves and magnetic fields are relatively harmless), it measures signals emitted by the body's own naturally occurring hydrogen atoms, and it offers very high sensitivity and tissue contrast. Risks and contraindications of MRI are relatively few. The most commonly encountered contraindications involve metallic objects or implants in the patient's body, including pacemakers, metallic prosthetic cardiac valves, aneurysm clips, and the like. Metalworkers such as welders may have metal fragments embedded in their bodies as a result of work exposure and can be permanently injured by the imposition of a strong magnetic field, especially if the metal fragments are located in the eyes.

Uses of magnetic resonance imaging

MRI can differentiate many elements of spinal anatomy, including delineation of the spinal cord, the surrounding cerebrospinal fluid, and the extradural structures such as the intervertebral disks. Changes in disk hydration and morphology due to disk degeneration are manifested by changes in signal intensity in the disk. MRI can also readily detect disk herniation, facet joint arthropathy, infection of the vertebral bone or disk, subluxation, spinal stenosis, fracture, neoplasm, vascular abnormalities, and so forth. The patency of neural foramina can be readily visualized with transverse images. (See *MRI of a lumbar disk herniation*, page 76, for an example of disk herniation revealed by MRI.)

Many joints throughout the body, such as the knee or the temporomandibular joint, can be evaluated by MRI, and it is now an essential technique for visualizing the face and neck, pelvis, retroperitoneum, mediastinum, and brain. When compared to CT of the brain, MRI provides greater contrast resolution, fewer artifacts from bone, and far clearer images of the brain stem and other structures in the posterior fossa. Additionally, MRI offers much greater ability to demonstrate the three-dimensional location of a lesion, such as a brain tumor, when compared to CT. Intravenous contrast agents can also be used with MRI to help further delineate lesions with abundant vascularity.

Ultrasound

Ultrasound establishes an image of internal structures by measuring their capacity to transmit or reflect high-frequency sound waves. A sound transmitter is applied to the patient's skin overlying the area of focus. The transmitter contains a detector that records the sound waves reflected from internal structures. The reflected sound waves are converted to an echogram that is displayed on a monitor.

Because of differences in reflective characteristics, collections of fluid such as those found in abscesses and in the gallbladder and renal collection system are easily distinguished from solid masses. In fact, ultrasound is now considered the best form of imaging for the initial evaluation of suspected gallbladder disease such as gallstones in cases of abdominal pain. Because bone does not transmit sound well, ultrasound has little use in the evaluation of musculoskeletal pain.

The advantages of this diagnostic tool are that it is relatively inexpensive and that exposure to sound waves poses little or no risk. Ultrasound is therefore ideal for children and pregnant women.

Bone scanning

Radionuclide bone scanning is used to reflect an increase in total body bone turnover, such as occurs in fractures, metastatic tumor, and infection. The high sensitivity of this imaging technique makes it especially useful in the detection of subtle lesions such as very small fractures that may be missed by other imaging modalities.

MRI of a lumbar disk herniation

This MRI reveals a right L4-5 paracentral disk herniation. It is shown here compressing the spinal fluid and
impinging on the nerve root as it exits the spinal column. This lesion could easily be missed with conventional X-ray.

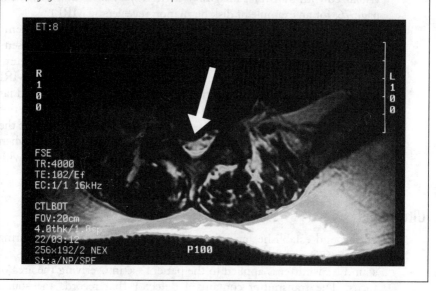

In a routine bone scan (see *Bone scan showing metastatic disease*), the patient first receives an I.V. injection of a bone-seeking radiopharmaceutical that emits gamma radiation. The radiopharmaceutical accumulates preferentially in any skeletal sites experiencing bone turnover and thus acts as a tracer. Approximately 2 to 3 hours later, a camera with gamma-sensitive film is used to obtain images of the entire skeleton or special areas of interest. Areas of tracer accumulation appear as "hot spots" on the images.

The advantage of bone scanning is that it does not rely on actual bone loss to demonstrate pathology but takes advantage of local bone repair processes, the sites at which tracer accumulates. Early stages of bone metastasis or infection that could be missed by conventional radiography are easily detected by bone scanning. Even small stress fractures or hairline fractures, commonly missed by other imaging techniques, are routinely demonstrated on bone scanning. However, even though bone scanning is known to be very sensitive, it is also nonspecific. While it adeptly demonstrates bone abnormalities, these abnormalities may not be clinically significant or be causing any difficulties for the patient. Even for those lesions

Bone scan showing metastatic disease

This bone scan reveals multiple sites of increased tracer uptake. These "hot spots" indicate that there is increased bone turnover, which is consistent with metastatic prostate cancer.

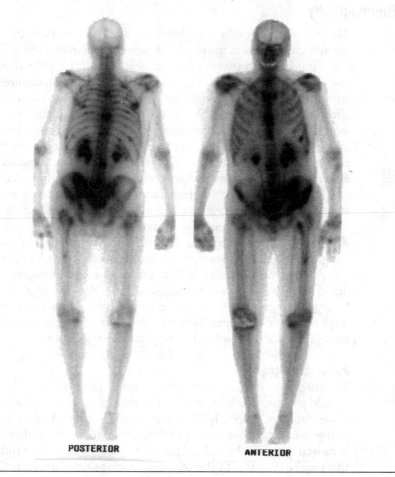

POSTERIOR   ANTERIOR

that are clinically significant, bone scanning usually cannot be used alone to specify the underlying etiology or diagnosis but must be used in conjunction with appropriate clinical information and other radiographic studies to reveal a specific diagnosis.

Uses of bone scanning
Beside the uses described above, bone scanning is routinely used in the evaluation and follow-up of metastatic disease to the bone; acute

osteomyelitis, which may not be detectable by conventional radiography even one week after onset; bone trauma such as occult fractures; and arthritis as well as other pathological processes that result in active bone turnover such as Paget's disease.

Thermography

Medical thermography diagnoses dysfunction by measuring and recording variations in the pattern of infrared radiation given off by the body. It is based on the premise that objects emit thermal radiation in characteristic patterns that depend in part upon the temperature of the emitting surface. Thermography can record localized temperature alterations on the body surface that perhaps indicate underlying physiological changes such as circulatory changes that are related to those alterations. It differs significantly from CT, MRI, and conventional radiography in that it reflects physiological processes rather than anatomical abnormalities, a characteristic it shares with bone scanning.

Patients undergoing thermography are first acclimated to a constant temperature for a set time period. Then the body area to be studied is exposed to an infrared-sensitive camera. An accompanying tele-electronic system converts the detected infrared radiation to electronic signals, which are displayed as a colored picture on a monitor.

A slightly different technique called contact thermography uses liquid crystals imbedded in flexible sheaths that are applied to the body part to be examined. The crystals assume different color patterns that are determined by the temperature of the patient's skin. A camera records the resultant color patterns for analysis.

Uses of thermography

Thermography is safe, noninvasive, relatively inexpensive, and appears to hold promise as a screening tool in various neuromuscular and soft tissue disorders, especially those that present with predominantly subjective complaints but few or no objective abnormalities that can be perceived during a physical examination. Some neuropathic syndromes that may be evaluated by thermography include reflex sympathetic dystrophy, radicular syndromes, peripheral neuropathies, carpal tunnel syndrome and other nerve entrapments, postherpetic neuralgia, thoracic outlet syndrome, and trigeminal neuralgia. Thermography has been used in the evaluation of myofascial syndromes such as fibromyalgia and lumbosacral strain. Circulatory disorders are also subject to evaluation by thermography, for example, peripheral vascular occlusive disease, vasospastic disease such as Raynaud's phenomenon, and venous insufficiency. Skeletal disorders, such as osteomyelitis, lumbar facet syndrome, rheumatoid arthritis, scoliosis, and postfracture extremity pain, also have been examined by using this technique.

The advantages of thermography are that it is noninvasive and painless and that it does not expose the patient to ionizing radiation, allowing for its safe use in children and pregnant women. However, the use of thermography and its clinical applicability are still controversial. It is by no means commonly used in the medical community in general nor in the pain management community specifically. Currently, thermography should be regarded as one possible source of information for findings that must be integrated with other available information in the physician's decision-making process.

Electrodiagnostics

Electrodiagnostic studies are commonly used to evaluate the functioning of nerve roots, peripheral nerves, and muscles. Painful conditions that lead to abnormal functioning in these structures and thus may be assessed by electrodiagnostic studies include nerve entrapment, radiculopathy, and peripheral neuropathy, to name just a few. These tests are relatively risk-free and provide reliable, reproducible results, two important reasons for their uniform acceptance and utilization throughout the medical community. Electrodiagnostic studies are almost always performed by physicians who have undergone special training to administer the procedures as well as to interpret the results. The most useful tests in electrodiagnosis are EMG and NCSs. Somatosensory evoked potentials (EPs) may also be helpful in evaluating patients with pain syndromes.

Electromyography

EMG records voltage changes within a muscle by means of a needle electrode (see *Typical wave forms seen in electromyography*, page 80). Usually, a monopolar needle electrode is used, and the electrical potential is measured between the tip of the needle inserted within the muscle and a surface electrode taped to the skin, the latter being the reference electrode. The electrical activity measured within the muscle is amplified and then displayed on an oscilloscope as well as monitored through a loudspeaker as the various types of muscle activity, normal or abnormal, make characteristic sounds. Various forms of electrical potentials are recognized as abnormal and indicate a pathological process in the muscle or the nerve supplying that muscle.

Electromyographic activity is measured during needle insertion, during complete rest of the muscle, which normally should show no electrical activity on the monitor, and during active muscle contraction. Abnormal electrical potentials seen in EMG testing include abnormal activity during needle insertion and abnormal spontaneous

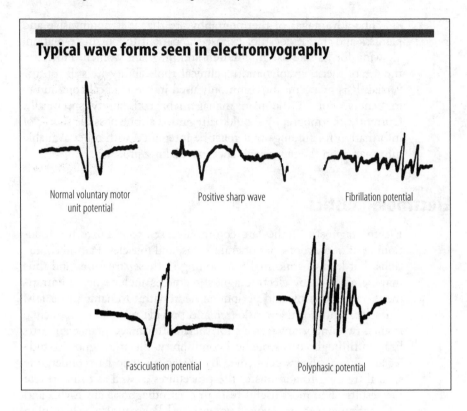

Typical wave forms seen in electromyography

Normal voluntary motor unit potential

Positive sharp wave

Fibrillation potential

Fasciculation potential

Polyphasic potential

activity of the resting muscle, which often occurs in three distinct patterns: fibrillation potentials, positive sharp waves, and fasciculation potentials.

Fibrillation is the spontaneous generation of an action potential in a resting single muscle fiber and characteristically occurs in muscle fibers that have had their nerve supply disrupted. Positive sharp waves also represent abnormal activity of resting single muscle fibers. They consist of a sharp change in potential toward the positive followed by a slowly developing negative potential of lower absolute amplitude. Fibrillation potentials and positive sharp waves are frequently encountered together and are often associated with radiculopathy and various peripheral neuropathies, such as disease of a nerve plexus or degenerative disease of nerve axons. In these disorders, muscle fibers have lost their normal innervation, allowing for their spontaneous depolarization. Fasciculation potentials represent the combined electrical activity generated by the spontaneous depolarizations of a motor unit, a group of muscle fibers innervated by a single nerve fiber. Although they are sometimes found in normal subjects, especially the elderly, their presence along with fibrillation potentials and positive sharp waves is considered further evidence of a neuropathic disorder.

After the muscle being examined has been studied at rest, the patient is asked to minimally contract the muscle with the needle electrode still in place, so that a single motor unit is activated. Under normal conditions, a motor unit potential contains up to four phases. A potential with five or more phases is termed "polyphasic." An increase in the percentage of polyphasic motor unit potentials is considered abnormal and may be indicative of either neuropathic disease or myopathy.

Nerve conduction studies

NCSs are used to determine the ability of a peripheral nerve to propagate an electric impulse along a portion of its length. Abnormalities in nerve conduction indicate a neuropathic process. This study can also be used to localize a lesion along the course of a nerve and is commonly used in the evaluation of nerve entrapment syndromes, such as ulnar nerve entrapment at the elbow. The nerve to be studied is stimulated electrically, and the measurement of various parameters allows determination of the nerve's functional status. Both the electrical stimulation of the nerve and the recording of transmitted potentials are usually done with surface electrodes placed on the skin overlying the nerve.

Motor NCSs are performed by electrically stimulating a nerve at some point along its course and recording the evoked response (contraction) from a distal muscle that it innervates. The muscle contraction is detected by a skin electrode placed directly over the muscle and converted to a visual waveform, which is recorded and analyzed on a monitor. Typically, measurement of impulse velocity, amplitude, and latency (the time interval between application of the electrical stimulus and generation of the muscle contraction) allow assessment of the nerve's ability to carry an impulse.

In determining the velocity of nerve conduction in a particular segment of a nerve, for example from the elbow to the wrist along the median nerve, the investigator electrically stimulates the nerve at the elbow and at the wrist and in each case measures the time required (the latency) for generation of an action potential at a specific muscle in the hand. This gives two different latencies: a distal latency (from wrist to hand muscle) and a proximal latency (from elbow to hand muscle). The conduction velocity of the median nerve segment between elbow and wrist is easily calculated by subtracting the distal latency from the proximal latency and dividing this difference into the distance between the two stimulus sites.

Sensory NCSs are performed by placing two electrodes, one for stimulation and one for recording, directly over the sensory nerve being examined. When the stimulating electrode is placed proximal to the recording electrode, it is termed antidromic conduction as the electric impulse is traveling in the opposite direction from the normal direction of impulses in a sensory nerve. When the stimulating electrode is placed distal to the recording electrode, the term orthodromic conduction is used. The time is measured between the onset of the stimulus at the stimulating electrode and its arrival at the recording electrode (determination of the latency). Dividing this time into the distance between the two electrodes yields the sensory conduction velocity. Sensory NCSs are valuable in the early detection of peripheral neuropathies because abnormalities may appear in these studies before the patient experiences significant symptoms of sensory loss.

Sensory nerves commonly studied include the median, ulnar, radial, lateral femoral cutaneous, sural, superficial peroneal, and tibial. Motor studies may be done on the median, ulnar, radial, tibial, peroneal, sciatic, and other nerves. More proximal neural structures such as the nerve roots may also be studied using specialized techniques.

Evoked potentials

Somatosensory EPs are the electrical signals recorded by skin electrodes along the normal course of sensory information flow. The route under study begins at a point where electrical stimulation is applied to a peripheral nerve, travels up the spinal cord through the brainstem, and terminates on the contralateral scalp overlying the sensory cortex. The nerves usually studied include the median, ulnar, tibial, and peroneal. By placing recording electrodes on the skin overlying the structures in the path described above, latencies between any two recording sites can be calculated and compared to established normal values. In this way, nerve function in both the peripheral and central nervous systems can be measured.

The most common uses for EPs testing currently are as an aid in the diagnosis of multiple sclerosis and in monitoring spinal cord function during neurosurgical procedures. EPs are not uniformly used in diagnosing painful neuropathies or radiculopathies or any of the other usual painful disorders commonly encountered in clinical practice. Theoretically, EP testing may be useful in more elusive diagnoses, such as plexopathies, thoracic outlet syndrome, or central pain syndromes (those associated with lesions in the spinal cord or brain).

Laboratory tests

The multitude of laboratory tests available to the clinician as well as the vast number of possible disease processes that may underly certain pain states make it difficult to present this subject comprehensively. Let it suffice to say that appropriate laboratory testing is an invaluable and indispensable tool for the diagnostician in the evaluation of most conditions that cause pain.

Many neurological diseases include pain as one of the presenting symptoms. Several of these disease states may have associated abnormalities that can be tested in the laboratory. Peripheral neuropathies, for example, account for a significant proportion of compaints of chronic pain and may be associated with a number of underlying pathological processes that can be discovered through laboratory tests. Examples include tests for serum glucose levels to screen for diabetes; certain nutrient levels, such as vitamin B_{12} and folate, to screen for malnutrition states that are commonly seen in alcoholism, gastrointestinal disease, and so forth; nerve-damaging toxins, such as arsenic and thallium; and protein analysis to look for dysproteinemias. Compression neuropathies such as carpal tunnel syndrome may indicate an underlying thyroid disorder that can be investigated by obtaining thyroid function tests from the blood. Neuropathic pain may also result from abnormal inflammatory states or autoimmune dysfunction that may be evaluated by obtaining laboratory tests such as an erythrocyte sedimentation rate (ESR) or levels of antinuclear antibodies (ANA). Components of the body other than blood may also be evaluated by laboratory testing, including urine and cerebrospinal fluid as well as biopsies of nerve and muscle.

Identification of an underlying disease is of paramount importance, because specific treatment of the disease is usually integral in the management of the pain symptoms arising from the disorder.

Diagnostic nerve blocks

Diagnostic nerve blocks are performed by injecting a local anesthetic into a nerve proximal to a presumed lesion that is generating the pain. Local anesthetics bind sodium channels and thus temporarily inhibit conduction of action potentials along the nerve. If pain relief follows application of local anesthetic to a particular nerve, a presumptive diagnosis is made. Three types of nerve blocks are performed in the diagnosis and management of chronic pain: peripheral, visceral, and central nerve blocks. Peripheral nerve blocks are performed by injecting local anesthetic into a peripheral nerve. For visceral nerve blocks, local anesthetic is injected into a ganglion or nerve plexus. A central nerve block employs local anesthetic injected spinally near the spinal cord at the dorsal root zone, into the epidural space, or into the subarachnoid space.

Peripheral nerve blocks

Peripheral nerve injuries can result from trauma or disease or can be complications after surgery. One common manifestation of peripheral nerve injury is pain. For example, a common presentation of carpal tunnel syndrome is pain in the hand. Although frequently not necessary for carpal tunnel syndrome, the diagnosis can be further clarified by performing a median nerve block proximal to the flexor retinaculum (the ligamentous band crossing the anterior carpus) where the median nerve is frequently entrapped.

Visceral nerve blocks

There are five classes of visceral nerve blocks: stellate ganglion block, celiac plexus block, lumbar sympathetic ganglion block, superior hypogastric plexus block, and ganglion impar block. The stellate ganglion block is performed to determine whether or not patients have sympathetically mediated pain of the upper extremities, upper thorax, or face. As a therapeutic modality, it is used in the treatment of acute herpetic neuralgia, sympathetically maintained pain, and vasoocclusive diseases. The celiac plexus block is performed to determine whether or not pain arises from the abdominal viscera. Celiac plexus blocks are also commonly performed for therapeutic pain relief in upper abdominal malignancies, including pancreatic cancer. Positive response to a diagnostic block of the celiac plexus implies a positive prognosis for several months of pain relief from celiac plexus neurolysis. A lumbar sympathetic ganglion block is performed to determine whether or not patients have sympathetically mediated pain of the lower extremities. A superior hypogastric plexus block is a recently described block that helps to determine whether or not there is a visceral etiology of pelvic pain. Finally, the ganglion impar block is a recently described block performed to help delineate the etiology of rectal pain.

Central nerve blocks

Central nerve blocks are usually performed by injecting local anesthetic into the epidural space of the spinal cord or onto selected dorsal roots in the attempt to discern whether pain is arising from a particular sensory nerve root. These nerve blocks are performed under fluoroscopic guidance with local anesthetic and occasionally with dye to assure proper needle placement and spread of the local anesthetic. If pain relief follows an appropriately performed block, the pain generator is presumably distal to the site anesthetized. If a correctly performed block results in numbness in the appropriate dermatomal distribution with no accompanying pain relief, the pain generator is considered to be proximal or collateral to the site anesthetized.

Differential epidural blocks

Some pain specialists perform differential epidural blocks as well as blocks within the subarachnoid space to help delineate whether the etiology of the pain is somatosensory (arising in the somatic nerves), sympathetic (arising in the sympathetic nervous system), or central (arising in the brain or spinal cord).

In the differential epidural, the procedure is begun by injecting a saline placebo into the epidural space. If the patient has pain relief following placebo injection, no further injection is made. If the placebo relief is long-lasting, the patient is presumed to have psychogenic pain. If the placebo produces no relief, three injections are given, each with a successively higher concentration of local anesthetic. If the patient obtains relief with the lowest concentration of anesthetic, the pain is determined to be sympathetically maintained, possibly due to reflex sympathetic dystrophy. If relief is obtained at the next level of anesthetic, the pain is presumed to be somatosensory. If the patient still has pain after the second injection of anesthetic, a third anesthetic injection is given, usually resulting in the patient's temporary loss of motor function. If this level of anesthetic does not provide relief, the patient's pain is assumed to be centrally maintained (originating in the central nervous system) or possibly psychogenic.

The use of diagnostic nerve blocks, including differential epidural blocks, is controversial. There are many variables to consider when interpreting negative and positive responses following local anesthetic blocks. False positive results can occur following a placebo response, systemically administered analgesics, or systemic uptake of local anesthetics, and there can be other nonspecific effects of needle placement and injection. It is not appropriate to label a patient as having solely psychogenic pain following a positive response to a placebo (Staats and North, *Perspectives in Neurosurgery*, in press).

Diagnostic facet blocks

Diagnostic local anesthetic blocks to the facet joints of the lumbar spine are commonly performed to help delineate the etiology of low back pain. This type of nerve block deserves special mention, because the disease, facet joint syndrome, is defined in part by the response to the diagnostic block. Clinically, the syndrome is characterized by continuous unilateral or bilateral pain in the lumbar region with absence of objective neurologic signs. The pain may radiate to the hips or, rarely, below the knee and is elicited with ipsilateral hyperextension of the spine.

In the cervical region, facet joint syndrome is characterized by reproduction of pain with ipsilateral rotation and extension of the cervical spine. Characteristic referral patterns have also been documented. For example, pain arising from the C2-C3 facet joints often radiates to the occiput, while the C5-C6 joints radiate to the shoulder.

Because degenerative changes noted radiographically are also seen in asymptomatic joints, radiographic features alone are inadequate to make the diagnosis of facet joint syndrome. Furthermore, other pathology in the spine, including discopathy, nerve root impingement, and myofascial disease, can present with similar symptoms. Facet joint syndrome is differentiated from other diagnoses by the response to radiographically guided injections of local anesthetics, either into the joints or into the respective posterior rami nerves. However, the same problems that exist with diagnostic nerve blocks also exist with diagnostic facet blocks; that is, a positive test with local anesthetic imperfectly predicts the outcome of permanent ablative or anatomic procedures.

Conclusion

Understanding the wide range of etiologies that give rise to chronic pain is the first step in developing a diagnostic plan. The tools presented in this chapter should help in the formulation of specific diagnosis in most chronic pain patients. Diagnosis leads to appropriate treatment of the underlying disorder and hopefully, resolution of the pain.

REFERENCES

Bonica, J.J. *The Management of Pain*, 2nd ed. Baltimore: Williams & Wilkins, 1990.

Chapman, C.R., and Turner, J.A. "Psychological and Psychosocial Aspects of Acute Pain." In Bonica, J.J. *The Managment of Pain*, 2nd ed. Baltimore: Williams & Wilkins, 1990.

Staats, P.S., and North, R.B. "The Role of Nerve Blocks, Facet Blocks, and Discography in the Management of Pain," in *Perspectives in Neurosurgery*. Edited by Hadley, M. In press.

Staats, P.S., et al. "Psychological Behaviorism's Theory of Pain: A Basis for Unity." *Pain Forum*. In press.

CHAPTER 4

Common pain syndromes

Michael G. Byas-Smith, MD

The sensation of pain makes it possible for people and animals to interface safely with the external environment and serves as a warning sign of internal abnormality. People who lack the ability to perceive pain suffer a variety of ailments, including joint deformities and repeated bacterial infections, and often have shortened life spans. Conceptual models of the nervous system's processing of acute pain signals from sensory nerve endings to the brain have not changed much for many decades and continue to be consistent with experimental evidence. Consequently, acute pain conditions have been relatively easy to research, particularly since sophisticated monitoring tools that track nerve potentials are commonplace and relatively inexpensive to purchase and maintain. These signals can be surveyed even after they have reached nuclei located deep in human brains, and it can be done in real time with the patients awake to comment on what they are feeling.

Despite the availability of this impressive technology, it has proven to be inadequate to explain the complexities of the pain experience. Most pain conditions require far more complicated neural processing than just the simple telegraphed message. If it were that easy, mastery over pain would have been achieved decades ago and this book would not be necessary. In addition to tracking the destination of nerve potentials generated during nociception, researchers are also studying cellular responses to nociceptive information. A variety of substances are produced by nerves in response to acute and chronic pain stimulation. The electrical and molecular responses to painful stimulation are intriguing, of course, but how are all those actions and reactions integrated to create pain, and to what extent can those components be controlled to alleviate pain?

The nociceptive component of a painful experience is accompanied by a variety of emotions, such as fear, anger, anxiety, and hopelessness. In fact, without these affective components, pain would not necessarily be distinguished from other sensations, such as soft, rough, wet, cool, or sticky. When someone says, "This is going to hurt," a person's reaction and preparation are very different from his response to "This will feel wet." In addition, the complex nature of pain is particularly compounded in patients with chronic pain.

Imagine that while you are cooking you splatter hot grease onto your hand and arm. Although the initial experience of such a burn can be quite painful, the sensation of pain usually diminishes in a short time and the intensity of the pain begins to decrease almost immediately. Suppose that instead of the normal chain of events, the painful sensation does not regress and, moreover, moving your arm or hand exacerbates the pain. Imagine that over time, the pain increases in intensity and spreads to areas not burned initially. Imagine that five months later, long after the burned tissue has healed, your pain has not diminished. Physicians have treated you with a variety of medications and procedures, none of which have helped you. A few of the many physicians whom you have visited think that you are faking pain or need psychiatric evaluation. What do you do? Who will help you? The original pain-inducing event may be different or even unknown, but many chronic-pain patients find themselves in a situation similar to what you have just imagined, and blocking the nerve impulses from the painful tissue may not be enough to provide relief.

In this chapter I will introduce a number of common pain conditions that parallel the circumstance that you imagined for yourself above. It would be impossible to discuss all the common painful conditions in this limited space; for additional information on each of the topics discussed here or for commentary on pain problems not covered, I recommend review of the reference section at the end of the chapter. I hope that each section of this chapter will provide a general understanding of the impact of a specific painful disease or disorder on patients, an outline of how each pain problem is managed, and a short description of possible mechanisms of the painful condition. Other chapters in this book and elsewhere provide greater detail and specifics on the pharmacology, physiology, and other aspects of pain.

A quick review of the drugs discussed in this chapter is presented in *Commonly used analgesics*. For many painful diseases and disorders, the drugs listed, as well as many other nonmedicinal approaches, provide effective treatment and are readily available. However, not all patients respond to standard therapy and many patients respond to them only some of the time. Not even morphine can be relied upon to relieve pain always, even in extremely high doses. After reading this chapter or book, no one should be left with the impression that we have licked the problem of pain. On the contrary, we are far

Commonly used analgesics

Drug class	Mechanism of analgesia	Conditions treated	Common side effects
Opioids Morphine Hydromorphone Methadone Oxycodone	Activate opioid receptors on nerve cells in the spinal cord and brain. The response is suppression of pain signals.	Effective in a variety of conditions, such as cancer pain, acute inflammatory pain. Often not effective in neuropathic pain.	Sedation, nausea, vomiting, hallucinations, constipation, respiratory depression, muscle twitching.
Nonsteroidal anti-inflammatory drugs (NSAIDs) Ibuprophen Naproxen Ketorolac Indomethacin	Inhibit prostaglandin synthesis. Pain associated with the inflammatory response is reduced.	Used for a variety of conditions but most effective in treating muscular pain, headache, and bone pain.	Gastrointestinal upset, including nausea, epigastric pain from mucosal irritation and ulceration, and GI bleeding. Inhibition of platelet aggregation leading to increased risk of bleeding. Loss of hearing and ringing in the ears in some patients.
Salicylates Aspirin Diflunisal Choline magnesium trisalicylate	Same as NSAIDs.	Same as NSAIDs.	Same as NSAIDs. Platelet aggregation inhibition exists for the life of the platelet.
Local anesthetics Lidocaine Mepivacaine Bupivacaine	Block sodium channels on nerve axons. No nociceptive signals can reach the CNS.	Used to block ongoing nociceptive information, such as in plexopathy.	Blockage of all sensory information, not just pain impulses. High doses in the blood stream associated with heart and nervous system effects, such as cardiac arrest, seizures.
Headache medications Ergotamine Sumatriptan	Act as agonists or partial agonists at serotonin receptors.	Used for acute treatment of vascular headaches.	Intense vasoconstriction; chest pain and shortness of breath due to ischemia.
Analgesic adjuvants **Tricyclic antidepressants** Amitriptyline Imipramine Desipramine Doxepin	Block re-uptake of serotonin and norepinephrine in CNS synapses.	Best results seen in neuropathic pain conditions.	Anticholinergic effects resulting in intensely dry mouth, constipation, orthostatic hypotension, and, rarely, cardiac conduction abnormalities. Sedation, particularly in elderly patients.
Aniticonvulsants Carbamazepine Phenytoin Sodium valproate	Unknown.	Same as the tricyclic antidepressants.	Dermatological disturbance. Marrow and liver suppression or inflammation (carbamazepine).

from it, and I encourage continued interest in and funding for research into this area of medicine and biology.

Head and facial pain

Among the most commonly occurring head and facial pain syndromes are headaches of various types, facial pain associated with neuralgia of the trigeminal nerve, and pain associated with disorders of the temporomandibular joint (see *Characteristics of common headaches*, pages 92-93).

Tension headache

"I feel as if my head is in a vice." "Sometimes it feels like my head is going to explode." These statements are common descriptions of the pain experienced with a tension headache (THA). A person with THA frequently describes a bandlike tightness around the head. On physical examination, the muscles located at the temples and the nape are frequently found to be tender to palpation. Mild depression and fatigue may accompany these symptoms as well. The symptoms are brought on or exacerbated by activities that are physically and psychologically stressful. There are no neurological deficits or physical changes that accompany these symptoms.

Pathophysiology of tension headache
The underlying pathophysiology of THA is uncertain, although for many years it was thought to be secondary to chronic muscle contractions about the head as a consequence of chronic physical and psychological stress. Indeed, many patients have demonstrable increases in action potential generation that correlate with painful muscles as measured by electromyography (EMG). Other patients with identical symptoms fail to show correlations between painful regions and muscle contractions, nor is there a correlation found between the chronicity of the headache and increased EMG potential. Although the evidence for the role of muscle contraction in THA is conflicting, technical improvements in EMG measurements may still reveal an effect of chronic muscle contraction in most people with THA.

Aberrations in serotonin metabolism is also considered a causative factor in THA. Platelet serotonin content and plasma serotonin levels have been found to be low in these patients, although a direct cause-and-effect link between serotonin levels and THA has yet to be established. At the very least, decreased serotonin levels may turn out to be a very important marker for a variety of pain problems, including THA. Other mechanisms have been proposed, but no single pathology has been accepted universally as the causative agent.

Treatment

Most patients self-treat their symptoms with over-the-counter preparations, and many are aware of the connection between increased stress and onset of headaches. Consequently, many patients practice relaxation techniques on their own, including exercise, meditation, and lightened work schedule. The patients who present themselves to the clinician for assistance are generally those whose chronic headaches are unresponsive to straightforward approaches and whose symptoms exceed their ability to cope with them. These patients are commonly given nonsteroidal anti-inflammatory drugs (NSAIDs) and assisted in developing coping strategies for dealing with stressful circumstances. Diet and behavioral modifications are also utilized to gain control of headaches. A psychologist may prescribe biofeedback and relaxation training techniques as well as psychotherapy. A physical therapist will prescribe exercises as a part of therapy. Patients are instructed to abstain from smoking and caffeine-containing food products. Modifications in the workplace might be the key to eliminating or reducing symptoms. As with other chronic pain conditions, alleviating chronic THA requires patients to be active participants in their own care.

Migraine headache

Migraine headaches, considered by many to be the most notorious of headaches, are common. Symptoms can be quite severe and debilitating. People commonly diagnose themselves as having migraine headaches if they develop severe headaches that are unusual relative to their previous experience. Sometimes they are correct, but in many cases the specific criteria needed to make this diagnosis are not met. Migraine headaches are categorized into two major divisions, migraine with aura and migraine without aura. Previously, classifications referred to these two groups as classical migraine and common migraine, respectively. The aura refers to specific nonpainful symptoms that patients experience prior to an attack. During the aura phase patients may experience visual disturbances, such as flashes of light and lost fields of vision. The aura usually precede the pain by less than one hour. The pain of the migraine comes on gradually and usually reaches its peak within one to two hours after the beginning of the attack, although some patients crescendo as much as 24 to 36 hours later.

Migraines are far more common in women than in men, and the age at onset of the symptoms is usually in the early 20s. Migraine headaches tend to run in families, and it is common for a physician to treat several members of the same family simultaneously. The

Characteristics of common headaches

Headache type	Symptoms	Pathophysiology	Treatment
Tension	Dull, aching tightness or constricting band around the head. Dizziness and fatigue are common.	Stress Chronic muscle tension Ischemic muscles Serotonin depletion	*Acute variety* Rest, removal of stressful triggers Paracetamol (acetaminophen) Nonsteroidal anti-inflammatory drugs *Chronic variety* Same as acute variety Discontinue habitual use of tranquilizers, sedatives, caffeine, narcotics Tricyclic antidepressants Beta-blockers Monoamine oxidase inhibitors (MAO Inhibitors) Biofeedback Relaxation therapy Physical therapy Transcutaneous Electrical Nerve Stimulation (TENS) Psychotherapy
Migraine	*Without aura* Usually unilateral pain, pulsating, moderate or severe intensity and aggravated by physical activity; pain may be associated with nausea, vomiting, photophobia, phonophobia. *With aura* Pain as without aura. Aura symptoms usually involve blurred vision, flashing lights, and missing area of visual field. Aura is fully reversible, lasting less than 1 hour. Headache follows aura within 1 hour.	Cortical spreading depression Trigeminal vascular activation Serotonin depletion	Dietary Changes Decreased stress and stressful triggers Biofeedback Relaxation therapy Psychotherapy *Acute Attacks* Acetylsalicylic acid (ASA) Paracetamol (acetaminophen) Nonsteroidal anti-inflammatory (NSAIDs) Ergotamine Dihydroergotamine (DHE) Metoclopramide or Domperidone ($5HT_3$ agonist) Sumatriptan ($5HT_1$ agonist)

Characteristics of common headaches *(continued)*

Headache type	Symptoms	Pathophysiology	Treatment
Migraine, *continued*			*Prophylaxis* Beta-blockers Calcium antagonists $5HT_2$ antagonists Valproic acid Amitriptyline
Cluster	No nausea or photophobia. Pain is not exacerbated by movement but is associated with lacrimation, rhinorrhea, ptosis. Pain is always unilateral and commonly located behind the orbit. Symptoms are exacerbated if unable to move or ambulate. Attacks occur in clusters followed by remissions lasting several months. Attacks commonly occur after onset of sleep (patient awakens).	Chronobiological changes Impaired autonomic activity Trigeminal vascular activation Hypoxia Histamine release	Dietary changes Decreased stress and stressful triggers Biofeedback Relaxation therapy Psychotherapy *Acute* Oxygen Indomethacin (NSAID) Sumatriptan Ergotamine tartrate *Prophylaxis* Corticosteroids Verapamil (calcium channel blocker) Lithium carbonate Chlorpromazine Ergotamine tartrate Valproic acid Methysergide

symptoms may vary considerably from one patient to another, even within a family. Some patients never experience the aura prior to the onset of pain. Some patients have a very good response to medications such as sumatriptan, whereas others experience only the side effects of the medication.

The pain of an attack is described as a throbbing, pulsating sensation, usually located behind the eye. The symptoms are generally unilateral, but in one-third of cases, patients complain of bilateral symptoms. Nausea and vomiting are frequently associated with the pain. Sound and light tend to worsen the symptoms, and frequently the physician finds the patient in the examination room lying quietly in the fetal position with the lights turned off. These particular observations are important in differentiating migraine headaches from others such as cluster headaches.

The duration of the pain of a migraine will be at least 1 hour and may last as long as 2 to 3 days. The intensity of the headaches will vary from episode to episode, but the majority of those with migraine headaches suffer pain intensity levels in the moderate range.

Pathophysiology of migraine headache

A variety of abnormal findings have been identified in patients with migraine headaches. Using brain blood-flow imaging techniques, neuroscientists have identified spreading hypoperfusion of blood across the cerebral cortex as a phenomenon seen in some migraine attacks. This change in cortical blood flow, termed cortical spreading depression (CSD), is thought by many to initiate the migraine attack and to account for the clinical features and observed changes that occur during the aura phase of a migraine attack. CSD also may explain the spreading oligemia (low blood flow) observed during cerebral blood-flow studies. During the aura phase of the classical migraine, vasoconstriction of the intracranial blood vessels can be demonstrated. During the pain phase, the blood vessels dilate. CSD can be experimentally induced by blocking nitric oxide synthesis. Nitric oxide is normally produced by blood vessels to help control vascular tone and blood flow. CSD leads to activation of the trigeminal nucleus caudalis, also called the spinal trigeminal nucleus caudalis, which is located in the lateral regions of the brain stem. Activation of the trigeminal ganglion leads to a release of the potent vasodilator calcitonin gene-related peptide (CGRP) into the external jugular venous blood. Presumably, release of this vasodilator causes blood vessel dilation and the onset of the pain phase of a migraine attack. Release of CGRP is blocked by treatment with sumatriptan (Imitrex).

Magnetic resonance imaging (MRI) studies of the brain have revealed low brain tissue levels of high-energy phosphates and magnesium in migrainous states. These changes render neural cells hyperexcitable; hence, the central neuronal hyperexcitability theory has been proposed to explain migraines. None of these theories can completely explain the pain and other aspects of migraine headaches, and appropriate research continues to progress in this area.

Treatment

For many years, ergot alkaloids have been the mainstay treatment for migraines along with opioid-containing medications such as Darvocet (propoxyphene with acetaminophen) for severe attacks. More recently, sumatriptan (Imitrex) has been introduced and has provided considerable improvement for many patients who suffer this disorder. Like the ergotamine preparations, sumatriptan affects the serotonin receptors, but it is more selective and tends to work primarily as an agonist at the $5HT_1D$ receptor, the serotonin receptor located in the brain.

Migraine patients generally treat themselves at home for 1 to 2 days prior to seeking the assistance of a medical professional. If the patient has not been successful by the time of the office or emergency room visit, no additional ergot or sumatriptan can be given, and the opioid medications are the usual alterative taken.

Cluster headache

Cluster headache is much less common than migraine or tension headache, but it has received considerable attention from practitioners and scientists over the decades. Periodic cluster headaches are characterized by the temporal clustering of attacks during periods lasting for 2 weeks to 3 months, separated by remission of at least 3 or 4 months. There is also a chronic cluster variety which will not be discussed here. Cluster headaches are more common in men, with a male-to-female ratio of 5 to 1. Cluster headaches can begin at any age, but they start most commonly between the ages of 20 and 40.

In addition to the clustering of attacks, other characteristics of cluster headache differentiate it from other headaches. Very commonly the headaches occur soon after the patient has gone to sleep. The attacks correspond with the first rapid eye movement (REM) period of the sleep cycle. The pain is always unilateral and almost always located behind one eye. In addition to pain behavior and complaints, the patient displays tearing and suffusion in the eye. Invariably, the patient also develops a ptosis (drooping) of the eyelid on the affected side along with a stuffy nasal passage and unilateral runny nose. This constellation of signs and symptoms is called a partial Horner's syndrome. A complete Horner's syndrome is not diagnosed when the pupil is not affected and sweating is normal.

Interestingly, most attacks occur in relation to seasonal photoperiod (length of day) changes, increasing in frequency during the seasons with diminishing or lengthening photoperiods. Most attacks occur during July and January, two weeks after the longest and shortest days of the year. Some people who move from northern regions of the United States to the southernmost regions, where seasonal changes in day length are less dramatic, have reported resolution of attacks. Other factors in the patients' lives changed as well, but anecdotal evidence supports the concept that environmental influences are at play.

Pathophysiology of cluster headache

The changes in the autonomic nervous system (partial Horner's syndrome) are coupled with the onset of symptoms and they remain until the headache is relieved. This has led researchers to believe that the cause of cluster headaches is related to abnormalities or imbalances in the autonomic nervous system. The vascular changes that occur during an attack also point to a defect in the autonomic system. Like the painful periods of migraine, cluster pain is associated with extracranial vasodilation. Cluster headaches can easily be differentiated from migraines, however. A typical migraine patient lies very still and avoids light and sound, but a cluster patient paces the floor, rubs the head and eye, and appears very anxious. With almost all other types of headache, the patient prefers to be as still as possible. There do not seem to be any theories that explain this phenomenon, but it is a very useful observation when the history is not clearly differentiating. Another nonspecific observation is that the cluster headache tends to be reported as excruciatingly severe, never mild or moderate. Fortunately, cluster headache is relatively uncommon compared to migraine and tension headache. During a cluster period, people suffer greatly with symptoms that are difficult to manage.

Treatment

The common analgesic medications are used to treat cluster headache but are generally limited in effectiveness, opioid medications included. Cluster headaches are unique in that supplemental oxygen can sometimes abort the headache, and steroids have been reported to relieve the symptoms. Smoking can trigger attacks and should be discontinued, if possible. Ergotamine as well as sumatriptan have both been used effectively. The fact that similar medications are used effectively to treat migraine and cluster suggests that the underlying pathophysiology may be similar; however, the differing clinical presentations suggest that there are major differences as well.

Trigeminal neuralgia

Trigeminal neuralgia (TN) is characterized by paroxysmal pain involving regions of the face innervated by the trigeminal nerve. Of the three branches of the trigeminal nerves (ophthalmic, maxillary, and mandibular), the mandibular division is the most commonly affected. TN most frequently afflicts women over 50. The pain is usually initiated with mechnical manipulation of the face. (See *A typical case of trigeminal neuralgia.*)

Trigeminal neuralgia is also called tic douloureux because patients sometimes have muscle spasms accompanying the pain. The other diagnoses that must be considered are atypical neuralgia, myofascial pain, temporomandibular facial pain, and cluster headache. The examining physician also must rule out local diseases in the sinuses, jaw, teeth, throat, and skull. Physical examination of TN patients may reveal a completely normal head, neck, and sinuses. The temporomandibular joint (TMJ) may rotate smoothly with full range, and the TMJ muscles may be normal and lack any ten-

A typical case of trigeminal neuralgia

Ms. Smith, a 45-year-old woman with a 1-year history of trigeminal neuralgia, had worked at the courthouse for 25 years and had never missed work due to sickness for more than 1 or 2 days at a time. During the 3 months following the first attack of pain, she missed several weeks of work and was not able to maintain her share of housework. She described the pain in the right side of her face as incredibly intense and also as similar to the pain that arises "when you hit your funny bone, but much worse."

Describing her first attack, which occurred very suddenly during lunch at work, she said, "It was like a bolt of lightning hit me." Her first pain lasted for 10 or 20 seconds and stopped as quickly as it had come on. She thought that a bee might have stung her. Five minutes passed, she resumed eating her meal, and the "jabbing," "shocking" pain returned. Again, it lasted only for 20 seconds or so, but the third, fourth, fifth,

and sixth attacks came much sooner after relief. This first cycle of on-and-off pain lasted for about an hour.

That night at dinner, the scenario was repeated. Initially, the pain was triggered only by eating, especially very cold or hot foods. After about a week, simply talking could trigger an attack. She tried putting ice, heat, pressure, and liniment on her face and lip, but all these approaches made her pain worse. She became afraid to wash her face or brush her teeth. The pain was located mostly in the right portion of her lip and a little along the right side of her face. Occasionally, severe shocklike pain occurred and the entire lower part of her face went into spasms. The only guarantee of relief was sleeping. The commonly used analgesics were ineffective.

After visiting her dentist and family practitioner, she was finally diagnosed as having trigeminal neuralgia. She was started on appropriate treatement and her symptoms resolved.

derness to palpation. As for the other disorders mentioned here, it is rare to find that pain is triggered by touch unless there is an obvious physical finding. Also, the quality of the pain of these other disorders is different from TN pain, with the exception of cluster headache, which can have similar quality and location. A very low percentage of patients with TN have multiple sclerosis (MS), and this diagnosis should be considered when the pain is bilateral.

Pathophysiology of trigeminal neuralgia

According to some authorities, TN is caused by damage of the trigeminal nerve as it passes from openings in the skull toward the facial muscles and skin. Chronic pressure on a nerve shreds its myelin sheath (demyelination). Myelin both insulates and provides nutrition to nerve axons. When the nerve fibers become diseased, inappropriate pain signals can be triggered and sent to the brain. In some patients the trigeminal nerve is compressed by an artery that travels along with the nerve. In those cases the nerve can be decompressed with surgery. Some researchers doubt that most patients have this problem. Other researches think that the pain is caused primarily by changes in neural tissues within the skull, where the nuclei of the trigeminal nerve live. Altered central nervous system processing of sensory information can result from damage to peripheral nervous tissue or changes within the brain. Regardless of the site of initial damage, the result is generation of pain impulses or misinterpretation of normal signals as pain.

Treatment

Some patients need surgery to address trigeminal neuralgia, but most are treated successfully with medications. All patients start with drug therapy before invasive therapy is considered. Carbamazepine (Tegretol) is the drug of choice for treating TN. At least two-thirds of patients report relief after initiating this therapy, and for many the relief is complete. As with all medications, side effects are possible. Carbamazepine can cause nausea, dizziness, somnolence, dermatitis, and, rarely, liver and bone marrow dysfunction. The patient's blood is tested periodically to avoid serious complications. Other drugs that have been reported to be helpful include phenytoin (Dilantin), baclofen (Lioresal), and chlorphenesin carbamate (Maolate). All of these drugs affect nervous tissues and can suppress aberrant nerve activity.

There are few alternative approaches to managing this problem if the drugs fail. Nerve blocks of the trigeminal ganglion can effectively relieve active symptoms and occasionally provide long-term relief. The mechanism for the long-term relief is unknown. Portions of the ganglion can be destroyed to provide relief, but the part of the face innervated by the nerve is left without sensation. It is the rare patient who fails to respond to at least one approach, and the long-term prognosis for these patients is usually good.

Temporomandibular joint disease

TMJ disease can be divided into four major categories:

- disease of the muscles of mastication
- internal derangement of the contents of the joint space
- degenerative joint disease
- invasion of the joint or surrounding tissues by tumor or inflammation.

Four patients, each representing one of these TMJ diseases, are described in *Four types of TMJ pain*. Most TMJ pain is not attributable to straightforward, diagnosable problems, and there is considerable overlap among groups of patients in terms of treatment and symptom presentation.

Four types of TMJ pain

The four case studies here illustrate four different diagnoses and treatment plans for TMJ pain.

TMJ muscle dysfunction

Kathy speaks: "During my freshman year in college I first noticed pain in my jaw and I started getting headaches. The headache pain was located mostly at my right temple. The jaw pain is there most of the time and is made worse with chewing or during stressful periods like final exam week. My roommate tells me that I grind my teeth when I sleep at night. Sometimes I have severe muscle spasms in my jaw muscles. This can be very painful and occasionally the pain extends to the muscles in my neck and shoulders."

Kathy has been prescribed an oral splint which she wears at night to prevent her from clenching her teeth. If a finger is placed over her right TMJ and she is asked to open her mouth maximally, a little clicking can be felt. More noticeable, the muscles (temporalis, masseter) around the joint feel tighter on the right than on the left and she is able to open her mouth only two fingerbreadths. Normally a person should be able to open his or her mouth at least three fingerbreadths. There was also considerable tenderness on palpation of these regions when she first sought treatment. Although the problem has not been completely resolved, wearing the splint, using NSAIDs regularly, and doing physiotherapy has helped Kathy reduce her pain significantly.

Derangement of joint contents

Jennifer speaks: "I had some of the symptoms that Kathy complains of. I did develop some headaches in the temple, but most of my pain was in the joint. At first all I noticed was a lot of clicking in my jaw, and when I opened my mouth, my jaw deviated to the left. As the pain developed, I was unable to open my mouth as wide as normal and the clicking changed to a cracking sound. After a trial with splints, aspirin, and steroid injections in the joint was not effective, an MRI scan of my TMJ was done and they found a displacement of the cartilage in the joint. Two months ago I had surgery to repair it, and so far I am well on my way to recovery. Occasionally I have a bad day, but I can open my mouth again without pain, and most of the clicking noise is gone."

Jennifer is an example of a patient with internal derangement of the joint space. In her case it was a displaced meniscus, a crescent-shaped cartilage that allows the joint components to glide smoothly over one another when the mouth is opened and closed.

Degenerative joint disease

Rebecca speaks: "Unlike Jennifer and Kathy, I never have pain unless I talk a lot or eat a meal continuously for more than a few minutes. Both of my TMJs are affected by my disease. It started with a crackling sensation in my jaws. As the sound became more intense, the pain started. It feels raw in the joint when I move it, as if the bones are rubbing together. Ibuprofen is useful, but I get my best relief by resting my jaws. I drink a lot of milk shakes and eat soft foods to avoid chewing, and I try to talk with my mouth closed when possible."

Rebecca has degenerative joint disease (DJD) in both TMJs. When her joints are felt as she opens and closes her mouth, crepitation, vibration produced by bone or irregular cartilage surfaces rubbing together can be felt. This is common in DJD. Regular X-rays of the joints reveal degenerative changes. Rebecca's therapy at this point is anti-inflammatory medications. Surgery is not indicated at this time.

Tumor of the TMJ

Sharon speaks: "I have pain similar to the pain of all these women. My pain is always there, even when I am not using my jaw. I have pain in the joint, chronic headaches, and muscle pain when I chew and talk. I have a tumor that has invaded my TMJ. The tumor

(continued)

Four types of TMJ pain *(continued)*

comes from somewhere else in my body, but the doctors have not found where. I have had infections in the joint and had to stay in the hospital for many days to get multiple debridements and intravenous antibiotics. Once the infection clears and if the tumor can be shrunk with radiation and chemotherapy, a reconstructive procedure will be attempted."

These cases of TMJ disease were relatively easy to diagnose, but many cases are much more difficult. Some patients endure years of agony and uncertainty without a specific diagnosis. In recent years surgical and dental reconstructive procedures have become more common treatments for these patients, even though there is little scientific evidence to support their efficacy.

The ratio of females to males with TMJ disease is six to one. Considerably more research is needed in this area to develop better diagnostic tools and treatments.

Low back pain

Low back pain is a very common among people in industrialized societies (see *Common sources of low back pain*). The etiology for most low back pain is undetermined. It continues to take its toll on this nation's productivity. The majority of people with low back pain never present themselves to physicians for treatment. Instead, these individuals usually self-treat the ailment or endure the pain as long as they can continue to function at work and play. The patients who do frequent the physician's office and emergency rooms are those with acute onset of severely painful symptoms or with severe exacerbation of chronic symptoms. The etiology for the pain in these patients is usually undetermined, but this group is more likely to have conditions that may require aggressive therapy.

Disk degeneration is one of the diagnoses that must be considered in patients with acute onset of severe pain, particularly when neurological deficits are identifiable. Unfortunately, the sensitivity (ability to detect disease when it is present) and specificity (ability to reject the presence of disease) are not perfect in any of the many tests available to evaluate these patients. Consequently, a number of patients will get procedures and therapies that are unnecessary. Only 1% of all low back pain problems require surgical intervention, but because low back pain is so pervasive in this society, a considerable

Common sources of low back pain

Arthritis

Diskitis

Facet joint disease

Intervertebral disk disease

Infection

Lordosis

Nerve root disease

Sacroiliac joint disease

Scoliosis

Spinal stenosis

Spondylolisthesis

Muscular disease

number of back surgeries will be performed each year. Intervertebral disk degeneration is one of the common indications for surgery.

Intervertebral disk degeneration and failed back syndrome are highlighted here, but they account for only a small proportion of low back pain sufferers.

Intervertebral disk degeneration

The intervertebral disks serve as shock absorbers for the axial skeleton. To some extent, all disks degenerate with age. When the disk contents are forced out of the normal anatomical location, they follow the path of least resistance. Because there is little or no potential space to accommodate the rupture, the surrounding soft tissues, including the nervous tissue in the area, are compressed. The pain experienced by patients with disk degeneration is most commonly the result of impingement of nerve roots as they exit the vertebral column. Certain parts of the disk compartment are also capable of generating painful sensations in the presence of inflammation. Although not always the case, it is quite common for people to experience the first symptoms of disk disease while performing physical labor, such as heavy lifting or pulling, in which the back musculature is required. Patients describe a "popping" sensation as a disk ruptures, and the ensuing pain leaves patients incapacitated. In short order, muscle spasms develop on top of the nerve irritation, which exacerbates the original pain. In addition, pain sensations often radiate into the tissue that is served by the nerve.

If the ruptured disk is in the lumbar region, pain can radiate down the posterior leg and even into the foot if the fifth lumbar disk is involved. Patients describe the pain as burning, shooting, and cramping. Any kind of movement worsens the symptoms, yet the patient usually cannot find a comfortable position, either sitting or reclining. The description of the location of the pain and the findings of the physical examination will help the examining physician to pin-point the location of the disk disease and allow formulation of an a priori hypothesis before ordering tests. It is important to form such a pretest hypothesis because of the likelihood of finding abnormalities on X-rays and scans that may have been present before the onset of pain. During the physical examination, the physician looks for neurological deficits such as loss of reflexes, muscle weakness, and loss of sensation. Raising the legs above the plane of the trunk while the patient is in the supine position will tug on the meninges and induce pain that replicates the ongoing complaints.

Treatment of disk degeneration

If the patient has evidence of neurological deficits, such as loss of reflexes, strength, or sensation, and there is evidence of nerve impingement on the computed tomography (CT) or MRI images, then the patient is recommended for laminectomy, a procedure in which the removal of a posterior vertebral arch allows removal of an associated herniated disk to decompress the affected nerve. If the patient has only pain, even with evidence of disk disease on the scans, a more conservative approach is taken, including bed rest, injection of steroids into the spinal canal, and symptom control with narcotic and nonsteroidal anti-inflammatory medications. If after many weeks the symptoms persist and the patient cannot resume normal activities, elective surgery may be considered. After the surgery, all or only some of the painful symptoms may be relieved. For patients with radicular pain (pain in a dermatomal distribution associated with nerve root compression) prior to surgery, the pain radiating down the leg, for example, may disappear, but the low back pain may remain. Several months might pass before a sense of normality is regained.

For the patient with no neurological deficits, surgery should be considered only as a last resort. There is no good evidence that early surgical intervention is better than conservative therapy. The use of epidural steroid therapy is controversial. Many physicians believe that the procedure is of little use and should not be practiced while many others continue to employ it, particularly when the patient has a radicular component to the low back pain. There has not been very good evidence that either rest or exercise makes a difference in the outcome of these patients. For several decades traction was used to control the acute episode of pain, but today this practice is not as widely used as in the past. The major advantage or accomplishment of surgery has been an earlier recovery of function, even though in the long run, the outcome may not be better than with conservative therapy. If no herniated disk is found during surgery, the success rate falls to about 40%. The differential diagnoses for low back pain are extensive, and very few cases are amenable to surgical therapy. When surgery is performed inappropriately, patients may experience even more pain and disability after the procedure.

Failed back syndrome

Many patients who undergo laminectomy procedures for low back pain fail to get sustained pain reduction afterwards. This circumstance is referred to as failed back syndrome. Surgery can fail to relieve back pain for three primary reasons:

- incorrect diagnoses
- improper or inadequate surgery
- complications of surgery.

When encountering patients with failed back syndrome, people tend to indict the surgeon for using poor judgment in patient selection or poor surgical technique. Careful examination of the preoperative and postoperative records can reveal possible etiologies of the pain.

Many of these patients have undergone not only one but two or more back surgeries to relieve pain. The first procedure is usually a lumbar laminectomy, followed by a second laminectomy or a fusion procedure to stabilize the spinal column. Once surgical indications have been exhausted and the spinal column is deemed to be stable, scar tissue is commonly identified as the cause of ongoing pain, and the patient is likely to remain with pain and disability for a considerable period of time. Another severe complication is arachnoiditis, inflammation of the arachnoid membrane of the spinal cord. Neither of these conditions is amenable to surgical intervention and neither of them responds to medicinal approaches. The only drugs that relieve the symptoms are the opioid-containing products, such as Lortab (acetaminophen with hydrocodone), Percocet (acetaminophen with oxycodone), and Tylenol #3 (acetaminophen with codeine). Unfortunately, because of concern about dependence on these medications, most physicians are unwilling to treat patients with such drugs for longer than a few weeks. Ultimately, many of these patients find themselves in a rehabilitation treatment program.

Because surgery has proven to be a mistake for a significant number of back pain patients, better screening techniques are necessary to separate unsuitable candidates from patients who really need surgery. Some of these patients do not respond to any form of therapy. The patient who has had ineffective surgery is doubly difficult to rehabilitate.

Neuropathic pain

Acute pain that arises in response to disease or tissue injury has the protective function of warning a person to take remedial action to avoid further injury or exacerbation of disease. Chronic pain that arises as a result of ongoing tissue damage or inflammation, such as the pain of rheumatoid arthritis or the pain of metastatic cancer, also is a normal nociceptive response that serves as a warning.

In contrast to normal nociception, which accompanies disease or injury and which confers a survival advantage, neuropathic pain may appear long after injury and subsequent healing of tissue are complete. Neuropathic pain appears to arise from damage to the nervous system itself. In many cases, neuropathic pain does not appear until weeks or months after an initial injury or insult to the nervous system.

Deafferentation pain syndrome

Deafferentation pain refers to neuropathic pain that arises due to loss of afferent input into the central nervous system. Damage to or disease of a nerve leads to the loss of the capacity to conduct afferent information. In deafferentation pain syndromes, damage to the nervous system can be demonstrated, and it is likely that nerve damage has resulted in a loss of somatosensory impulse transmission. For example, a patient who suffers an accidental severance of an intercostal nerve during a thoracotomy (surgical procedure to open the chest) and subsequently develops persistent pain would be considered to have a deafferentation pain syndrome. In this case, the dorsal root ganglion serving that nerve as well as the spinothalamic tract neurons that transmit information to the brain have been deafferentated, or deprived of afferent signals from the intercostal nerve. Trigeminal neuralgia would not be considered a deafferentation pain syndrome despite the derangement in neural function as there is usually no evidence of deafferentation.

Like many other terms used in pain medicine, deafferentation pain syndrome is a general description that covers a variety of conditions. Deafferentation terminology is used when the pathophysiology of the disease is being considered. More specific names are used to describe the various problems in the clinic. If the deafferentation is caused by diabetes, it is referred to as painful diabetic peripheral neuropathy. If a cerebral infarct is the culprit, it might be called thalamic pain syndrome. Deafferentation pain syndromes involving the peripheral nervous system are by far the most common and, therefore, are the focus of this section.

Pathophysiology of deafferentation pain

Many factors cause the painful sensations associated with nerve deafferentation. Once a peripheral nerve is cut and cannot be reattached, a major contributor to pain generation occurs, ironically, when the damaged nerve attempts to regenerate itself. The nerve fibrils grow haphazardly in an attempt to reconnect with the severed distal segment. These regenerating nerve endings no longer have the usual protective covering of an intact nerve and are abnormally exposed to a variety of molecules and stresses. Macro- and micro-neuroma (nodules composed of axon sprouts at the site of the regenerating axon) are formed as a consequence of this activity. In a descriptive sense, the system has been short-circuited and action potential generation is out of control and unpredictable.

Patients with deafferentation syndromes experience painful sensations that are present at rest and exacerbated with activity and mechanical manipulation of the diseased tissue. In addition to deranged activity in the peripheral nervous system, the central processing sites have altered their activity as well. Nerve cells broaden their receptive fields and respond to nonpainful sensations as if a painful stimulus had been applied. The mechanism for these central alterations seems to be related to activation of N-methyl-D-aspartate (NMDA) receptors. Blocking these receptors in animal models of deafferentation pain prevents and reverses pain behavior. Research using NMDA receptor antagonists is under way.

For a summary of various treatment approaches for deafferentation pain, see *Symptoms and treatments for deafferentation pain syndromes*, page 106.

Dorsal root avulsion

Damage to the dorsal roots of sensory neurons is often caused by trauma or malignancy. This problem is particularly difficult to manage. The pain and dysesthesia (distressing sensations that are not painful) are so intense and constant that it is next to impossible for these patients to concentrate enough even to participate in everyday social activities. Commonly, these patients become socially withdrawn and despondent, living in extreme emotional states of depression, anger, or frustration. Seldom does any treatment approach provide complete relief of pain and normalization of sensations.

Nerve roots involving an upper extremity and the neck are common sites of injury. Because these nerves supply innervation to the shoulder, arm, hand, head, and neck, patients experience pain in these regions of the body. Symptoms may begin shortly after the injury or may be delayed. Burning, pins and needles, and electricity-like sensations are common descriptors for the pain these patients

Symptoms and treatments for deafferentation pain syndromes

The more distal the lesion the better the prognosis. For all these syndromes recovery is a long process. Often opioid medications are ineffective in relieving symptoms. Physicians may be unwilling to prescribe opioids for prolonged periods.

Location	Causes	Symptoms	Treatment
Peripheral nerve	Diabetes Acquired immuno-deficiency syndrome (AIDS) Alcoholism Amyloidosis Fabry's disease	Burning pain, intermittent electricity-like pain, or stabbing pain. Severe pain may be elicited by lightly touching the skin (allodynia). Mildly painful stimulation (a pinprick) may induce unexpected severe pain. (hyperalgesia).	*Drug Therapy* Opioids Tricyclic antidepressants Neuroleptics Carbamazepine Propranolol Local anesthetics (mexiletine)
Spinal cord	Traumatic spinal cord injury Demyelinating disease Necrotizing myelitis Syringomyelia Spinal cord ischemic injury Arteriovenous mal-formation		*Surgery* Excision of neuroma Sympathectomy Rhizotomy Cordotomy Dorsal column stimulation Midbrain lesions Thalamotomy Prefrontal lobotomy Cortical ablations
Brain stem	Vascular injury Surgical procedures Demyelination		*Psychological Treatment* Psychotherapy
Thalamus	Vascular injury to ventroposteriolateral (VPL) and ventro-posteriomedial (VPM) nuclei		Biofeedback Relaxation Hypnosis Stress management
Cortex	Injury to parietal cortex and subcortical white matter that interrupts sensory pathways		

experience. The constant pain tends to worsen at night, and frequently it is exacerbated by extreme paroxysms of pain that might be triggered by some special circumstance or might strike without warning. In many cases the exacerbation of pain can be controlled. The remaining goal is to lessen the ongoing pain. Suicide will be a consideration for many of these patients, particularly after several months or years of disease, feelings of loss of self-worth, and despair.

The medications and procedures for treating damage to dorsal roots are numerous. Opioid medications are rarely effective as pain relievers, but patients use them for other effects, such as sedation and relaxation. Placing these patients on chronic opioid regimens is risky, because most patients require very high doses to get any analgesic benefit. Commonly, depression becomes a major component of the patient's experience, and some patients require aggressive treatment, including electroconvulsive therapy and high doses of antidepression medications. If the medication approach is unsuccessful, invasive procedures, such as dorsal column stimulation (see Chapter 7, Medical and Surgical Pain Management Techniques), intraspinal infusion of opioids, and surgical ablative procedures, become the next option for relief. Behavioral techniques such as psychotherapy can be helpful but generally are not.

Surgical procedures designed to deal with this problem involve destroying nerve tissue further upstream, for example at the spinal cord entrance of the dorsal roots, to block the incoming nociceptive impulses. Many of the patients who undergo these procedures get good relief initially, but if they live long enough, the pain returns with equivalent or greater intensity. These procedures are usually used only as a last resort and commonly are reserved for patients with terminal illness.

Postherpetic neuralgia

Postherpetic neuralgia (PHN) is a complication of shingles. Shingles, also called acute herpetic neuralgia (AHN) or zoster eruption, is characterized by pain and vesicular eruptions of the skin along the course of a nerve due to inflammation of the dorsal roots and dorsal root ganglia. Shingles is caused by the varicella-zoster virus, the same virus that causes common childhood chickenpox. In fact, an individual can contract chicken pox if exposed to a patient who has shingles. After a person recovers from chicken pox, the virus lies dormant within the dorsal root ganglia. In patients with AHN, the virus has become activated later in life after there is a diminished immunity to the virus. Why shingles often involves the chest and the ophthalmic branch of the trigeminal nerve area is a mystery. (The ophthalmic branch of the trigeminal nerve innervates the forehead and eye region). Most cases involve two or fewer dermatomes and almost always involve only one side of the body. Patients with severely depressed immune systems, such as AIDS patients, are at risk of multiple dermatome involvement and systemic infection.

The pain during the acute stages of herpes zoster infection is limited to the dermatomes served by the dorsal root ganglia that are infected by the virus. The skin lesions will begin to crust after the second to third week, and by six weeks healing is well on its way. For most patients the pain and analgesic requirements have subsided by then. If the pain persists for one month after the skin lesions have healed, the diagnosis of postherpetic neuralgia may be considered.

Unlike the pain of acute herpetic neuralgia, the pain of postherpetic neuralgia is not caused by the varicella zoster virus. This pain is the result of the damage caused by viral invasion of the nerve and the resultant deafferentation. The likelihood of developing postherpetic neuralgia after suffering a zoster eruption is mostly dependent on the age at which the shingles develops. Patients over the age of 50 have a much higher incidence of postherpetic neuralgia than their younger counterparts.

The symptoms of PHN are somewhat similar to those of AHN. Patients have a raw sensation along the affected dermatone. There are hypersensitivity and frankly painful sensations in response to mechanical stimulation in multiple areas along the dermatome. Scarring of the skin from the acute infection is frequently identifiable, and the painful locations are usually pigmented areas of skin surrounding pale, scarred tissue that is insensitive to painful and nonpainful stimuli. Patients describe the pain as jabbing, electric, shouting, or burning, to name a few. Wearing clothing over the painful area may be impossible without inducing considerable pain and discomfort. Sleeping at night is problematic and sexual activities become nearly impossible.

The good news for patients with a short history of PHN is that most patients improve within a few months, with gradual resolution of the pain. Patients who continue to have symptoms after twelve months may continue to have pain for years to come. PHN is the number one reason given for committing suicide among patients over age 80.

Diabetic neuropathy

Approximately 10% of diabetic patients will develop a neuropathy during the course of their disease. Many of these patients will develop pain as a consequence of their neuropathy, which translates into thousands of patients developing painful neuropathy every year because diabetes is so prevalent in this society. Painful diabetic neuropathy is broadly categorized into mononeuropathies, or focal neuropathies, and symmetrical polyneuropathies. Symmetrical polyneuropathies are the most common, occuring in patients with poorly controlled diabetes and in those who have only slight elevations in their glucose levels.

The typical patient with symmetrical polyneuropathy pain has had diabetes for several years before the pain begins, but a significant number of patients will present with painful extremities before they develop objective evidence of hyperglycemia, or diabetes. (See *A case of diabetic neuropathy*, page 110, for a typical presentation of a patient with painful symmetrical polyneuropathy.)

In contrast to symmetrical polyneuropthy, patients with mononeuropathy generally have had long-standing diabetes that has not been controlled, although this is not always the case. As the name suggests, these patients develop painful symptoms in a territory innervated by a single major nerve. They may develop the pain anywhere in the body, including the eye, the chest, or a single extremity. Their symptoms come on much more rapidly than do the symptoms of patients with symmetrical polyneuropathy and symptoms tend to be more intense and disabling. Hypersensitivity to touch can be intense, and the patient will even avoid clothing at times to avoid stimulation of the area affected. Like polyneuropathy patients, these patients also have burning and numbing pain, but electric, shooting pain is much more prevalent and sometimes the central complaint. The duration of the pain is shorter than in most cases of symmetrical polyneuropathy.

A small population of diabetic patients develop intense mononeuropathy pain after correction of severe hyperglycemia. Generally, this is seen in patients with long-term, very poorly controlled diabetes that is then suddenly brought under control with intravenous insulin. These patients may have very severe pain that is unresponsive to most of the recommended therapies. Their symptoms are short-lived and will resolve if the glucose is maintained under control for 3 to 4 weeks.

Diabetic neuropathy can be traced to several pathological circumstances. Excess glucose and abnormal glucose metabolism will result in damage to peripheral nerves. These patients might also develop vascular disease of the small blood vessels that are responsible for supplying the peripheral nerves with blood. One of the prevailing theories to explain the observation that polyneuropathy patients first develop symptoms in their distal extremities is that the longer nerves are most susceptible to the ischemic changes resulting from small blood vessel disease and so are the first to manifest symptoms of disease. Over time, the shorter nerves also succumb to the ischemic changes and multiple regions in the body then show evidence of the neuropathic changes. With respect to abnormal glucose metabolism, all nerves in the peripheral system should be affected equally.

Mononeuropathy patients develop acute onset and escalation of symptoms, suggesting an acute process underlying the pain. For those

A case of diabetic neuropathy

Mr. Jones, age 55, was diagnosed 5 years ago with diabetes. His disease has been controlled with oral medications to date, and his glucose levels never exceed 200. Approximately 1 year ago, Mr. Jones began to notice a feeling that pebbles were in his shoes whenever he walked. He found himself frequently taking off and emptying his shoes to remove any contents that might be pressing against the ball of his foot. He tried a variety of shoe types to alleviate this annoying problem.

After 2 or 3 months, he began to notice numbness in his toes and soles. About that time he also began to experience a burning sensation in his toes. The intensity and location of all these symptoms were symmetrical. Weekly, the patient noticed increases in the intensity of the burning sensation, which began to spread symmetrically from his toes into his soles and up into his ankles. Despite the burning sensation, the patient also continued to experience worsening of the numbing, which he described as painful. His symp-

toms are exacerbated when he walks, particularly on hard surfaces for long periods of time.

Approximately 4 to 5 months into the symptom development, he began to notice hypersensitivity to touch in his feet. Specifically, he noticed that the sheets or blankets on his bed caused severe pain. Consequently, he slept with his feet outside the covers. Soaking his feet in warm water and a massage are nightly routines. Deep pressure stimulation relieves the symptoms rather than exacerbates them.

Currently, Mr. Jones has numbness that extends to the level of his knees bilaterally. He has recently begun to experience some tingling and some numbing pain in his upper extremities, primarily in his fingertips. During the past month, the hypersensitivity has diminished, but he continues to have numbing pain and ongoing burning pain. His symptoms and history of diabetes prompted his doctors to do a vascular evaluation which showed normal blood flow in the extremities.

patients who develop severe pain after bringing their glucose under control, normalization of the metabolic milieu may be the reason. Under normal blood glucose conditions, the nerves are able to respond to the insult of the disease and the patient experiences pain.

When the peripheral nerves of both types of patients are viewed under a microscope, the larger fibers are seen to have been damaged considerably, and the smaller fibers, which transmit painful sensation, are left intact or are only slightly depopulated. This imbalance between the small-fiber and the large-fiber population seems to put patients at risk for developing painful neuropathy, although the etiology for the development of pain in both types of patients is probably multifactorial.

The management of this form of pain is similar to the management of deafferentation pain syndrome, but control of glucose and normalization of metabolism are the first steps toward improvment. Unlike patients with acute onset mononeuropathy pain, patients with symmetrical polyneuropathy whose glucose levels are extremely elevated will see improvement in their pain symptoms when their glucose levels are brought under control. Opioid medications have been shown to be effective for pain relief in these patients, but higher doses than are currently acceptable for long-term use in nonmalignant syndromes will be required to maintain an effect. Consequently, opioids are not often used in these patients. Just as for postherpetic neuralgia, a variety of creams and jellies are available for application directly to the painful areas, and they provide successful resolution of symptoms in some patients.

The tricyclic antidepressants can be quite effective in relieving the symptoms of diabetic neuropathy, but their use is frequently limited by their side effects. The side effects of the various tricyclic antidepressants vary in intensity and type, but the analgesic effect for diabetic neuropathy patients seems to be the same for all of them. Therefore, the physician has some room to tailor medication to a patient's specific needs. For example, a patient who is having insomnia would benefit from a tricyclic that provides nighttime sedation. A patient who is hindered by the sedating effects of tricyclic antidepressants can be placed on a tricyclic that causes minimal sedation yet still provides analgesia. NSAIDs generally are not effective in relieving this kind of pain. As a rule, significant improvement in quality of life is possible after 12 to 18 months of treatment if the blood glucose levels and general health of the patient can be controlled and normalized.

Phantom limb pain

Phantom limb pain seems to the patient to originate in an extremity that has been amputated. It can be one of the most troublesome and intellectually stimulating syndromes to treat and manage. How is it possible to treat pain in an extremity that does not exist? What causes these disturbing phantom sensations? The many descriptive cases in the literature discuss patients who have had traumatic loss of a limb. Although not a prerequisite for development of this syndrome, pain in the extremity prior to amputation has been experienced by many of these patients. The phantom pain may begin immediately after recovery from the surgical anesthetic or may take days to weeks to manifest. Commonly, the pain is most intense in or is limited to the most distal part of the phantom extremity, for example the hand or foot. The patient may experience multiple painful symptoms. The muscles are likely to feel tight or cramped continuously. A discrete area of the phantom part may feel as if it is on fire. If there was ongoing pain prior to the amputation, the pain intensity, quality, and location may persist in the phantom limb.

Treatment of phantom limb pain extends to the perioperative period, if possible. To the extent that painful preamputation symptoms contribute to postamputation pain, control of pain before the amputation will lessen the pain afterwards. This can be accomplished by providing the patient with ample opioid availability. At some centers, epidural analgesia is started in the preoperative period. During surgery, the epidural block can be deepened to anesthetic levels and continued in the postoperative period. During the postoperative period, adequate analgesic medications in the form of regional analgesia, systemic opioid medications, and NSAIDs should be provided. Aggressive analgesic therapy seems to make a difference in the control and prevention of phantom pain sensations.

If the patient develops or continues to experience phantom limb pain after the surgical wound has healed, the opioid medications and NSAIDS have little pain-relieving effect. Initial acute inflammatory pain seems to exacerbate phantom pain, but phantom pain is neuropathic and does not depend upon the presence of acute inflammation to manifest. Therapy for chronic phantom pain includes a variety of medications. Because phantom limb pain can be exacerbated by inflammation in the stump, any ongoing nociceptive areas in the stump should be extinguished if possible. This might include local injection of steroids and anesthetics, corrections in prosthesis, or control of local muscular spasms. TENS units can be beneficial as well.

Musculoskeletal pain

Chronic pain and tenderness involving muscles is probably the most common pain problem humans experience. Both myofascial pain syndrone (MPS) and fibromyalgia, the two common musculoskeletal disorders discussed here, have a poorly understood pathophysiological basis. Diagnosis is based primarily on the patient's pattern of symptoms and pain. As yet, there are no objective physical signs, laboratory results, or radiographic findings that consistently characterize these disorders. Patients who are diagnosed with either of them may also have a coexisting disease such as osteoarthritis that contributes to the musculoskeletal symptoms. (See *Differentiating fibromyalgia from myofascial pain syndrome* for a comparison of diagnostic features).

Myofascial pain syndrome

Most low back pain complaints are related to muscle problems, and many low back pain patients will be given a diagnosis of MPS. Although any muscle group can be affected, the buttocks, lower back, upper back, and shoulders are the most common areas of complaint.

PAIN MANAGEMENT PRINCIPLES

Differentiating fibromyalgia from myofascial pain syndrome

Both of these syndromes cause pain in the musculoskeletal system, but careful attention to the patient's history and symptoms will allow an alert examiner to distinguish between them.

Diagnostic criteria for MPS
- Pain localized to a single muscle group
- Referred pain upon palpation of the trigger points
- Palpable taut muscle bands that are tender to palpation
- Measurable decreased range of motion
- Local twitch of muscle after snapping muscle
- Pain alleviated by stretching muscle

Diagnostic criteria for fibromyalgia
- Widespread pain (above and below the waist)
- Painful axial skeleton (cervical spine, anterior chest, thoracic spine, or low back)
- Pain in 11 of 18 specific sites on palpation such as bilateral at the midpoint of the upper border of the trapezius, bilateral at the suboccipital muscle insertions, and so forth.

Additional characteristics
Pain in fibromyalgia is at the muscle-tendon junction. Pain in MPS is in the muscle belly. Fibromyalgia pain is localized at key points described in the diagnostic criteria above; in MPS, palpation of tender trigger points causes pain to be referred to other areas distant from the trigger point. In addition, fibromyalgia patients complain of severe sleep disturbance and widespread pain and stiffness that peaks upon rising in the morning; MPS patients suffer mild to moderate sleep disturbance and experience constant, localized pain that does not vary in intensity with the time of day. Although both disorders occur predominantly in females, males are more likely to suffer myofascial pain than fibromyalgia. The ratio of female to male patients is 10 to 1 in fibromyalgia, but 2 to 1 in myofascial pain.

People diagnosed with MPS note spontaneous pain at rest but, more importantly, they have severe incident pain with movement and upon palpation of small areas of the muscles. These tender zones, called trigger points, are the defining feature of MPS. They are usually associated with fibrous bands in the muscles. Classically, the pain produced by palpation of the trigger point is not limited to the point of local stimulation but radiates predictably to remote regions. For example, palpation of a trigger point located over the scapula may cause pain in the shoulder or neck. Although trauma is a common initiating event, the initiating injury does not have to be severe. Stressful physical and psychological circumstances exacerbate the pain and often are more significant to the history of the pain than is the initial traumatic event.

Test results are invariably normal and are not useful in making the diagnosis except to rule out other diseases that might mimic MPS. For example, a cervical disk herniation could present as an

MPS and resolve with correction or resolution of the disk disease. In the physical examination, the doctor looks for sustained localized muscle contractions within the belly of the muscle upon palpation or pinching of the muscle. Stretching the painful muscle group relieves the pain in most patients, while repeated contractions frequently exacerbate the pain and spasm. Patients may complain of sleep disturbance, but this is not a universal finding.

The cause of MPS is speculative at best. Precipitating causes vary and can include trauma, muscle fatigue from repetitive use, poor posture, local ischemia, and psychological distress. No consistent pathophysiologic findings have been determined. One theory is that the initiating event, for example, trauma, sets up a cycle of pain and debilitation. The debilitation sets up more muscle spasm and pain, which leads to further disability. Muscle biopsies of the tender bands have revealed no consistent abnormalities.

Treatment of myofascial pain syndrome

Low-potency narcotics may be administered immediately after the acute episode, but are almost never used on a long-term basis. If patients get relief and can tolerate the side effects, NSAIDs and tricyclic antidepressants are given. Chronic use of braces should be abandoned if no bona fide indication is present. For many patients, injection of trigger points with saline or local anesthetic is useful in relieving the symptoms. Some patients may even obtain relief from simple insertion of a dry needle into the trigger point. This procedure is thought to provide relief by inducing relaxation of the taut muscle bands and by breaking the pain cycle. TENS, too, is commonly prescribed for these patients.

Maintenance of physical activity seems to be critical to improvement of this condition. Consequently, the physical therapist will play an important role in the patient's management. Without stretch and strengthening exercises, these patients usually get worse. No single therapeutic approach is adequate to manage MPS alone, and a multidisiplinary approach, including psychological evaluation and treatment, is needed. The prognosis for patients with MPS is good, and patients should be able to return to normal life after several months in a rehabilitation program.

Fibromyalgia

MPS is diagnosed more commonly than is fibromyalgia, even though the local complaints may be very similar. The criteria for fibromyalgia are much more stringent than for MPS. Fibromyalgia syndrome is a common pain disorder characterized by generalized muscular aching, stiffness, fatigue, and sleep disturbance.

Fibromyalgia is a long-term problem that is very difficult to manage. Patients have frequent exacerbations of their pain and are resistant to most approaches. Fibromyalgia symptoms are similar to those of rheumatological syndromes: complaint of early morning stiffness and difficulty in getting activated. As the day progresses, the stiffness lessens. The diagnosis hinges on the physical findings, however. Among the criteria for making the diagnosis of fibromyalgia is that the patient demonstrate painful points at 11 of 18 specific regions of the body.

Low potency narcotics may be administered immediately after the onset of fibromyalgia, but they soon lose their effectiveness. If the patient tolerates and gets relief from NSAIDs and tricyclic antidepressants, these medications are frequently used for extended periods. Some patients receive a series of local injections with local anesthetics into the most painful trigger points, but unlike myofascial pain, fibromyalgia pain tends to be less affected by trigger point injections, and in many cases such injections will worsen the symptoms. They are tried because the procedure is relatively risk-free and any pain exacerbation is usually short-lived. Occasionally, the patient will get considerable relief.

There are reports of histologic changes in muscles of patients with fibromyalgia but, as in MPS patients, the changes are not consistent and repeatable. Neuropeptide changes have also been reported, including alterations in serotonin and catecholamine metabolism. Fibromyalgia commonly accompanies both the rheumatic and nonrheumatic autoimmune diseases, and psychological disturbance seems to be a consequence of the syndrome rather than a marker of the disease.

A variety of medications have been used for treatment, including amitriptyline (Elavil), cyclobenzaprine (Flexeril), alprazolam (Xanax), dothiepin (a tricyclic similar to amitriptyline), and s-adenosyl-methionine (SAMe). Some patients have responded to regional sympathetic block, biofeedback, cardiovascular fitness programs, and cognitive behavioral therapy. Local anesthetic injections, TENS, steroids, and many other commonly used analgesic techniques do not seem to be effective. Psychological intervention that employs a cognitive behavioral approach is becoming more popular. A multidisciplinary approach to fibromyalgia combines medical, psychological, social work, physiotherapy, occupational therapy, and nursing interventions to assist patients in developing active, resourceful self-management skills for coping with fibromyalgia.

Cancer pain

One common reason for cancer pain is the development of various neuropathies that arise as a result of tumor invasion of nervous tissue or that develop as a side effect of chemotherapy or radiation therapy. Another common cause of cancer pain is tumor invasion of bones, which causes pain for a number of different reasons. (See *Cancer-related pain conditions*.)

Bone metastasis

Bone metastasis is probably the most common chronic pain condition in cancer patients (see *Several approaches to metastatic bone pain*, page 118). The most troublesome area for bone metastasis is the spinal column. Significant metastasis to these bones results in loss of normal bone integrity, compression fractures of the spinal column, and subsequent nerve root compression, which in turn may cause loss of motor and sensory functions, as well as urinary and fecal incontinance.

Both the fractures themselves and the nerve root compression cause significant pain. The mechanism for the pain caused by the fractures or tumor invasion is related to the periosteum (the layer of connective tissue that covers all bones), which is highly innervated, such that any invasion of that tissue stimulates or activates the pain fibers. Such tumors secrete substances that activate pain fibers. The mass compression from the tumors also generates pain.

A variety of palliative treatments are available to deal with these problems. Patients will sometimes undergo fusion procedures to stabilize the spine, reduce dislocation, and prevent compression of the spinal cord. Various forms of chemotherapy and radiation are used to shrink bony metastases, not so much to cure the patient as to relieve some of the pressure on the spinal cord and nerve roots that has been generated by the growth of the tumor. This can be very effective in relieving the pain. Pain from bony metastases also responds well to NSAIDs, but some patients cannot tolerate the side effects of these drugs. Steroids sometimes can be helpful in shrinking tumors, and most patients respond very well to the pain-relieving effects of the opioid medications.

Neuritis

Neuritis commonly complicates treatment of patients with a variety of cancers. It is difficult to describe in a direct manner because neuritis always accompanies other painful conditions. A common cause of neuritis is radiation therapy.

Cancer-related pain conditions

Class of problem	Description
Bony metastases	
Spine	Metastases or local invasion of the spine will induce localized pain secondary to nerve and bone destruction. Patient may have extensive spread of disease but only localized symptoms.
Long bones	Disease of the long bone will have characteristics similar to other bony invasion sites, but the extent of invasion usually is consistent with the area of painful complaints.
Skull	Skull metastases are mostly painful when the lesions are located near the base of the skull. Extensive lesions above the base may not induce significant symptoms.
Neural invasion	
peripheral nerve, plexus, spinal cord	Invasion of nervous tissue at any of these sites can result in pain limited to the area of tissue innervated by the nerve. Neurologic deficits usually accompany the painful symptoms, such as weakness and loss of reflexes. If deficits are not present and there is evidence of neural impingement, patient must be monitored for first signs of defects so that appropriate steps can be taken to prevent further morbidity.
Visceral invasion	
Obstruction	Obstruction of a hollow viscus will cause a cramping, colicky pain along with loss of normal functioning of the affected organ. Surgery may be required to remove the obstruction, as this is a life-threatening condition.
Organ invasion	Tumor growth within a solid viscus causes pain usually when the capsule of the affected viscus is stretched. Organ capsules contain the pain-signaling fibers.
Treatment side effects	
Postsurgery-related	Painful conditions are common sequelae of surgical palliative procedures for cancer. Nerves sometimes must be resected in order to remove diseased tissues. Scar formation is another common source of pain.
Chemotherapy-related: peripheral neuropathy, aseptic necrosis, mucositis	In addition to destroying cancer cells, chemotherapy affects normal tissue. Damaged tissues, including nerves, bone, and mucous membranes, may respond with pain and malfunction.
Postradiation therapy-related: neuritis, myelopathy, tissue fibrosis	Like chemotherapy, radiation is not selective to cancer cells. Nerves within the field of radiation are particularly vulnerable to radiation effects and are liable to induce chronic pain because neural tissues lack the resilience of other tissues.

PATIENT HISTORY

Several approaches to metastatic bone pain

Ms. Ward, a 47-year-old businesswoman and mother of five children, has been a very difficult patient to manage. Essentially, she has bony metastasis to almost every bone in her body. The most troublesome area is the spinal column where most of the bony substance has been eaten away, resulting in multiple compression fractures. In addition to the pain of the compression fractures, her unstable spinal column has resulted in painful nerve root compression at multiple levels.

In an effort to shrink the tumors and relieve pressure on her spine, she received her full compliment of radiation therapy and no longer can receive additional doses. An initial trial of NSAIDs was discontinued because the drugs caused ringing in her ears and temporary loss of hearing. Those symptoms resolved after discontinuation of those medications.

What is left for relieving this patient's pain is opioid medications. Initial intraspinal infusions of morphine provided very effective relief, but because of other problems, that mode of therapy was discontinued. She is now receiving a systemic infusion of morphine, which reduces her pain; but she suffers the usual side effects of opioids, including significant sedation, confusion, hallucinations, nausea and vomiting, and constipation.

As an example, patients with rectal cancer frequently require radiation therapy to the rectum to control or cure their disease. In many circumstances a cure is achieved, but the patient must contend with ongoing pain as a consequence of the radiation therapy. These patients complain of severe burning, itching, and muscle cramping in the rectum. The pain usually does not begin until 2 to 3 months after radiation therapy is complete. Mechanical manipulation commonly exacerbates the pain. For the rectal cancer patient, this means that defecation will result in severe pain not only during the bowel movement, but often for several hours afterward. Such a patient will attempt to avoid bowel movements and, as a consequence, constipation frequently develops. The constipation will make the pain much worse when the patient can no longer delay defecation or, worse than that, the bowel can become impacted.

Pathophysiology of neuritis

The mechanism for generation of neuritis pain is not different from the neuropathic pain conditions described earlier in this chapter. The peripheral nerves that serve the radiated region are damaged. As they repair themselves, neuroma form, and the damaged nerves depolarize, both spontaneously and in response to biochemical and mechanical influences. The signals are perceived as painful, even if normal physiologic activity is taking place. Neuritis will also result in abnormal functioning of the viscus. In the case of rectal cancer, the dam-

spread after initial response to radiation therapy and, unfortunately, the amount of radiation that can be administered is limited. For many patients palliative procedures to reduce tumor size will do more harm than good, and symptom control becomes the main therapy.

Treatment of cancer pain

The opioid medications are the mainstay therapy for control of cancer pain. Most cancer patients do not require very high doses of morphine or other opioid-containing products to control their pain. Many patients do, however, become tolerant to a pain medication and may then require very high doses to control their symptoms. Escalating the opioid dosing will overcome the tolerance to the medication and the patient will get pain relief. A significant number of patients will have such severe pain or opioid-resistant pain combined with their tolerance to the medications that they do not get significant relief, and when this occurs, more aggressive therapy will be required. For example, opioids administered directly onto the spinal cord can provide good analgesia. Analgesic potency is directly related to the concentration of opioid at spinal cord receptor sites; therefore, greater analgesia results if the opioid is introduced directly into the spinal canal. Intraspinal opioids also have the advantage of providing localized analgesia as well as analgesia mediated by the central nervous system. Opioids given systemically must be given in very high doses in order to provide high concentrations of the drug at the spinal level. Such high doses invariably cause side effects, such as constipation, nausea, itching, sedation, and so forth. Intraspinal administration of opioids can result in better pain control with fewer side effects.

In addition to the opioids, local anesthetics can be used to block nerves and provide pain relief, because much of the pain from metastatic cancer is nociceptive in nature. Often, these patients will have a combination of nociceptive pain and neuropathic pain. As mentioned earlier, neuropathic pain generally does not respond well to opioids, and alternative approaches will be required. Drugs such as carbamazepine, tricyclic antidepressants, and neuroleptic medications are commonly used to combat this problem and can be quite effective.

Mucositis

Mucositis, another painful complication related to chemotherapy and radiation therapy, occurs as a consequence of sloughing of the oral mucosa along with inflammation and irritation of peripheral nerve endings. The mucosal lesions are usually accompanied by superinfection with bacteria, and often these patients develop viral eruptions such as herpes simplex.

Bone marrow transplant

Mucositis is a common problem for patients undergoing bone marrow transplant. The onset of the mucositis generally occurs 1 to 2 weeks after the bone marrow transplant and peaks in intensity around the 20th to 25th day. This patient population is particularly difficult to manage because of limitations in the kinds of drugs that can be employed. NSAIDs cannot be used because the patient's below-normal platelet count already carries an increased risk for bleeding. Any NSAID-related gastrointestinal irritation could induce severe bleeding and death. The intensity and acuteness of the mucositis pain makes it unlikely to respond to drugs like tricyclic antidepressants and carbamazepine; therefore, the opioid-containing medications are the only options left. Commonly, these patients are managed with patient-controlled analgesia (PCA) (see Chapter 2, Pharmacology of Pain Management). Often these patients report that the medication is not very effective in relieving their pain, but it does induce sedation and calming, which helps patients to cope better with the condition.

Because bone-marrow transplant patients have ongoing mucositis pain for several weeks and sometimes months, tolerance to opioids does develop, so higher doses are required to provide analgesia, even though the severity of mucosal injury seems to be at a steady state. Some pain caused by the mucositis may also be resistant to opioid analgesia. Other approaches to managing the problem include topical agents such as local anesthetic preparations and phenol, which provide temporary numbing of the peripheral nerve endings. This approach is complicated by the fact that these patients suffer nausea and vomiting. Any increased secretions worsens the patient's ongoing nausea and induces vomiting. The acid vomitus causes further sloughing and desolation of the mucosal membranes in the esophagus, throat, and mouth.

Pain from the oral mucosa is only part of the story. All of these patients experience a major depression of mental and body functions, which is described by many patients as being as near death as possible without actually dying. The severe malaise and extremely low energy level make mundane activities such as going to the bathroom tremendously difficult. Unrelieved pain only serves to compound this experience of general illness. Because of the swollen mucosal membranes, severe nausea, vomiting, and pain, these patients are unable to consume any oral fluids or food during some period of their bone marrow transplant. Most patients are fed intravenously, and continued mucositis near the later part of their treatment becomes the limiting factor in hospital discharge and full recovery. Once the mucositis comes under control and the patient is able to eat and swallow fluids, then peripheral alimentation can be discontinued and the patient is more likely to be discharged. Therefore, control of the patient's mucositis pain becomes more important than just the provision of symptom relief. Indeed, relief of mucositis symptoms may allow patients to leave intensive care sooner than expected.

Conclusion

At this time, a limited armamentarium exists for dealing with complex, chronic pain problems. No single or multidimensional approach is a panacea, and too frequently drugs are ineffective or induce nasty side effects, including the risk of death. The charge given to the physician is to provide care without doing harm. Only constant struggle keeps the benefit/risk ratio above one. Stomach irritation and bleeding, nausea, vomiting, constipation, sedation, hallucinations, and drug dependence are just a few of the common obstacles to pain relief through drug administration. Despite a difficult battle, the medical profession is learning to use drugs more wisely, and combining various therapies is the rule rather than exception. Certainly, to do nothing is not an option, because making that choice guarantees morbidity for the patient. New drug classes are in the pipeline, and more selectively acting medications may lessen side effects and increase analgesic efficacy. Continued research in pain control is a must, at the bench and in the clinic. Greater interest and funding are necessary to support these efforts.

REFERENCES

Bonica, J. J. *The Management of Pain*, 2nd ed. Baltimore: Williams & Wilkins, 1990.

Cailliet, R. *Low Back Pain Syndrome*, 5th ed. Philadelphia: F.A. Davis, 1995.

Cady, R.D., and Fox, A.W. *Treating the Headache Patient*. New York: M. Dekker, 1995.

Davar, G., and Maciewicz, R. J. "Deafferentation Pain Syndromes," *Neurologic Clinics*, 7(2): 289-304, 1989.

Foley, K.M. "Pain Syndromes in Patients with Cancer," *Medical Clinics of North America*, 71(2): 169-84, 1987.

Rachlin, E.S. *Myofascial Pain and Fibromyalgia: Trigger Point Management*. St. Louis: Mosby-Year Book, 1994.

Wall, P., and Melzack, R.:*Textbook of Pain*, 3rd ed. New York: Churchill Livingstone, 1994.

CHAPTER 5

Psychological aspects of pain

Dennis C. Turk, PhD

Pain has existed since time immemorial. Perhaps the first recorded mention of pain is found in the Ebers papyrus, a 4th century B.C. document that notes the use of opium as a headache treatment. Since that time pain has been the focus of philosophical speculation and scientific attention.

The phenomenon of pain is present from birth. From the earliest awareness, everyone is familiar with the acute pain of a cut, a sunburn, or a bruised knee. Acute pain associated with superficial injuries is self-limiting and will disappear on its own or with over-the-counter analgesic medication and rest in a reasonably short period of time, usually hours, days, or a few weeks.

Three categories of pain

In acute pain, nociception has a definite purpose. It acts as a warning signal that directs immediate attention to the situation, it promotes reflexive withdrawal, and it fosters other actions that prevent further damage and enhance healing. For example, if a person places a hand on a hot stove, he or she quickly removes it to avoid being burned. Acute pain also signals that an injury or disease is present, as in the case of a broken leg or appendicitis. In these instances, acute pain serves an important protective function, announcing that it is time to take steps to prevent additional problems and, if necessary, seek medical attention.

There is another type of pain that does not fit nicely into the classification of acute pain. A number of pain diagnoses, for example, migraine headaches or temporomandibular disorders, although of relatively brief duration, tend to recur with or without an identifiable provocation. For example, migraine headaches, a particularly severe form of headache, may last for several hours and then remit even without any medical treatment. The migraine sufferer may be headache-free for days or weeks only to have another migraine episode and, after the headache runs its course, another headache-free period until recurrence of yet another episode.

Other recurrent pain syndromes do have an identifiable cause; for example, an episode of acute pain in sickle cell disease that's associated with vasooclusive crisis. Migraine headaches, sickle cell disease, and other painful conditions with similar episodic characteristics may be viewed as recurrent acute pain. In these disorders, pain-free periods are punctuated by pain episodes. In the case of some conditions such as migraine headache, recurrent acute pain seems to serve no useful purpose because there is no protective action that can be taken, nor is there necessarily any tissue damage that can be prevented. In the case of sickle cell disease, the acute pain episodes may serve a useful function by encouraging the sufferer to seek medical treatment. One hallmark of both types of recurrent acute pain is their episodic nature.

Chronic pain, unlike acute pain and acute recurrent pain, persists and can last for months or even years beyond any expected period of healing. The average duration of pain noted for patients treated at clinics specializing in the treatment of pain exceeds 7 years, with durations of 20 to 30 years quite common. In chronic pain, for example, trigeminal neuralgia or low back pain, the adaptive function of pain plays a significantly smaller role, and often no obvious useful function can be determined. Pain that is chronic or recurrent can significantly compromise quality of life and, if unremitting, may actually produce physical harm by suppressing the body's immune system.

All three categories of pain, acute, recurrent acute, and chronic, are prevalent. Consider a sample of some available statistics:

- After upper respiratory infections, pain is the second most common reason people visit physicians, accounting for over 70 million office visits each year (National Center for Health Statistics, Koch 1986).
- Over 23 million surgical procedures were performed in the United States in 1989 and most of them involved acute pain (Peebles and Schneidman 1991).
- Acute recurrent and chronic pain affect over 70 million Americans with over 10% reporting the presence of pain over 100 days per year (Osterweis, et al. 1987).
- Over 11 million Americans suffer from recurring episodes of migraine headaches, over 30 million experience chronic or recurrent

back pain, and 37 million have pain associated with arthritis (Stewart, et al. 1991; Holbrook, et al. 1984; Lawrence, et al. 1989).
• Approximately 3.5 million people in the United States have cancer. Bonica estimated that moderate to severe pain is reported by 40% to 45% of patients initially following the diagnosis, by 35% to 45% at the intermediate states of the disease, and by 60% to 85% in advanced stages of cancer (Raj 1990; Bonica 1979).

Furthermore, pain is an extremely costly problem for society in terms of health care expenditures, disability costs, and lost productivity. It has been estimated that chronic pain alone costs the American people approximately $65 billion a year. With such astronomical figures, it is all too easy to lose sight of the incalculable suffering accompanying pain for both the individual and his or her family.

Given the lengthy history of pain and the statistics on its prevalence, it might be assumed that pain is well understood and successfully treated. Despite advances in the understanding of anatomy and physiologic processes, and despite new and sophisticated pharmacologic, medical, and surgical treatments, pain continues to be a perplexing puzzle for health care providers and a source of significant distress for individuals. No treatments currently available consistently and permanently relieve pain in all individuals.

Characteristics of patients with persistent pain

Patients with chronic pain unrelated to a known disease and those with recurrent acute pain often feel rejected by the very elements of society they need for support. They may become frustrated with and lose faith in a medical system that initially promises a cure and then becomes indifferent when treatments prove ineffective. While the likelihood of returning to work and earning a full income becomes more elusive, medical bills for unsuccessful treatments mount up. In time, people with chronic pain may begin to feel they are being blamed by their physicians, employers, and even family members when their pain condition does not respond to treatment. Third-party payers may even suggest that the individual is faking pain in order to receive financial gain.

Thus, the emotional distress that is commonly observed in chronic pain patients may be attributed to a variety of factors, including fear, inadequate or maladaptive support systems and other coping resources, treatment-induced (iatrogenic) complications, overuse of potent drugs, inability to work, financial difficulties, prolonged litigation, disruption of usual activities, and sleep disturbance. Moreover, the experience of "medical limbo," (the presence of an undiagnosed, possibly life-threatening, painful condition that is also labeled psychogenic or malingering) is itself a source of stress and can initiate psychological distress or aggravate a premorbid psychiatric condition. In the case of cancer, the stress of pain is superimposed on the general fear of living with and possibly dying from a potentially fatal disease.

Although acute pain patients often receive relief from primary health care providers, people with persistent pain complaints, especially those whose pain seems unrelated to a known disease, become enmeshed in the medical community as they go from doctor to doctor, laboratory test to laboratory test, and imaging procedure to imaging procedure in a continuing search for diagnosis and treatment. For many patients pain becomes the central focus of their lives. In an elusive quest for relief they withdraw from society, lose their jobs, and alienate family and friends. Thus, it is hardly surprising that many pain patients feel anxious, demoralized, helpless, hopeless, frustrated, angry, depressed, and isolated.

Uncertainty in pain diagnosis

How can a problem as prevalent, costly, and devastating as pain be so poorly understood and managed? A significant factor contributing to the current situation is diagnostic uncertainty. The diagnosis of pain is not an exact science. Pain is a subjective, or internal, state and, although everyone knows what pain is, there is no pain thermometer that can accurately measure the amount of pain an individual feels.

It can only be inferred from indications, such as the amount of tissue damaged, verbal complaints, and nonverbal behaviors (such as limping or guarded movements). Even with tissue damage, it is impossible to specify how much pain is being experienced. For example, should a cut that is 1/2″ long and 1/4″ deep hurt twice as much as a cut that is 1/4″ long and 1/8″ deep?

Nociception is a sensory process. In contrast, the experience of pain is a perceptual process that requires attention and interpretation of the nociceptive input. Thus, nociception and pain are not synonymous. This chapter reviews the most common theoretical models of pain, examines the role of psychological contributors in the etiology and exacerbation of pain, and describes integrative models that attempt to combine the physiologic and psychological variables of pain perception. The final sections describe the range of psychological-assessment methods and therapeutic interventions that have been used with recurrent acute and chronic pain patients. Although discussed in the context of chronic pain and recurrent acute pain, many of these methods have also been successful with acute pain.

Conceptualizations of pain

The concept of pain has undergone multiple transformations throughout history. However, only in the past quarter-century has there been a significant shift in thinking based on the gate control theory developed by Ronald Melzack, a psychologist, and Patrick Wall, a physician and anatomist (Melzack and Wall 1965). This theory will be examined later. First, let us examine the traditional sensory model that has dominated thought since it was first proposed by Descartes in the 15th century.

Unidimensional sensory model

Historically, pain has been viewed from the perspective of Cartesian mind-body dualism as a sensory experience dependent on the degree of noxious sensory stimuli impinging on the individual. This sensory model posits two ends of a pain pathway similar to two ends of a telephone transmission line. According to this view, intense stimuli represent a pull on one end of a string that activates a pain-signaling bell located somewhere in the brain.

Sensory models of pain postulate that pain is a specific sensation uniquely different from other sensations. The production of pain is traced to specific peripheral pain receptors that respond exclusively to nociceptive stimuli. It is assumed that tissue damage will biochemically excite these pain receptors at the injury site, initiating pain-specific nerve impulses that are transmitted along specific afferent pain pathways to specific pain centers in the brain.

Sensory models propose that the amount of pain experienced is a direct result of the amount, degree, or nature of sensory input or physical damage. Pain is explained in terms of specific physiologic mechanisms. Clinically, it is expected that the report of pain will be directly proportional to the amount of pathology. Based on this model, assessment should focus on identifying the cause of the pain, and treatment should involve removal of the cause or cutting or blocking the specific pain pathways by surgical or pharmacologic means.

The sensory model has continued to be endorsed by many due to its logic and simplicity, even though it fails to account for a number of observations, such as these:

- Patients with objectively determined, equivalent degrees and types of tissues pathology vary widely in their reports of pain severity.
- Surgical procedures that cut the neurologic pathways believed to transmit the pain signals may fail to alleviate it.
- Patients with equivalent degrees of tissue pathology treated with identical pain alleviation methods respond differently.

Unfortunately for those with chronic pain, the underlying causes of many painful conditions remain largely unknown despite the use of sophisticated diagnostic imaging procedures, such as the CT scan and MRI. For some conditions such as recurrent headaches, diagnostic procedures do not reveal any pathology that is sufficient to account for the pain reported. This does not mean that no cause exists but that currently available diagnostic methods are unable to detect it.

Even when diagnostic procedures identify physical abnormalities, the degree of pathology is not necessarily proportional to the amount of pain experienced. For example, for some patients with chronic back pain, CT scans reveal arthritic degeneration of vertebrae and bulging disks; however, many other individuals who show similar degeneration do not report persistent back pain. In such cases it is unclear why two individuals with the same abnormal test results respond so differently. Obviously, something other than physical pathology alone is influencing patients' reports.

Psychogenic perspectives

As is frequently the case in medicine, if the pain reported by patients is believed to be disproportionate to observed physical pathology or if pain is recalcitrant to appropriate treatment, then it is assumed that psychological factors must be involved, even if not causal.

It is important to recognize that there is no objective way to determine how much pain is proportionate. How much should a given amount of tissue pathology hurt? Similarly, determination of appropriate treatment is not totally objective. Different health care providers might recommend widely different treatments for patients with the same presenting symptoms. For example, treatments for patients with TMJ disorders have been as diverse as surgery and psychotherapy.

A number of psychogenic models have been proposed. For example, a model of a pain-prone personality that predisposes individuals to experience persistent pain was originally described by George Engel and later extended by Dietrich Blumer and Mary Heilbronn as pain-prone disorder, a variant of depression (Engel 1959; Blumer and Heilbronn 1982). Among the many features of pain-prone disorder, the investigators noted denial of emotional and interpersonal problems, inability to deal with anger and hostility, craving for affection and dependency, and a family history of depression, alcoholism, and chronic pain. Engel proposed that once the psychic organization necessary for pain has evolved, the experience of pain no longer requires peripheral stimulation.

Lawrence Beutler and his colleagues proposed a model similar to that of Blumer and Heilbronn (Beutler et al. 1986). The authors suggest that difficulty in expressing anger and controlling intense emotions in general are the predisposing factors linking chronic pain and the experience of negative effect. They view chronic pain and depression as similar disturbances, both characterized by the failure to process intense emotion, for example, prolonged blocking or inhibition of intense interpersonal anger.

Little additional research has been reported that supports the causal role of effect inhibition in chronic pain states. Dennis Turk and Peter Salovey critically examine both the hypothesis of a pain-prone disorder and the empirical support for it. These commentators find the hypothesized pain-prone disorder to be flawed conceptually, circular in reasoning, with the definition itself tautological and the explanatory model lacking in parsimony. In addition, they claim the purported empirical support for the pain-prone disorder is invalid (Turk and Salovey 1984).

Recently, the American Psychiatric Association has created two diagnoses associated with pain, as noted in the fourth edition of the *Diagnostic and Statistical Manual of Mental Disorders* (American Psychiatric Association 1994):

- Pain Disorder Associated with Psychological Factors
- Pain Disorder Associated with Both Psychological Factors and a General Medical Condition.

The second diagnosis recognizes that both psychological factors and a general medical condition have important roles in the onset, severity, exacerbation, and continuation of pain. These two diagnoses are so broadly defined, however, that virtually all patients with persistent pain could be diagnosed as suffering from a psychiatric disorder.

Sensory models present pain as entirely somatogenic (caused by physical factors); psychogenic models posit psychic disorder or psychic disease as the primary cause of chronic pain. The dichotomy between these two views forms the basis for attempts to classify pain as "functional" (psychogenic) or "organic" (somatogenic) as well as for references to pain having a "functional overlay." When psychogenic models are posed as alternatives to purely somatogenic models, dichotomous reasoning prevails. Any pain report not confirmed by observed pathology becomes, ipso facto, pain with a psychological component.

Motivational view

A variation on the dichotomous somatic-psychogenic approach is the suggestion by many insurance companies and other third-party payers that pain unsubstantiated by observed physical pathology is an expression of symptom exaggeration or outright malingering. The assumption here is that patients are motivated primarily by financial gain.

This belief has resulted in attempts to catch malingers using surreptitious observation and sophisticated biomechanical machines geared toward identifying inconsistencies in functional performance. However, the validity of inconsistent findings obtained on mechanical apparatus has been seriously challenged. Moreover, no studies have demonstrated dramatic improvement in pain reports subsequent to receiving disability awards.

Although there appears to be little question that psychological factors play an important role in pain perception and response, the above models portray physical and psychological factors as being mutually exclusive. Before examining models that attempt to integrate psychological factors with somatic factors, it will be useful to understand the nature of the psychological factors involved.

Psychological contributors to pain

Psychologists have made important contributions to understanding pain by demonstrating the importance of psychosocial and behavioral factors in the etiology, severity, exacerbation, and maintenance of pain. Several effective treatments have been developed based on these factors.

Operant learning mechanisms

By the early 20th century, the effects of environmental factors in shaping the experience of pain had been acknowledged. A new era in thinking about pain began in 1976 with psychologist Wilbert Fordyce's extension of operant conditioning to chronic pain (Fordyce 1976).

In the the operant conditioning model, behavioral manifestations of acute pain, such as withdrawal, avoidance of activity believed to exacerbate pain, and attempts to escape from noxious sensations, are thought to be subject to the principles of operant conditioning, namely, positive reinforcement (repetition of specific behavior that elicits positive consequences or a reward of some type), negative reinforcement (cessation of specific behavior in order to obtain a positive consequence or reward), and avoidance learning (efforts on the part of an individual to avoid some negative consequence or loss of reward).

The operant view proposes that acute pain behaviors, such as avoidance of activity to prevent painful sensations, may be controlled by external contingencies of reinforcement (consequences that either promote or discourage repetition of a particular behavior). Pain behaviors may be positively reinforced, for example, by receiving attention from others as a positive consequence of limping or grimacing, or negatively reinforced, for example, the reduction of pain as a positive consequence of inactivity. Pain behaviors may also be maintained by the escape from noxious stimulation through the use of drugs or rest (negative reinforcement) or the avoidance of undesirable activities such as work (avoidance learning). In addition, "well behaviors," such as activity and working, may not be positively reinforced, so the more rewarding pain behaviors may, therefore, be maintained. (See *Operant conditioning model of pain*.)

For example, when back pain flares up, a woman may lie down on the floor and hold her back. Her husband may unknowingly positively reinforce his wife's pain behaviors by spending extra time with her, rubbing her back, or bringing her something to eat. Another powerful way he may reinforce her pain behaviors is by permitting her to avoid undesirable activities, such as suggesting they cancel the evening plans with his brother, an activity that the sufferer might have wished to avoid anyway. This is not to suggest that the pain sufferer consciously communicates pain to elicit attention or avoid undesirable activities. Rather, reinforcement of pain behaviors is more likely the result of a gradual process that neither person recognizes.

The pain behavior originally elicited by injury or disease may come to occur, totally or in part, in response to reinforcing environmental events and may persist long after the initial cause of the pain is resolved or greatly reduced.

It is important to avoid mistaking pain behaviors for malingering. Malingering patients consciously fake symptoms such as pain for some gain, usually financial. In the operant conditioning model there is no suggestion of conscious deception, only the unintended performance of pain behaviors resulting from environmental reinforcement. Patients are not aware that the behaviors are being displayed and are not consciously motivated to obtain positive reinforcement from the behaviors. The operant conditioning model concerns itself less with the initial cause of pain (the nociceptive event) than with patients' behavioral responses. It considers pain an internal, subjective experience secondary to the experience of nociception. This internal experience cannot be directly assessed and may be maintained even after the initial physical basis of the pain has been resolved.

The operant view has generated effective treatment for select samples of chronic pain patients. Treatment focuses on the elimination of pain behaviors by withdrawal of attention from others and an increase in well behaviors through positive reinforcement. Treatment based on operant conditioning will be discussed later in this chapter.

Flaws in the operant view

Although operant factors undoubtedly play a role in the maintenance of disability, exclusive reliance on the operant conditioning model has

Operant conditioning model of pain

The operant conditioning model of pain posits that pain behaviors are perpetuated by reward. Reward can be either positive reinforcement of a pain behavior (receiving extra attention from a loved one as a response to grimacing) or negative reinforcement of a pain behavior (escape from an unpleasant chore as a positive consequence of lying down).

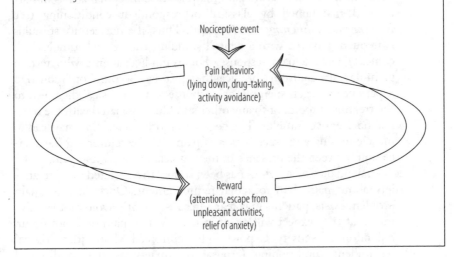

Nociceptive event

Pain behaviors
(lying down, drug-taking,
activity avoidance)

Reward
(attention, escape from
unpleasant activities,
relief of anxiety)

been criticized for its narrow focus on motor pain behaviors, failure to consider the emotional and cognitive aspects of pain, and failure to treat the subjective experience of pain. This model presents problems for pain associated with cancer because stoic behaviors in these patients are not helpful in promoting recovery. For possibly fatal diseases, behaviors such as talking about pain and requesting medication are encouraged, and they are even essential to inform health care providers about disease progression.

Another fundamental problem with the operant approach is the emphasis on overt behaviors and the use of them as the sole basis for understanding pain, distress, and suffering. However, there is no way of determining whether a particular behavior results from pain, from a structural abnormality, or from a coping response. Limping, for example, is viewed from the operant perspective as a pain behavior. Limping could, however, result from an anatomical alteration in the hip joint and have no direct association whatsoever with pain, distress, or suffering. Consequently, attempts to extinguish the putative pain behavior by ignoring it will be fruitless and inappropriate. Similarly, lying down during the day, also labeled a pain behavior, may be a relaxation practice recommended by a mental health pro-

fessional or a regular rest period associated with activity pacing recommended by an occupational therapist. In such situations, lying
down during the day would not be a pain behavior at all, but adherence to care recommendations.

Respondent learning mechanisms

Chronic or recurrent acute pain may also be conceptualized as initiated and maintained by classical or respondent conditioning (see
Respondent conditioning model of pain). Thus, if a nociceptive stimulus
is frequently paired with a neutral stimulus, the neutral stimulus will
come to elicit a pain response. For example, patients who receive
painful treatment from a physical therapist may become conditioned to
experience a negative emotional response to the physical therapist, to
the treatment room, or to any other stimulus associated with the original nociceptive stimulus. The negative emotional reaction may lead to
muscle tensing and exacerbation of pain, thereby reinforcing the association between the presence of the physical therapist and pain.

Avoidance of activities has been shown to be related more to anxiety about pain than to actual reinforcement. Once an acute pain
problem exists, patients may fear and subsequently avoid motor activities that they expect will result in pain. When pain does not occur,
reduction of activity is powerfully reinforced. Thus, the original
respondent conditioning (arousal of anxiety as the conditioned
response to the conditioned stimulus of activity) may be followed by
an operant learning process (activity avoidance that is reinforced by
reduction of activity-associated anxiety). Over time, however, anticipatory anxiety related to activity may develop and act as a conditioned stimulus for sympathetic activation that may be maintained
after the original, unconditioned stimulus (the injury) and unconditioned response (pain and sympathetic activation) have subsided.

Eventually, more and more triggers, such as people, physical
locations, leisure, work, sexual activity, may be seen as eliciting or
exacerbating pain and will be avoided. This is known as stimulus generalization. In addition to avoidance learning mechanisms, patients
may experience exacerbation and maintenance of pain in certain situations due to anxiety-related sympathetic activation and muscle tension. Thus, psychological factors may directly affect nociceptive stimulation and need not be viewed as only reactions to pain. This point
will be revisited later.

Corrective feedback

Continued avoidance of specific activities reduces the opportunity for
corrective feedback, the experience that an activity does not produce
an anticipated level of pain. The prediction of pain promotes pain-

Respondent conditioning model of pain

The respondent conditioning model presents acute pain as an unconditioned stimulus. Any stimulus that the patient associates with the pain (a conditioned stimulus) may elicit the conditioned response and subsequent anticipation of pain.

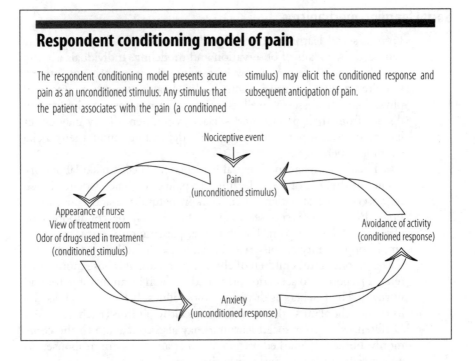

avoidance behavior and overpredictions of pain promote excessive avoidance behavior. By contrast, repeatedly engaging in behavior that results in less pain than predicted encourages more accurate subsequent predictions which, in turn, promote reduction of avoidance behavior.

From a respondent conditioning perspective, through stimulus generalization, patients may have learned to associate increases in pain with all kinds of stimuli. Sitting, walking, engaging in cognitively demanding work or social interaction, sexual activity, or even thoughts about these activities may increase anticipatory anxiety and concomitant physiologic and biochemical changes. Subsequently, patients may display maladaptive responses to many activities other than those that initially induced pain. Physical abnormalities associated with chronic pain, such as distorted gait, decreased range of motion, and muscular fatigue, may actually be secondary to maladaptive behavior changes initiated through learning. As pain becomes associated with more and more situations and activities, they will be avoided, resulting in greater physical deconditioning, isolation, physical and emotional disability, and ultimately more pain. Pain will increase due to greater nociception associated with decreased muscle strength, flexibility, and endurance and by the patient's preoccupation with symptoms and personal plight.

Social learning mechanisms

From a social learning perspective the acquisition of pain behaviors can occur by means of observation and modeling. Individuals acquire new behavioral responses by observing the responses of others. Children acquire attitudes about health, health care, symptoms, and physiologic processes as well as appropriate responses to injury and disease from their parents and social environment. They may either ignore or overrespond to symptoms, depending upon their social learning experiences.

There is ample experimental evidence from controlled laboratory studies of the role of social learning in pain and some evidence based on observations of patients' behaviors in naturalistic and clinical settings. Physiologic responses to pain stimuli may be conditioned by observing others in pain. For example, patients on a burn unit have ample opportunity to observe the responses of other patients with burns. In one study, children of chronic pain patients chose more pain-related responses to scenarios presented to them by an investigator and were rated by teachers as displaying more illness behaviors such as visits to the school nurse than children of healthy controls (Richard 1988). Differences in prior social learning may also contribute to the commonly observed, marked variability in pain behavior responses to objectively similar degrees of physical pathology.

Role of cognitive factors

A great deal of research has consistently demonstrated that patients' attitudes, beliefs, and expectations of themselves, their coping resources, and the health care system affect the entire spectrum of pain behavior.

Beliefs about pain

Patients may differ greatly in their beliefs about pain. Behavior and emotions are influenced by interpretation of events, not simply by the facts of those events. Patients who believe their pain results from ongoing tissue damage or a progressive disease are likely to experience more suffering and behavioral dysfunction than those who view their pain as resulting from a stable, manageable problem. A person who awakes with a headache believing that the pain is due to excessive alcohol consumption responds very differently from someone who believes that the pain signals a brain tumor.

Certain beliefs may lead to maladaptive coping, increased suffering, and greater disability. People's beliefs, appraisals, and expectations regarding the consequences of an event and their ability to affect the outcome are understood to impact functioning in two ways: through a direct influence on mood and on coping efforts.

For example, low back pain patients have demonstrated poor behavioral persistence in various exercise tasks and that their performance of these tasks was independent of physical exertion or actual self-reports of pain. Instead, performance was related to previous pain reports (Schmidt 1985). The patients' negative view of their abilities and expectation of increased pain upon exercise form a rationale for avoiding exercise. The expectation of exercise-related pain reinforces patients' beliefs regarding the pervasiveness of their disability. Patients who believe that disability is a necessary reaction to pain and that activity is dangerous are likely to experience a vicious circle of disability, with the failure to perform activities reinforcing the perception of helplessness and incapacity.

The presence of pain may change the way individuals process pain-related and other information, for example by focusing attention on all types of bodily signals. David Spiegel and Joan Bloom reported that the pain severity ratings of cancer patients could be predicted by their affective state and by their interpretations of pain. Patients who attributed their pain to a worsening of the underlying disease experienced more pain than patients with more benign interpretations, despite comparable levels of disease progression (Spiegel and Bloom 1983).

Once cognitive schemata (beliefs and expectations about a disease) are formed, they are difficult to modify. Patients tend to avoid experiences that could invalidate their beliefs and they guide their behavior in accordance with these beliefs. Consequently, as noted in the discussion of respondent conditioning, they do not receive corrective feedback.

Beliefs about pain are also important elements in disability, response to treatment, and adherence to self-management activities. Successful rehabilitation appears to be accompanied by an important cognitive shift from beliefs about helplessness and passivity to belief in the ability to function regardless of pain. Clearly, patients with chronic and recurrent acute pain must learn to de-emphasize the role of experienced pain in their regulation of functioning. In fact, results from numerous treatment outcome studies have shown that changes in pain level do not parallel changes in activity level, medication use, return to work, ability to cope with pain, or pursuit of further treatment.

Self-efficacy

Closely related to the sense of control over aversive stimulation is self-efficacy expectation, the personal conviction that one can successfully execute a course of action to produce a desired outcome. This variable has been demonstrated as a major mediator of therapeutic change. Self-efficacy judgments are based on four sources of information, listed in descending order of impact:

- one's own past performance of the task or of similar tasks
- the performance of those who are perceived to be similar to one-self
- verbal persuasion by others that one is capable
- the experience of physiologic arousal, which is, in turn, partly determined by prior efficacy estimation.

Performance mastery experience can be encouraged through subtasks that are increasingly difficult or close to the desired behavioral repertoire. From this perspective, coping behaviors, the basis of self-efficacy, are seen as arising from individuals' belief that the situational demands do not exceed coping resources. For example, James Council and his colleagues asked patients to rate their self-efficacy as well as their expectation of pain in relation to the performance of movement tasks. Patients' performance levels correlated highly with their self-efficacy expectations, which appeared to be determined by their expectation of pain levels (Council et al. 1988).

Coping strategies

Self-regulation of pain and its impact depends on an individual's specific ways of dealing with pain and its accompanying distress. This set of responses composes a person's coping repertoire. Coping consists of spontaneously employed, purposeful acts and is assessed in terms of overt and covert behaviors. Overt coping strategies include rest, medication, and use of relaxation. Covert coping strategies include distraction, reassuring oneself that the pain will diminish, seeking information, and problem solving. Coping strategies may alter the perception of pain intensity and promote the ability to manage or tolerate pain and to continue everyday activities.

Studies have found active coping strategies (efforts to function in spite of pain or to distract oneself from pain) to be associated with adaptive functioning, and passive coping strategies (depending on others for help in pain control and restricting one's activities) to be related to greater pain and depression. However, beyond this, there is no evidence supporting the greater effectiveness of one active coping strategy compared to any other (Fernandez and Turk 1989). A particular strategy may be adaptive in one situation and not so in a different situation, maladaptive or effective for some individuals at some times, but not necessarily for all individuals all of the time.

A number of studies have demonstrated that patients instructed in the use of adaptive coping strategies experience a decrease in pain intensity and an increase in pain tolerance. The most important factor in poor coping appears to be catastrophizing (extremely negative thoughts about one's plight) rather than differences in the nature of specific adaptive coping strategies.

Direct effects of psychological factors on pain

Psychological factors may act directly on pain and disability by reducing physical activity and consequently reducing muscle flexibility, strength, tone, and endurance. Fear of re-injury, fear of loss of disability compensation, and job dissatisfaction can also influence return to work.

People in pain may develop avoidant coping strategies that in the short run seem adaptive but that in the long run foster chronic pain and disability. For example, following a back injury, individuals may cease activities that exacerbate pain and restrict movements to avoid pain. As a result, they may lose muscle strength, flexibility, and endurance, thus creating a vicious circle of activity avoidance and increased disability. In addition, the distorted movements and postures that individuals assume to prevent pain may cause further pain unrelated to the initial injury. For example, limping protects muscles on one side of the back, but the overactive muscles on the other side can develop painful conditions of their own.

In addition, people with chronic pain who have had limited success in controlling it perceive pain to be outside of personal control and are unlikely to attempt new pain-management strategies. Instead, they feel frustrated and demoralized when uncontrollable pain interferes with rewarding recreational, occupational, and social activities. Such people commonly resort to passive coping strategies, such as inactivity, self-medication, or alcohol to reduce emotional distress and pain. People who feel little personal control over their pain are also likely to catastrophize situations that exacerbate pain as well as about the impact of a pain episode itself.

If psychological factors can cause maladaption to pain, they can also have a positive effect. Individuals who have a number of successful methods for coping with pain may suffer less than those who feel helpless. Later in this chapter we will consider some effective psychological interventions that help people with persistent pain to eliminate their pain or, if that is not possible, to reduce their pain, distress, and suffering.

Indirect effects of psychological factors on pain

Several studies have suggested that psychological factors may indirectly affect the physiologic parameters of nociception. Cognitive interpretations and affective arousal may influence physiology by increasing autonomic sympathetic nervous system arousal, promoting endogenous opioid (endorphin) production, and fostering elevated muscle tension.

Effects of thoughts on autonomic arousal

Chronic and excessive sympathetic nervous system arousal is the immediate precursor of increased skeletal muscle tone (hypertonicity) and may set the stage for hyperactive muscle contraction and muscle contraction persistence, all of which are proximate causes of muscle spasm and pain. People who exaggerate the significance of their problems, whether consciously or unconsciously, may influence sympathetic arousal and thereby predispose themselves to further injury or otherwise complicate the process of recovery.

The direct effect of thoughts on muscle tension response was demonstrated by Herta Flor, Dennis Turk and Niels Birbaumer. These investigators interviewed patients with back pain disorders, patients with other pain disorders, and healthy individuals. While muscle activity was monitored with sensors, patients recalled and described recent personal episodes of extreme pain or severe stress. The study found that during recall, back pain patients had significantly elevated back muscle tension but not elevated forehead or forearm tension. However, resting back pain patients not engaged in pain or stress recall had back muscle tension levels no higher than that of patients in the other groups. Neither the patients with other pain disorders nor the healthy individuals showed elevations in muscle tension when discussing severe stress. Thus, back pain patients showed pain-site-specific muscular response simply to thinking or talking about pain and stress (Flor et al. 1985). Similar results have been observed in studies with patients who had chronic arm and shoulder pain and temporomandibular disorders.

Effects of thoughts on biochemistry

Albert Bandura and his colleagues directly examined the role of central nervous system opioids in cognitive control of pain. They provided cognitive training in which subjects received instructions and practice in using different coping strategies for alleviating pain. They demonstrated that:

- expectations about the ability to control pain and disability (self-efficacy) increased with cognitive training.
- self-efficacy predicted pain tolerance.
- naloxone, an opioid antagonist, blocked the pain-alleviating effects of cognitive coping.

The latter result implicates the direct effect of thoughts on the endogenous opioids, endorphins. Bandura et al. concluded that self-efficacy may influence pain perception at least partially via the endogenous opioid system (Bandura et al. 1987).

Ann O'Leary et al. provided stress management treatment (described below) to rheumatoid arthritis (RA) patients. RA, an autoimmune disease that may result from impaired functioning of the suppressor T-cell system, causes inflammation of many different serous membranes, especially the synovial membranes, resulting in joint pain and stiffness, among other symptoms. In the O'Leary study, those with higher self-efficacy and greater self-efficacy enhancement displayed greater numbers of suppressor T-cells, a direct effect of self-efficacy on physiology. Significant effects were also observed in relation to self-efficacy vs the degree of pain and joint impairment (O'Leary et al. 1988).

Integrative models of pain

An integrative model of pain, including chronic pain and acute recurrent pain, incorporates the interrelationships of physical, psychosocial, and behavioral factors and the changes that occur in these relationships over time. A model that focuses on only one set of factors will inevitably be incomplete.The physiologic model proposed by Ronald Melzack and Patrick Wall (Melzack and Wall 1965) mentioned earlier can be contrasted to the more psychological, cognitive-behavioral model proposed by Dennis Turk and his colleagues (Turk et al. 1993). Melzack and Wall focus primarily on the basic anatomy and physiology of pain, whereas Turk et al. emphasize the influence of psychology on the physiology underlying the experience of and response to pain. Yet both models incorporate physical and psychological factors to account for the experience of pain.

Gate control theory

More than thirty years ago Ronald Melzack and Patrick Wall proposed gate control theory, a new integrative model that included both physiologic and psychological factors (Melzack and Wall 1965). Perhaps the most important contribution of gate control theory is its creative rethinking of pain perception. This model postulates three systems that together process nociceptive stimulation and contribute to the subjective experience of pain: sensory-discriminative, motivational-affective, and cognitive-evaluative.

The gate control theory proposes that the dorsal horn substantia gelatinosa of the spinal cord contains a spinal gating mechanism that inhibits or facilitates transmission of peripheral nerve impulses to the brain, depending on the diameters of the active peripheral fibers and the influence of certain brain processes. It postulates that the spinal gate is influenced by the relative amount of excitatory activity in afferent, large-diameter (myelinated) and small-diameter (unmyelinated) nociceptive fibers converging in the dorsal horns. It further proposes that activity in A-β (large-diameter) fibers tends to inhibit transmission of nociceptive signals (close the gate), while primary afferent activity in small diameter A-δ and C fibers tends to facilitate transmission (open the gate). The balance of activity of small diameter (A-δ and C) and large-diameter (A-β) fibers influences the level of nociceptive input that reaches the brain.

Ascending and descending biasing mechanisms

Melzack and Wall postulate further that efferent neural impulses descending from the brain influence the spinal gating mechanism. They propose that a specialized system of large-diameter, rapidly conducting A-β fibers (the central control trigger) activates selective cognitive processes that then influence, by way of descending fibers, the spinal gating mechanism. They also suggest that the brain stem reticular formation functions as a central biasing mechanism inhibiting the transmission of pain signals at multiple synaptic levels of the somatosensory system.

According to gate control theory, large-diameter fibers play an important role in pain by inhibiting synaptic transmission in dorsal-horn cells. When large-fiber input is decreased, mild stimuli that are not typically painful trigger severe pain. Loss of sensory input to the spinal cord, such as occurs in neuropathies, causalgia, and phantom limb pain, tends to weaken inhibition and lead to persistent pain. Herniated disk material, tumors, and other factors that exert pressure on these neural structures may cause pain by imposing an input loss. Emotional stress and medication that affect reticular formation may also alter the biasing mechanisms and, thus, intensity of pain.

The gate control model contradicts the notion that pain is either somatic or psychogenic and instead postulates that both factors potentiate or moderate pain perception. In this model, for example, pain is not understood to be the result of depression or vice versa. The two are seen as evolving simultaneously. The gate control theory's emphasis on ascending and descending modulation of dorsal horn input and the dynamic role of the brain in pain processes and perception fosters inclusion of psychological variables, such as past experience, attention, mood, and other cognitive activities, into current research and therapy. Prior to this formulation psychological processes were largely dismissed as reactions to pain.

After the proposal of gate control theory, pain could not be viewed exclusively in terms of peripheral factors. As additional knowledge has accumulated since the original formulation in 1965, specific points have been disputed, revised, and reformulated. Overall, however, the gate control theory has proved remarkably resilient and flexible in the face of mounting scientific data and challenges to various parts of the model. This theory has had enormous heuristic value in stimulating basic research. It has also spurred new clinical treatments, including neurosurgical procedures such as analgesia through electrical stimulation of peripheral nerves and of collateral processes in the spinal cord dorsal columns, pharmacologic advances, behavioral treatments, and interventions to modify pain perception.

Although the gate control theory provides a physical basis for the role of psychological factors in pain, it does not address psychological factors in depth. The cognitive-behavioral model offers a thorough consideration of psychological factors as potent variables in pain perception, pain experience, and response.

Cognitive-behavioral model

The cognitive-behavioral model incorporates many of the psychological variables of operant and respondent learning, namely, anticipation, avoidance, and contingencies of reinforcement. However, the model suggests that cognitive factors, particularly expectations, rather than conditioning factors are of central importance. The cognitive-behavioral model suggests that so-called conditioned reactions such as experiencing anxiety and pain at the prospect of exercise are largely self-activated on the basis of learned expectations rather than being automatically evoked responses to conditioned stimuli. The critical factor for the cognitive-behavioral model, therefore, is not that events occur together in time, but that people learn to predict them and to engage in anticipatory anxiety and avoidance behaviors.

The cognitive-behavioral perspective suggests that behavior and emotions are influenced by personal interpretations rather than solely by the objective characteristics of an event. This model emphasizes that the experience of pain is influenced by the ongoing reciprocal relationships among physical, cognitive, affective, social, and behavioral factors. Patients' experience of pain is shaped by personal attitudes, beliefs, and schemata that filter and interact reciprocally with emotions, social influences, and behavioral responses as well as with sensory experience. Moreover, patients' behaviors elicit responses from significant others that can reinforce both adaptive and maladaptive modes of thinking, feeling, and behaving. Thus, a reciprocal and synergistic model is proposed.

In pain management strategies based on the cognitive-behavioral model, five central assumptions operate (Turk and Meichenbaum 1994):

- *People actively process information; they do not merely react to environmental contingencies.* To make sense of stimuli, people filter information through organizing attitudes (schemata) derived from prior learning and general information processing strategies. People's responses are based on these appraisals and subsequent expectations and are not totally dependent on the actual consequences of their behaviors. The anticipated consequences are as important in guiding behavior as the actual consequences.

- *Thoughts can elicit or modulate affect and physiologic arousal, both of which may influence behavior. Conversely, affect, physiology, and behavior can influence thinking.* Causal priority may be of less concern than the view that thoughts, feelings, physiologic activity, and behavior interact continuously and reciprocally.
- *Successful interventions to alter maladaptive behavior focus on people's maladaptive thoughts and feelings as well as behaviors and not on one to the exclusion of the others.* Changing only thoughts, only feelings, or only behaviors does not necessarily mean the other two will follow suit.
- *Behavior is reciprocally determined by both the environment and the individual.* Individuals not only passively respond to their environment but also elicit environmental responses by their behavior. In a very real sense people create their environments. Patients with symptoms who decide to seek medical attention initiate a set of circumstances different from those that arise if the same individuals choose instead to self-medicate.
- *Since people develop and maintain maladaptive thoughts, feelings, and behaviors, they can also change those maladaptive modes of responding.* Despite their common beliefs to the contrary, patients with chronic pain, no matter how severe, are not helpless pawns of fate. They can and should learn and carry out more effective modes of responding to their environments and their plights.

In the cognitive-behavioral model, people with pain are viewed as having negative expectations about their own ability to control the pain experience or to engage in certain activities without pain. These negative appraisals and expectations are postulated to lead to a reduction in coping efforts and activity, which may in turn contribute to psychological distress (helplessness) and subsequent physical limitations.

Over time, biomedical factors associated with the original pain experience play less of a role in disability. Meanwhile, secondary problems associated with deconditioning may exacerbate and maintain the pain. Inactivity leads to increased preoccupation with the body and pain, and these cognitive-attentional changes increase the likelihood of overemphasis on symptoms and the perception of oneself as disabled. Reduction of activity, fear of reinjury, pain, loss of compensation, and an environment that perhaps unwittingly supports the pain-patient role can impede pain alleviation and successful rehabilitation.

Cognitive schemata

People respond to medical conditions in part based on their subjective representations of illness and symptoms (schemata). People's beliefs about the meaning of pain and about their own ability to function despite discomfort are important aspects of schemata about pain. For example, a schema that one has a very serious, debilitating condition, that disability is a necessary aspect of pain, that activity is dangerous, and that pain is an acceptable excuse for neglecting responsibilities will likely result in maladaptive responses. Through stimulus generalization, such patients may avoid more and more activities and become more physically deconditioned and more disabled.

Many interdependent factors facilitate or disrupt patients' sense of control: personal beliefs, appraisals, and expectations about pain; coping ability and social supports; the nature of the disorder; the medico-legal system; the health care system; the response of employers. These factors also influence patients' investment in treatment, acceptance of responsibility, perceptions of disability, adherence to treatment recommendations, and support from significant others.

Cognitive interpretations also affect how patients present symptoms to significant others, including health care providers and employers. Overt communication of pain, suffering, and distress may lead physicians to prescribe more potent medications, order additional diagnostic tests, and, in some cases, perform surgery. Family members may express sympathy, excuse the patient from responsibilities, and encourage passivity.

Integration of three treatment perspectives

The cognitive-behavioral approach integrates the operant conditioning emphasis on external reinforcement with the respondent view of learned avoidance within the framework of information processing. According to the cognitive-behavioral model, people's negative, maladaptive appraisals of their situations as well as disavowal of personal efficacy in controlling pain and pain-related problems lead to reduced coping efforts and increased psychological distress.

From the cognitive-behavioral perspective, assessment and treatment of patients with persistent pain requires a broad strategy that addresses all relevant psychosocial and behavioral factors in addition to biomedical ones. This pain management perspective provides patients with techniques to regain personal control over the life-changing effects of pain as well as the skills to modify the affective, behavioral, cognitive, and sensory facets of the pain experience. During treatment, patients discover that they are more capable than they had assumed, thus increasing their sense of personal competence. Cognitive techniques help to place affective, behavioral, cognitive, and sensory responses under the patient's control. Treatment that increases perceived personal control over pain and decreases catastrophizing is associated with reduced pain severity ratings and functional disability (Jensen et al. 1994; Tota-Faucette et al. 1993). Treatment based on the cognitive-behavioral model assumes that long-term maintenance of behavioral changes occurs only if patients attribute success to their own efforts. Treatment based on this approach will be described following a discussion of chronic pain assessment strategies and methods.

Assessment methods

Appropriate treatment of patients whose primary symptom is pain begins with a comprehensive history and physical examination. Despite the ready availability of physical examinations and sophisticated laboratory and imaging techniques, pain assessment is complicated by the psychological, social, and behavioral characteristics of individual patients. An adequate assessment also requires evaluation of these myriad nonmaterial factors.

Quantifying the pain experience

Pain, a complex, subjective phenomenon, is unusually difficult to assess because it is uniquely experienced by each individual. Patients suffering from apparently identical pathology vary widely in their descriptions of the severity, quality, and impact of the pain. In addition, the patient's unique views and frame of reference may complicate communication between patient and caregivers and prevent direct comparisons among patients with different backgrounds and experiences. Patients' pain descriptions are also colored by cultural and sociological influences.

Physical contributors

Physical and laboratory abnormalities correlate poorly with patients' pain complaints. Difficulties in assessing the physical contributions to chronic pain are well recognized, and no universal criteria exist for scoring the presence or importance of a particular sign, such as positive radiographs or limitation of spinal mobility, quantifying the degree of disability, or associating these findings with treatment outcome. Interpretation of biomedical findings relies on clinical judgments and medical consensus based on a physician's experience and in some instances on quasi-standardized criteria. However, both the performance of physical examinations and the interpretation of diagnostic findings contain unavoidable subjective elements.

The inherent subjectivity of physical examinations is most evident when it is noted that agreement among physicians is better for items of patient history than for some items of the physical examination. The reproducibility of physical evaluation findings, even among experienced physicians, is low. For example, the interobserver agreement in physical examination of spinal motion and muscle strength, even when using standard mechanical assessment devices such as dynamometers, has been shown to be surprisingly poor.

The discriminative power of common objective signs of pathology has also been questioned. For example, the prevalences of leg-length differences, increased lumbosacral angles, spondylisthesis, transitional lumbosacral vertebrae, and spina bifida occulta in back pain patients do not differ significantly from those of an asymptomatic control group. Thus, there is no direct relationship between the amount of detectable pathology and the reported pain intensity.

For significant numbers of patients, no physical pathology can be identified. Even with sophisticated advances in imaging technology, a less than perfect correlation exists between identifiable pathology and reported pain. For example, magnetic resonance imaging (MRI) has identified structural abnormalities commonly associated with back pain in up to 30% of healthy, asymptomatic populations.

In sum, routine clinical assessment of chronic pain patients is frequently subjective and unreliable, making precise pathological diagnosis or even identification of the anatomical origin of the pain impossible. Despite these limitations, the patient's history and physical examination remain the bases of medical diagnosis and may be the best defense against overinterpreting results from sophisticated imaging procedures. For a recent discussion of some of the complexities involved in interpreting objective findings, see *Handbook of Pain Assessment* (Turk and Melzack 1992).

Psychosocial contributors

Any identified physical abnormalities may be influenced by coexisting psychosocial factors. The complexity of pain is especially evident when it persists over time because a range of psychological, social, and economic factors interact with physical pathology to modulate both patients' pain reports and the impact of pain on their lives. In chronic pain cases, health care givers should investigate not only the physical sources of the pain but also the patient's moods, fears, expectations, coping efforts, and resources, as well as the responses of significant others and the impact of pain on the patient's life. In short, evaluation must focus on the whole patient, not just on the cause of the pain.

Dennis Turk and Donald Meichenbaum have suggested that three central questions should guide pain assessment (Turk and Meichenbaum 1994):

- What is the extent of the patient's disease or injury (physical impairment)?
- What is the extent to which the patient is suffering, disabled, and unable to enjoy usual activities?
- Does the patient's behavior seem appropriate to the disease or injury, or is there evidence of symptom amplification for any of a variety of psychological or social reasons?

The remainder of this chapter focuses on the second two questions, specifically, the extent of patients' disabilities and the behavioral influences on patients' pain, distress, and suffering.

Interview techniques

When interviewing chronic pain patients, health care professionals should not focus only on factual information but also on patients' and significant others' specific thoughts and feelings, and they should observe specific behaviors. During the interview, it is important to adopt the patient's perspective. Attention should focus on the patient's reports of specific thoughts, behaviors, emotions, and physiological responses that precede, accompany, and follow pain episodes or exacerbations, as well as on the environmental conditions and consequences associated with all of the patient's typical responses to these situations. The interviewer should note the temporal association of these cognitive, affective, and behavioral events—their specificity versus generality across situations—and the frequency of their occurrence. The interviewer will then use this information to help the patient develop appropriate goals, alternative responses to pain episodes, and possible reinforcements for these alternatives.

Self-monitoring prior to or following the initial interview is also useful because it introduces patients to the active role they will be required to play in treatment. A sample self-monitoring form is contained in *Self-monitoring record of symptoms, feelings, thoughts, and actions.*

The health care provider should be alert for red flags that indicate the need for more thorough evaluation by other pain specialists (see *Screening questions for interviews with patients*, page 150). Positive responses to only a small number of these questions is not sufficient cause for referral for more extensive evaluation, but when a preponderance of responses are positive, referral should be considered.

In addition to interviews, a number of assessment instruments designed to evaluate patients' attitudes, beliefs, and expectancies about themselves, their symptoms, and the health care system have been developed. Standardized assessment instruments have advantages over semistructured and unstructured interviews. They are easy to administer, require less time, and provide a means of discovering

Self-monitoring record of symptoms, feelings, thoughts, and actions

A self-monitoring record (pain diary) helps patients understand the active role they must play in any pain management plan. Patients may be asked to keep such a diary prior to or following an initial interview with a pain management specialist.

Name: _____

Date/Time	Symptoms (How bad, 0 to 10?) Situation (What were you doing or thinking?)	How did you feel? (How bad, 0 to 10?)	What were you thinking?	What did you do? With what result?

important issues to be addressed during an interview. Several representative assessment instruments are described below.

Self-report measurement of pain

Often patients are asked to quantify their pain by providing a single, general rating, for example, by rating pain as mild, moderate or severe or by assigning it a number value, typically between 0 and 10, where 0 equals no pain and 10 equals the most severe pain imaginable. More valid information may be obtained by asking about the current level of pain or pain over the past week and by having patients maintain daily diaries of pain intensity. A number of simple methods can be used to evaluate current pain intensity—numerical scales, descriptive ratings scales, visual analog scales, and box scales. (See *Examples of pain intensity rating scales*, page 151.)

In most current thinking, pain is usually viewed as containing three components: a sensory-discriminative component (severity); a

▶ᒡ

PAIN MANAGEMENT PRACTICE

Screening questions for interviews with patients

These questions help care providers identify patients who may need referral to pain management specialists.

Clinical issues

- Has the pain persisted for 3 months or longer despite appropriate interventions and in the absence of progressive disease?
- Does the patient report nonanatomical changes in sensation such as glove anesthesia?
- Does the patient seem to have unrealistic expectations of the health care provider or of the treatment offered?
- Does the patient complain vociferously about treatments received from previous health care providers?
- Does the patient have a history of previous painful or disabling medical problems?
- Does the patient have a history of substance abuse?
- Does the patient display many pain behaviors such as grimacing or moving in a rigid and guarded fashion?

Legal and occupational issues

- Is there litigation pending?
- Is the patient receiving disability compensation?
- Was the patient employed prior to pain onset?
- Was the patient injured on the job?

- Does the patient have a job to which he or she can return?
- Does the patient have a history of frequent changing of jobs?

Psychological issues

- Does the patient report any major stressful life events just prior to the onset or exacerbation of pain?
- Does the patient demonstrate inappropriate or excessive depressed or elevated mood?
- Has the patient given up many activities (social, recreational, sexual, occupational, physical) because of pain?
- Is there a high level of marital or family conflict?
- Do the patient's significant others provide positive attention to pain behaviors such as taking over patient's chores or rubbing patient's back?
- Is there anyone in the patient's family who has chronic pain?
- Does the patient have no plans for increased or renewed activities if pain is reduced?

From Turk and Marcus (1994), "Comprehensive Assessment of Chronic Pain Patients," *Seminars in Neurology*, 14:206-212. Adapted with permission.

motivational-affective component (distress); and a cognitive-evaluative component. The scales described above focus only on severity. Similar methods can be used to evaluate distress by modifying the instructions and using appropriate anchors. For example, 0 = no distress and 10 = extreme distress.

The McGill Pain Questionnaire (MPQ), one of the most frequently used assessment instruments, includes a descriptive scale (Present Pain Intensity) with numbers 1 through 5 assigned to each of five adjectives (1 = mild and 5 = excruciating). The second part shows a human figure outline on which patients indicate the location of their pain. Finally, a pain rating index is derived from patients' selection of various adjectives that reflect the sensory, affective, and cognitive components of pain (Melzack 1975). The MPQ provides a

Examples of pain intensity rating scales

These scales help patients to quantify their current levels of pain. Additional information may be obtained by having the patient keep a pain diary over a period of days or weeks.

Visual analogue scale*
Place a line on the scale that indicates your current level of pain.

No pain |_____| Pain as bad as it can be

Descriptive pain intensity scale*
Place a line on the scale that indicates your current level of pain.

|_____|

No pain   Mild   Moderate   Severe

Numeric pain intensity scale
Circle the number below that indicates your current level of pain.

No pain | 0   1   2   3   4   5   6   7   8   9   10 | Pain as bad as it can be

Box pain intensity scale
Place an X through the number that indicates your current level of pain.

0	1	2	3	4	5	6	7	8	9	10

No pain   Most severe pain

*a 10-cm line is recommended

From Turk and Marcus (1994), "Comprehensive Assessment of Chronic Pain Patients," *Seminars in Neurology*, 14: 206-212. Adapted with permission.

great deal of information, but it takes much longer to complete than the simple ratings of pain severity. The MPQ may be inappropriate when frequent pain ratings are required, for example hourly ratings following surgery. A short form of the MPQ is available. In many cases the simple scales may be adequate.

Assessment of functional activities
The traditional measures of function performed as part of the physical examination cannot directly confirm symptoms or quantify func-

tion but are only approximations that may be influenced by patients' motivation to communicate pain, distress, and suffering to their physician. Common physical examination maneuvers, such as muscular strength and range of motion, as well as diagnostic tests such as radiography have been shown to have little value for predicting the long-term functional capacity of patients.

The questionable reliability and validity of physical examination measures has led to the development of self-report functional status measures that seek to quantify symptoms, function, and behavior directly, rather than having physicians infer them. Self-report measures allow assessment of individuals' reports of their abilities to perform a range of functional activities, such as walking up stairs, sitting for specific periods of time, lifting specific weights, and performing activities of daily living as well as assessments of reports of pain severity experienced upon performance of these activities. Some of the commonly used functional assessment scales include the Roland-Morris Disability Scale (Roland and Morris 1983), the Sickness Impact Profile (Bergner et al. 1981), and the Oswestry Disability Scale (Fairbank et al. 1980). The questions elicit specific information. One item on the Oswestry Disability Scale asks patients to indicate whether their pain prevents them from sitting at all, sitting for more than 10 minutes, sitting for more than 30 minutes, sitting for more than an hour, or whether they are able to sit for as long as they wish.

Despite the obvious limitations of self-report instruments, they have several advantages: economy, efficiency, and utility for assessment of a wide range of patient behaviors, some of which may be private such as sexual relations or unobservable, such as thoughts and emotional arousal. Although the validity of self-reporting is often questioned, studies have revealed fairly high correspondence among self-reports, disease characteristics, physicians or physical therapists' ratings of functional abilities, and objective functional performance.

Assessment of overt expressions of pain

Patients display a broad range of responses that communicate to others their pain, distress, and suffering. Some of these pain behaviors are controllable but others are not. For example, in acute pain, autonomic activity such as perspiring may indicate the presence of pain. Over time, however, these physiologic signs habituate and their absence cannot be taken as an indication of significant reduction or absence of pain.

Overt pain behaviors include verbal reports; other vocalizations such as sighs and moans; motor activity; facial expressions; body postures and gesturing, such as limping or grimacing; functional limitations, including reclining for extensive periods; and actions to reduce pain such as taking medication. Reinforcement of these behaviors through personal attention or avoidance of undesirable activity may lead to maintenance of the pain behaviors, even when the initial cause of pain is no longer present.

One way to assess pain behaviors is to have patients keep diaries in which they record the amount of time or the number of times they perform specific pain behaviors, such as reclining, sitting, taking medication, and so forth, as well as the circumstances surrounding the behavior. For example, a patient might note that he took medication after an argument with his wife and that upon seeing him take the medication, she expressed sympathy. In this case, recognizing the consequences of the pain behavior helps to identify a pattern of medication use that may be associated with factors other than pain per se. For this patient, a significant other may be providing positive reinforcement for the taking of analgesics thereby unwittingly encouraging increased medication use.

Health care professionals can attempt to quantify pain behaviors while observing patients in the waiting room, during the interview, or during a structured series of physical tasks. Several investigators have used the Pain Behavior Checklist (see *Pain behavior checklist*, page 154) and have found a significant association between self-reports by patients and observations by professionals.

Assessment of psychological contributors

The failure to find a consistent correlation between pathology and reports of pain has led some investigators to classify pain that is reported in the absence of physical findings as psychogenic. All people experience pain, and it would be naive to assume that individual differences in personality and prior learning are irrelevant in the decision to seek treatment for pain. However, it is equally important to acknowledge that pain induces emotional distress, which may be the result and not necessarily the cause of pain. Regardless of the initial cause of nociception, a range of cognitive and affective factors can modulate the experience and report of pain.

The use of traditional psychological measures, for example, the Minnesota Multiphasic Personality Inventory (MMPI), to identify specific individual differences associated with reports of pain must be approached with caution as most of these tools were not developed for or standardized on samples of medical patients. Recently a number of assessment instruments have been developed for use specifically with pain patients. One of these, which assesses both psychosocial and behavioral factors associated with chronic pain, is the West Haven-Yale Multidimensional Pain Inventory (WHYMPI), a 60-item, 3-part questionnaire (Kerns et al. 1985). The first part assesses

PAIN MANAGEMENT PRACTICE

Pain behavior checklist

Pain behaviors have been characterized as interpersonal communications of pain, distress, or suffering. Place a check in the box next to each behavior you observe or infer from the patient's comments.

- ❑ 1. Facial grimacing
- ❑ 2. Holding or supporting affected body area
- ❑ 3. Asking "Why did this happen to me?"
- ❑ 4. Distorted gait
- ❑ 5. Frequent shifting of posture or position
- ❑ 6. Requesting excuse from tasks or activities
- ❑ 7. Taking medication (when on a prn schedule)
- ❑ 8. Moving extremely slowly
- ❑ 9. Limping
- ❑ 10. Sitting with a rigid posture

- ❑ 11. Moving in a guarded or protective fashion
- ❑ 12. Moaning
- ❑ 13. Using a cane, cervical collar, or other prosthetic device
- ❑ 14. Requesting help in ambulation
- ❑ 15. Stopping frequently while walking
- ❑ 16. Lying down during the day
- ❑ 17. Being irritable
- ❑ 18. Avoiding of physical activity
- ❑ 19. Sighing
- ❑ 20. Clenching teeth

From Turk and Marcus (1994), "Comprehensive Assessment of Chronic Pain Patients," *Seminars in Neurology* 14:206-12. Adapted with permission.

patients' perceptions of pain severity, the impact of pain on various areas of life, affective distress, feelings of control, and support from significant others. The second section assesses the patients' perceptions of significant others' reponses to their pain complaints. The third section examines changes in patients' functional activities, such as household chores and socializing. The WHYMPI and many other assessment measures are reviewed and critiqued in the *Handbook of Pain Assessment* (Turk and Melzack 1992).

When objective physical findings do not substantiate the complaints of pain or when reports of its severity seem excessive in light of physical findings, health care professionals face difficulty in making a comprehensive evaluation. Caregivers must decide when it is appropriate to refer patients for psychological or psychiatric assessment by someone who specializes in chronic pain evaluation. (See *Sample topics for a psychological assessment interview.*)

Because pain is subjective, suffering and disability are difficult to prove, disprove, or quantify. Pain is influenced by cultural conditioning, expectancies, social contingencies, mood, and perceptions of control as well as physical pathology. The central point is this: the patient who reports the pain is the subject of evaluation, not the pain itself.

PAIN MANAGEMENT PRACTICE

Sample topics for a psychological assessment interview

A mental health professional specializing in pain management conducts an initial assessment interview with each new patient. The interview would probably explore the points below:

- What the patient thinks is wrong with him or her
- What the patient thinks about the causes, treatments, and future impact of the pain
- What worries the patient, such as progression of the condition or exacerbation of pain
- Problems the patient has confronted because of the presence of pain, such as vocational, marital, or financial circumstances
- Situational fluctuations in intensity, duration, and frequency of pain
- Common features associated with fluctuations such as time of day, connections with specific activities, presence of certain people
- How the patient expresses pain; how others know when the patient's pain is intense or present
- What effect the patient believes the pain is having on others
- What family, friends, coworkers, employers think about the patient's pain

- How others respond to the patient's pain complaints, other pain behaviors, and functional limitations
- Secondary gains such as attention and avoidance of undesirable activities
- Pattern of medication use and substance abuse (current and previous)
- Current mood, sleep, appetite disturbances
- What the patient tries or has tried to do to alleviate pain
- Work history: frequency of change, satisfaction, interactions with coworkers and supervisors
- Patient's expectations of health care providers and treatments
- Views of previous health care providers and treatments
- Prior history of pain in patient or family members
- Prior and current stressful life events
- Family (marital) relations (current and past)
- Motivation for rehabilitation and self-management

From Turk and Nash. "Psychological Issues in Chronic Pain." In *Pain Management: Theory and Practice.* Portenoy and Kanner (eds.) F. A. Davis Co., 1996. Adapted with permission.

Preparing patients for psychological referral

Patients with chronic pain often resist referral to psychologists because they fear that referral indicates that the health care provider believes they are weak, incompetent, emotionally disturbed, psychologically abnormal, exaggerating, or malingering. They may fear it implies that they are being abandoned by current caregivers as a hopeless case. Patients with known physical bases for pain usually believe that psychological assessment is irrelevant and that cure of the disease or elimination of the symptoms is all that is required. Conversely, patients who are convinced that an undiagnosed, untreated medical disorder causes the pain will reject any implication that psychological factors may contribute to the symptoms.

Candidates for psychological referral may be particularly defensive and express it as reticence, hostility, or an overly positive presentation meant to project an image of psychological well-being that disavows even minimal psychological distress or difficulty. Even if no concern is raised by patients, referring health care providers should assume that resistance is a potential problem and should explain the reasons for the referral, the specific nature of the referral question, how the results of the consultation will be used, and who will have access to information discussed with the mental health professional.

Patients should be informed that mental health professionals are clinical team members who are trained to help people with chronic pain and that they teach patients coping techniques that may help reduce pain-related suffering. In addition, the health care provider can acknowledge that long-standing pain and any accompanying disability, role alterations, or life-style changes often create psychological distress as well as loss of self-esteem and emotional well-being and note that mental health professionals help patients deal with these issues.

Psychological referral interview

The first tasks of the mental health professional are to ask patients about their reactions to referral, to correct misconceptions, and to allow the patients to ask questions.

A description of what will take place during therapy sessions should be made within a positive framework and with the expectation of success. It is critical to solicit questions and comments from patients and significant others. Many patients tend to be nonassertive in health care professionals' offices. For patients who do not ask questions, it is worthwhile saying something such as, "Although it may not have occurred to you, many people with problems similar to yours are concerned about seeing a mental health professional. This is quite natural." Patients may believe that because the interviewer is a mental health professional, he or she can help only with psychological problems, not with physical ones. The psychological therapist must address all of the patient's concerns and fears, including unspoken ones. If not addressed, these fears and concerns will inhibit participation in the treatment.

Treatment goals and therapeutic approach

The psychological therapist and patient must cooperatively establish treatment goals. Collaboration is essential because it helps patients to assume responsibility for adherence to the requirements as well as the outcome of treatment. A helpful strategy is to generate specific goals by asking questions such as, "How would your life be different if your symptoms (physical impairments) could be relieved?" Treatment goals should be specific and measurable. For example, the goal of feeling better is not specific enough. Patients need to specify concretely what they will be able to do that would indicate such improvement. Treatment goals typically include symptom reduction, improved physical, recreational, and vocational functioning, and reduction in use of the health care system.

Therapeutic approaches originally used in the treatment of psychological problems have been adapted for use with people in pain. Two commonly used approaches are the operant learning approach and the cognitive-behavioral approach.

Operant learning approach

Treatments based on operant learning focus on decreasing pain behaviors such as time spent lying down and increasing well behaviors such as engagement in activity, irrespective of pain levels. To reach these goals, attention is withdrawn from pain behaviors and focused on well behaviors. Typically, treatment promotes the well behavior of physical activity by establishing exercise quotas and providing positive reinforcement for exercise by means of rest and verbal praise or encouragement from others. When the patient engages in activity, the therapist and significant others provide corrective feedback or reassurance that pain based on movement need not signal injury. As the patient's activities are positively reinforced, pain behaviors are ignored, eventually leading to the extinction of the learned maladaptive behavior patterns.

The reinforcing aspect of medication is diminished by altering schedules from an as-needed basis to an interval basis so that medication becomes time-contingent and not pain-contingent. The amount of medication is then reduced according to a specific schedule.

Operant learning programs are usually conducted on an inpatient basis because it allows better control of external contingencies of reinforcement. The participation of family members and significant others is generally required because they will be the most important reinforcers of the new behavior patterns in the home. Occupational and physical therapy are important components of an operant learning program because they emphasize increased activity levels. For more detail on the operant approach to treatment, see *Behavioral Methods for Chronic Pain and Illness* (Fordyce 1976).

Cognitive-behavioral approach

Cognitive-behavioral therapy helps patients to identify, evaluate, and correct maladaptive conceptualizations and dysfunctional beliefs about themselves and their predicaments. Additionally, patients are taught to recognize the connections linking cognition, affect, and behavior, along with their consequences. Patients are encouraged to notice and monitor the impact of negative thoughts and feelings on their symptoms and maladaptive behaviors. Therapists are concerned not only with how patients' thoughts maintain or exacerbate disability and symptoms, but also with the nature and adequacy of patients' behavioral repertoires.

The strategy of cognitive-behavioral intervention is to help patients relinquish the belief that illness or disability is exclusively a medical problem that precludes personal control. Cognitive-behavioral intervention approaches the patient optimistically, emphasizing both the effectiveness of the intervention and the patient's ability to alleviate much personal suffering, even if he or she cannot completely control the disease and physical limitations.

Therapists enourage discussion of symptoms and physical limitations and their impact on the lives of patients and significant others. The patient must be willing to work with the therapist and other members of the rehabilitation team, who emphasize that they will not do anything to the patient. This discussion should take place with significant others present so that their concerns can be addressed as well.

The cognitive-behavioral approach is a highly collaborative endeavor that attempts to foster an increased sense of self-efficacy and self-motivation. During treatment, patients learn a range of cognitive and behavioral skills that assist them in dealing with maladaptive thoughts and feelings as well as with noxious sensations that may precede, accompany, or follow symptoms and thereby escalate emotional suffering. Both behavioral techniques (reinforcement, exposure) and cognitive techniques (cognitive resconceptualization, problem-solving training, coping skills training) are used. Other techniques based on these models, such as biofeedback, extinction of inappropriate illness behaviors, and reinforcement of activity, provide opportunities for patients to ask questions, reappraise, and acquire self-control over maladaptive thoughts, feelings, behaviors, and physiologic responses, as well as to develop adaptive skills. (See *Characteristics of the cognitive-behavioral approach to pain management.*)

Components of cognitive-behavioral intervention

Each component of cognitive-behavioral treatment for people with chronic pain should be directed toward accomplishing five objectives (see *Goals of the cognitive-behavioral approach to pain management,* page 160). Treatment is based on four interrelated components:

PAIN MANAGEMENT PRINCIPLES

Characteristics of the cognitive-behavioral approach to pain management

- Focuses on solving specific problems created by chronic pain (problem-oriented approach)
- Teaches self-management, problem-solving, coping, and communication skills (educational approach)
- Fosters teamwork between patient and health care provider (collaborative approach)
- Combines clinical and home practice to consolidate skills and identify problem areas (holistic approach)

- Encourages expression and then control of feelings that impair rehabilitation (affect-control approach)
- Addresses the relationship of thoughts, feelings, behavior, and physiology (integrative approach)
- Anticipates setbacks and lapses in newly acquired skills and teaches patients how to deal with them (self-management approach)

- reconceptualization
- skills acquisition
- skills consolidation
- generalization and maintenance.

Cognitive reconceptualization

People's thoughts can greatly influence their moods, their behaviors, and some of their physiologic processes. Conversely moods, behaviors, and physiologic activity can influence thoughts. Thus, it is important for people who are in pain to notice thoughts and feelings associated with episodes of pain. Cognitive reconceptualization, also called cognitive restructuring, is a means of encouraging people to identify and change the stress-inducing thoughts and feelings associated with their pain.

Many people with persistent pain find it hard to accept the idea that their thoughts and emotions can actually affect their bodies. To convince patients of this fact, it is useful to have them use a pain diary to self-monitor the thoughts and feelings that precede, accompany, and follow an episode or flare-up of pain. For example, patients may find that they have some of the following thoughts:

- I feel as though I can't take it any more.
- I can't do anything when my pain is bad.
- I don't see how this pain is ever going to get better.

These types of maladaptive thoughts can increase the perceptions of pain by increasing muscle tension and preventing efforts to cope with the situation. Once specific, pain-associated thoughts and emotions

Goals of the cognitive-behavioral approach to pain management

1. Educate patients about the nature of pain and the relationships among pain, suffering, and disability.
2. Modify maladaptive thoughts, images, and feelings associated with emotional distress, such as exaggerated perception of danger or loss, poor self-esteem, and anger. Combat demoralization.
3. Teach patients how and when to use coping techniques for specific challenges, for example,

symptom-coping skills, practical problem-solving skills, and self-control and self-management skills to diminish emotional distress.
4. Foster a sense of self-control and power to effect change to counteract feelings and perceptions of helplessness and hopelessness.
5. Teach patients to anticipate problems and deal with them as they arise, thus preventing relapse.

are identified, patients can consider alternative thoughts and strategies that might be used in similar circumstances. They can try these alternative thoughts and record the effects. For example, when a patient is reminded by his wife of growing financial pressures, he may think he has failed because of his inability to provide for the family financially. Labeling himself a failure leads to feelings of helplessness and hopelessness that can exacerbate his pain and depression. Many different thoughts and techniques can replace these distorted, self-defeating ones, such as changing the thought that his wife is blaming him to the thought that she is trying to get them to develop a plan to manage their finances. By viewing the situation realistically, he can limit the impact of stress on pain and depression.

The crucial element in successful treatment is effecting a shift from habitual and ineffective responses to systematic problem solving and planning, control of affect, behavioral persistence, or disengagement when appropriate. Reconceptualization continues throughout treatment to continually challenge patients' beliefs about their helplessness in the face of their symptoms. Patients learn to view symptoms and impairments as experiences they can differentiate, modify systematically, and control personally. Reconceptualization of the maladaptive view of physical symptoms provides incentive for patients to develop various coping skills to control symptoms (see *Functions of cognitive reconceptualization*).

Techniques for cognitive reconceptualization
Cognitive reconceptualization helps patients to identify anxiety-engendering and other maladaptive appraisals and expectations and

PAIN MANAGEMENT PRINCIPLES

Functions of cognitive reconceptualization

- Provides a more benign view of problems than the patients' original views.
- Translates patients' physical and psychological symptoms into specific, addressable problems, rather than problems that are vague and uncontrollable.

- Recasts problems in forms that are amenable to solutions and thus fosters hope, positive anticipation, and expectation of success.
- Prepares patients for treatment interventions that are directly linked to the conceptualization proposed.
- Creates a positive expectation that the treatment being offered is appropriate to the problem.

subsequently to consider more appropriate interpretations (see *Steps in cognitive reconceptualization*, page 162).

Using these steps, the therapist encourages the patient to test the adaptiveness rather than the so-called rationality of individual thoughts, beliefs, expectations, and predictions. During the process of reconceptualization, the patient and therapist collaborate to perform the following:

- elicit the patient's thoughts, feelings, and interpretations of events
- gather evidence for or against the patient's interpretations
- identify and test the validity of the patient's habitual statements, images, and appraisals
- identify automatic thoughts that set up escalating streams of negative, catastrophizing ideations
- help the patient examine how habitual thoughts exacerbate stress and interfere with adaptive coping.

A number of additional techniques assist patients in congitive reconceptualization.

Therapists encourage self-monitoring of stress. As patients gain skill in self-monitoring they learn to identify low-intensity cues for emotional arousal and to defuse the automatic connection between certain events and arousal or distress. Therapists help patients to discriminate between functional symptoms like hyperventilation-induced chest pain and disease-based symptoms like angina upon exertion and to respond appropriately to each. Therapists may ask patients to monitor symptoms but not to overreact by assuming that all unusual or noxious sensations indicate worsening of disease.

Therapists construct an atmosphere of trust. In a trusting therapeutic alliance patients are free to express troublesome thoughts and con-

PAIN MANAGEMENT PRACTICE

Steps in cognitive reconceptualization

Cognitive reconceptualization assists patients in altering habitual maladaptive thoughts that prevent effective coping with pain. The technique calls for the care provider to coach the patient through these steps:

1. Explanation of the rationale for cognitive reconceptualization and an overview of the procedures
2. Identification of maladaptive thoughts during problematic situations such as exacerbations of pain, emotional arousal, and stress

3. Introduction and practice of coping thoughts
4. Shift from self-defeating to coping thoughts
5. Introduction and practice of positive or reinforcing thoughts
6. Home practice and follow-up

From Turk and Nash. "Psychological Issues in Chronic Pain." In *Pain Management: Theory and Practice.* Portenoy and Kanner (eds.) F. A. Davis Co., 1996. Adapted with permission.

cerns and then critically challenge the validity of their own beliefs. Rather than suggesting alternative thoughts, the therapist attempts to elicit competing thoughts from the patient and then reinforce the adaptive nature of these alternatives. Only after repetitive practice in cuing competent interpretations and evaluations will patients come to change their conceptualizations.

Therapists allow, even urge, the patients' expressions of concern, fear, and frustration. Patients may need to express anger with the health care system, insurance companies, employers, social system, family, fate, and perhaps themselves. Failure to address these issues will inhibit motivation and success. Oftentimes, other caregivers have been inattentive to or dismissive of such concerns, and an expression of genuine interest will help to forge a connection.

Common ground can be established by discussing the role of stress in medical conditions. Stress has little effect on some patients' physical symptoms but a noticeable impact on their emotional distress. In these cases, a somewhat different explanation of the role of stress in eliciting symptoms would be presented. In either case, therapists can point out that individuals can do a great deal to control their levels of arousal and emotional distress once they are identified as problematic. Control is presented in a way patients can understand, using personally relevant examples.

Therapists promote discussion of ways in which significant others respond to patients' increasingly adaptive conceptualization. Therapists should attempt to ascertain whether significant others inappropriately attempt to alter patients' increasingly adaptive responses to stress or pain. If this is the case, patients may benefit by rehearsal, role playing, and discussion of the issue. Patients who identify such opposition should be encouraged to discuss the issue with the nonsupportive individual.

Therapists encourage recall of situations associated with symptom exacerbation. Patients may be asked to relive recent experiences of stress as if they were viewing a movie in slow motion, eliciting the thoughts and feelings around specific events and responses. A recent conflict with a spouse might be examined to determine whether distress had any effect on the physical or psychological symptoms experienced. Imaginal presentation or recall of previous symptomatic exacerbations can be especially useful. With the help of their therapists, patients can discover the impact of thoughts and feelings on the experience of symptoms.

Identification of cognitive errors

Maladaptive thoughts typically fall within a common set of cognitive errors that affect pain perceptions and disability. A cognitive error may be defined as a negatively distorted belief about oneself, one's situation, or the future. (See *Common cognitive errors made by patients with pain*, page 164.) Cognitive errors commonly observed in those with chronic pain can be related to emotional difficulties associated with living with pain. Some have suggested that the cognitive error of catastrophizing is the most important factor in poor coping, rather than differences in specific adaptive coping strategies.

Once cognitive errors contributing to pain perception, emotional distress, and disability are identified they become the target of intervention. Patients are usually asked to generate alternative, adaptive ways of thinking and responding. For example, they might choose to say, "I'll just take one day at a time," or "I'll try to relax and calm myself down," or "Getting angry doesn't accomplish anything, I'll try to explain how I feel." Patients will usually be asked to practice these adaptive thoughts at home and to review them during therapy sessions. Therapists should applaud their patients for learning to change. Because changing habitual thought patterns takes time, therapists should also encourage patients to reinforce themselves simply for making the effort to change, not just for attaining results.

Home assignments and practice

An important feature of the cognitive-behavioral approach is the active involvement of patients and significant others in home assignments and practice. Patients and therapists mutually establish home practice goals for accomplishing targeted, observable, manageable tasks, starting with those that are most readily achievable and progressing to more

PAIN MANAGEMENT PRINCIPLES

Common cognitive errors made by patients with pain

- **Overgeneralizing:** Extrapolation from the occurrence of a specific event or situation to a large range of possible situations. For example, "The failure of this coping strategy means none of them can work for me."
- **Catastrophizing:** Focusing exclusively on the worst possibility, regardless of its likelihood of occurring. For example, "This pain in my back means my condition is degenerating and my whole body is falling apart."
- **All-or-none thinking:** Considering only the extreme "best" or "worst" interpretation of a situation without regard to the full range of alternatives. For example, "If I am not feeling perfectly well, I cannot enjoy anything."

- **Jumping to conclusions:** Accepting an arbitrary interpretation without a rational evaluation of its likelihood. For example, "The doctor is avoiding me because he thinks I am a hopeless case."
- **Selective attention:** Selectively attending to negative aspects of a situation while ignoring any positive things. For example, "Physical exercises only serve to make me feel worse than I already do."
- **Negative prediction:** Assuming the worst. For example, "I know this coping technique will not work" or "If I lose my hair as a result of chemotherapy, my husband will no longer find me attractive."
- **Mind-reading:** Making assumptions about the thoughts behind another person's words or actions. For example, "My family members do not talk to me about my pain because they don't care about me."

difficult ones. The purposes of graded tasks are to enhance patients' sense of competence and to reinforce their continued efforts.

Experiences of mastery gained through accomplishments have the greatest impact on establishing and strengthening expectations because they provide the most information about actual capabilities and thereby challenge maladaptive beliefs about the lack of self-control and self-efficacy. Home practice assignments provide important feedback to both patients and therapists. Successful completion of these assignments can be reinforced, and maladaptive patterns that inhibit rehabilitation can be identified and addressed directly. *Home practice for patients with pain* summarizes factors to consider when developing and implementing home practice assignments.

Self-management strategies

A wide variety of self-managment techniques have been shown to help patients reduce suffering and disability while living with pain. Some of these techniques foster self-regulation or control of pain-associated physiologic responses, such as relaxation training, biofeedback, and attention diversion. Others use stress-management skills such as problem solving to promote control of the stress-inducing thoughts, behav-

PAIN MANAGEMENT PRACTICE

Home practice for patients with pain

Cognitive-behavioral pain management requires the patient to complete specific tasks between each scheduled visit with the care provider. To promote optimum participation, consider these factors when assigning tasks to patients.

- *Customize* the task to the patient's needs and style. To increase patient commitment, whenever possible, set the task collaboratively with the patient.
- Design the practice tasks so they are *appropriate* for the patient's level of education, gender, and physical and psychological abilities.
- Try to create a *no-lose situation* to ensure success. Set standards slightly below what you believe the patient can reasonably do. Increase task demands as the patient succeeds. For example, if walking 300 yards is the upper limit, begin with a task of walking 150 yards for two days increasing to 200 yards for two days, 250 yards for two days, and so on until an appropriate limit is reached.

- *Explain* the rationale for each home practice task.
- Make instructions for home practice tasks as *concrete and specific* as possible. For example, practice relaxation exercises for 10 minutes once at 8:00 in the morning and once at 8:00 in the evening.
- Ask the patient to *write down* each home practice task, to read them back to you, and to explain the rationale.
- Ask the patient to *anticipate* what factors, including thoughts and feelings, might interfere with his or her ability to complete the home practice successfully.
- Ask the patient what he or she *can do* if impediments to successful completion of home practice arise.
- Ask the patient to *record* the time of practice and what occurred. Ask him or her to bring the recording sheets to the next session.
- *Review* the home practice at the next session. Modify requirements as needed.

iors, and emotions that trigger pain and maladaptive responses. With self-management techniques, instead of being passive recipients of medical intervention, individuals play active roles in learning and applying skills to manage episodic or persistent pain problems. As patients learn to self-regulate physiologic responses and manage stressful situations, their increased sense of personal control over pain and factors that influence pain combats demoralization.

Skills acquisition

In all rehabilitation, whether physical or psychological, it is essential for patients to understand the rationale for learning specific skills and performing specific tasks. Patients who do not understand the rationale for treatment components or who have not had the opportunity to address personal issues or sources of confusion are less likely to persevere in the face of obstacles, benefit from therapy, or maintain therapeutic gains.

Cognitive-behavioral treatment employs a range of techniques and procedures to help patients alter their perceptions of situations, moods, and behaviors as well as their abilities to modify their own psychological processes. Techniques such as progressive relaxation training, problem-solving training, distraction skills training, and communication skills training, to name only a few, have all been incorporated within the general cognitive-behavioral framework.

Several publications have described in detail some specific techniques, and interested readers should consult them (Bernstein and Borkovec, 1973; Kanfer and Goldstein, 1986; Turk et al., 1993). Perhaps more important than the specific tactics chosen are the strategic goals of enhancing self-control and intrinsic motivation. The manner in which the various skills are described, taught, and practiced may be more important than the skills per se.

It is essential for therapists to focus on patients' perspectives and perceptions of each skill and assignment. Without a satisfactory therapeutic alliance, treatment will grind to a halt. Treatment should not be viewed as a rigid process with fixed techniques but should be individualized, even though the rationale remains constant.

Problem solving

Problem solving, an important part of cognitive reconceptualization, consists of six steps, each of which is related to specific questions or actions (see *Problem solving as a cognitive behaviorial technique for coping with chronic pain*). The first step is to identify situations associated with pain. Use of a pain diary identifies pain-associated thoughts and feelings.

Once a set of problems has been identified, patients can generate a set of solutions and evaluate the likely outcome of implementing each possible solution. Patients may then try their strategies and evaluate the outcomes. If they are not satisfied with the first strategy, they can try another. There is no one perfect solution, but at a particular time some are more effective than others. Through successful problem-solving, individuals gain confidence in their abilities to handle stressful situations.

Relaxation

The most common and practical techniques for modifying pain are controlled breathing and deep muscle relaxation. Because relaxation exercises are easy to learn and appear to patients to be physically oriented and thus credible, they should be introduced early in treatment. The teaching and practice of relaxation not only helps patients circumvent muscle tension but also helps them develop a behavioral skill useful for any situation requiring adaptive coping. Relaxation

PAIN MANAGEMENT PRACTICE

Problem solving as a cognitive-behavioral technique for coping with chronic pain

First review the six steps in solving any problem. Then apply these steps to the problem of alleviating pain-associated stress.

Six steps in problem solving

Steps	Questions/actions
1. Problem identification	1. What is the concern?
2. Goal selection	2. What do I want?
3. Generation of alternatives	3. What can I do?
4. Decision making	4. What is my decision?
5. Implementation	5. Do it!
6. Evaluation	6. Did it work? If not, rethink.

How to apply problem solving to pain-associated stress

- Define the source of distress or stress reactions as a problem to be solved.

- Set realistic concrete goals by stating the problem in behavioral terms.
- Generate a wide range of possible courses of action to reach each goal.
- Imagine how others might respond if asked to deal with a similar problem.
- Evaluate the pros and cons of each proposed solution and rank the solutions from least to most practical.
- Rehearse strategies and behaviors by using imagery, role-reversal, or behavioral rehearsal.
- Try out the most feasible solution.
- Expect some failures, but reward yourself for having tried.
- Reconsider the original problem in light of the attempted solution.
- Rethink if necessary.

From Turk and Nash. "Psychological Issues in Chronic Pain." In *Pain Management: Theory and Practice.* Portenoy and Kanner (eds.) F. A. Davis Co., 1996. Adapted with permission.

practice strengthens patients' beliefs that they can exert some control during periods of stress and symptom arousal and that they are not helpless or impotent.

Therapists should discuss with patients how to identify bodily signs of physical tension, awareness of the stress-tension cycle, how occupying their attention can short-circuit stress, how relaxation reduces anxiety through the experience of exerting control, how relaxation and tension are incompatible states, and finally, how unwinding after stressful experiences can be therapeutic. Relaxation can be used for its direct effects on specific muscles, for reduction of generalized arousal, for its cognitive effects as a distraction or attention-diversion strategy, and for its value in increasing patients' sense of control and self-efficacy. Relaxation skills are generic and include a wide variety of techniques, for example, biofeedback, imagery, and controlled breathing. Relaxation skills also involve active efforts, such as aerobic exercise, walking, and engaging in a range of pleasurable activities.

Therapists presenting relaxation training should clearly indicate to patients that these techniques have a high success rate, are clinically indicated, and are within patients' capabilities to achieve.

Controlled breathing is a simple relaxation technique that may be used in situations that arouse acute exacerbations of pain (see *Controlled breathing exercise*).

Progressive muscle relaxation is useful because it has face validity, it is a concrete procedure, easy to recall and practice at home, and it is more resistant than passive techniques to distractions caused by symptom or cognitive intrusions. Slight symptomatic exacerbations that often accompany muscle tensing clearly demonstrate to patients the role of muscle activity in symptom exacerbation. If muscle tension increases symptoms, patients discover for themselves that the converse, muscle relaxation, reduces symptoms. Also, the results of even the first relaxation training session are often inherently reinforcing because generalized arousal is reduced. Therapists can build on this initial success to predict the potential benefits that will come with practice. Instructions for progressive muscle relaxation exercises appear in *Progressive Relaxation Training* (Bernstein and Borkovec, 1973).

Throughout the practice of relaxation techniques, therapists act as their patients' collaborators. Assuming that role helps patients to conceptualize relaxation as a *self*-management skill for self-control of stress, affective distress and, at times, physical symptoms. Through frequent statements about patients' efforts and progress, therapists should foster the perception of success. Failure during the initial stages of treatment can seriously undermine the patients' confidence and motivation.

Following each session, patients should receive specific home practice assignments to perform, self-monitor, and record. At the beginning of each subsequent session, therapists should review the self-monitored practice records with patients to identify problems and to reinforce effort as well as success.

After patients have become proficient in relaxation, they are encouraged to visualize themselves employing relaxation skills in various situations of stress or conflict. Therapists may also describe how other patients have reported overcoming difficulties in trying to relax. In this way, patients learn that they can overcome problems that might arise and that they are not alone in experiencing difficulties. Therapists should point out that relaxation is a skill that requires practice. In subsequent sessions, therapists should emphasize the importance of relaxing with activities, such as exercise (walking, swimming), hobbies (knitting, gardening), and so forth, in addition to practicing the formal skills of progressive relaxation and controlled breathing.

PAIN MANAGEMENT PRACTICE

Controlled breathing exercise

Controlled breathing helps patients cope with pain by promoting both relaxation and a sense of self-control. To teach controlled breathing, follow these steps:

1. The patient should sit or lie down in a comfortable, relaxed position.
2. Instruct the patient to inhale slowly and deeply through the nose.
3. Instruct the patient to count up to five at 1-second intervals and then to slowly exhale.
4. Instruct the patient that between each count to think of a single word, such as "calm" or "peace," to help reduce distracting or stressful thoughts.

5. Instruct the patient to hold the breath for 5 seconds and then to exhale slowly through the mouth, counting backwards from five to one and silently thinking of the chosen word. While exhaling, instruct the patient to let the chest and stomach muscles relax and, if seated, to drop the shoulders.
6. Repeat this cycle at least three times, but continue for 3 to 5 minutes.
7. If the patient reports feeling light-headed, suggest alternation of a few shallow breaths between the deep breaths.
8. After the exercise is over, ask the patient about the experience and whether any difficulties arose.

Because many pain problems have musculoskeletal or neuromuscular components, learning to reduce and control muscle tension can be effective for several reasons. Where pain is due to muscle spasm, muscle relaxation may reduce pain by decreasing spasm. In addition, muscle relaxation may also reduce the anxiety and distress that accompany persistent pain or trigger pain episodes. Relaxation can improve sleep, which may have secondary benefits; it is much easier to cope when rested than when fatigued due to lack of sleep. Muscle relaxation may also serve to distract the patient from noxious sensations.

All too often, therapists fail to understand that relaxation is a state of mind as well as body. Mental relaxation may be as important as physical relaxation. There are many types of relaxation and no one approach has been demonstrated to be more effective than any other. With assistance, most patients will be able to find several effective methods.

Biofeedback

Biofeedback has been used to treat a number of chronic pain states, such as headaches, back pain, and temporomandibular joint pain. Biofeedback procedures teach individuals to exert control over physiologic processes such as muscle tension, processes of which they normally have only marginal awareness. Quite simply, biofeedback equipment converts the readings of physiologic responses into visual or auditory signals. While attending to the signal feedback, patients develop voluntary control over physiologic responses by altering their thoughts or breathing. The sounds or lights may increase or become brighter, for example, as muscles become more tense and become softer or dimmer as muscle tension decreases.

Two types of biofeedback procedures are commonly used for pain problems. The most common type, electromyographic (EMG) biofeedback, monitors electrical signals arising from muscle tension, allowing patients to become aware of and control muscle tension that contributes to pain. Thermal biofeedback, which is most frequently used in the treatment of migraine headache, monitors skin temperature, usually of a finger, as an indication of changes in peripheral blood flow.

As individuals progress, they can control physiologic activity without the need of the biofeedback apparatus. With practice most people can learn to control important physiologic functions that may be associated directly with pain and stress.

The mechanisms by which biofeedback produces its positive effects are unknown. Early investigators believed that biofeedback directly reduced maladaptive physiological processes associated with pain. However, several studies have demonstrated that biofeedback can be beneficial when no physical changes occur, or even when patients learn to increase levels of muscle tension. One possible explanation is that for some individuals the biofeedback does actually lead to reduction in maladaptive physiologic activity, whereas for others the biofeedback serves to instill the belief that they can exert some control over their bodies and their symptoms. This belief might lead to other coping behaviors that reduce emotional distress and ameliorate the pain problem. Regardless of the mechanism, biofeedback, usually in conjunction with other modalities such as cognitive reconceptualization, appears to benefit some people with chronic pain.

Cognitive coping skills

Coping consists of purposeful and intentional acts employed in order to assume control over a stressful experience. It can be assessed in terms of covert and overt behaviors. Cognitive coping strategies for pain include various means of distraction from pain, reassurance about personal capabilities or the likelihood that the pain will diminish, seeking information, and problem solving. Effective coping strategies are thought to alter both the perceived intensity of pain and the ability to tolerate pain while continuing daily activities. Studies have suggested that there is no one best coping skill to manage pain and disability. Rather than teach only a specific coping strategy, it may be more helpful to introduce patients to many different coping skills, which they may combine as needed.

Attention diversion

Patients experiencing pain are often preoccupied with symptoms, but they also try to distract themselves by reading books, watching television, engaging in hobbies, listening to music, or using thoughts and imagination. This is not a new idea; there are numerous personal accounts of the use of distraction to control pain. For example, the philosopher Immanuel Kant described focusing on the works of classic philosophers whenever he was unable to sleep because of gout pain.

Attention diversion, also called cognitive distraction, includes a number of cognitive strategies for coping with pain and is best used during episodes of pain or symptom exacerbation. A great deal of research has examined the role of attentional focus in determining the relative efficacy of various cognitive distraction techniques. Ephrem Fernandez and Dennis Turk classified these techniques into five different groups:

- attentional focus on the environment rather than on the body
- attentional focus on neutral images
- attentional focus on dramatized images in which the painful part was included in the image, for example, imagining that one is a wounded spy who is trying to escape
- attentional focus on pleasant images
- involvement in rhythmic activity, for example, humming a song.

Each of these strategies has been shown to be effective for mild to moderate pain. Fernandez and Turk concluded that no one coping strategy was consistently more effective than any other, but imagery strategies as a set seemed to be more effective than those that did not include any imagery (Fernandez and Turk 1989). It is important to personalize the images. Patients should identify specific situations that they find pleasant and engaging and then create a detailed image that incorporates one or more of these valued situations. Some people may have difficulty generating a particularly vivid visual image and may find it helpful to listen to a taped description or to focus on a picture as a way of assisting imagination. It seems to be important to involve all sensory paths—sight, sound, touch, smell, and taste (see *Attention diversion using a pleasant image*, page 172).

Obviously, no one would suggest that people in pain should be physically inactive and do nothing but fantasize about pleasant situations. Rather, imagery is most useful when people are tired or alone, such as during periods of insomnia. It is a distraction skill that improves with practice. Imagery and other cognitive coping strategies are usually combined with other techniques, such as cognitive reconceptualization, relaxation, and problem solving and would not be suggested as the sole treatment approach for dealing with persistent pain.

PAIN MANAGEMENT PRACTICE

Attention diversion using a pleasant image

Attention diversion is a technique that encourages the patient to focus his thoughts on a pleasant image or memory as a means of reducing the stress of coping with pain. As an aid to attention diversion, the therapist or the patient may record and later replay an audio-taped description of a pleasant scene. Here is a script suitable for such an audio tape.

Picture yourself standing by the shore of a large lake, looking out across an expanse of blue water and beyond, to the far shore. Immediately in front of you stretches a small beach and behind you a grassy meadow. The sun is fierce and very hot, bathing the landscape in a shimmering brightness. It is a gorgeous summer day. The sky is pale blue, with a few soft, fluffy clouds gently drifting by. The breeze is blowing gently, just enough to make the trees sway and to make ripples in the grass. Feel the wind on your cheeks. It is a perfect day, and you have it entirely to yourself, with nothing to do and nowhere to go.

You have a blanket, a towel, and a can of lemonade with you, and you walk off with them through the meadow. You find a spot, spread the blanket and lie down on it. It is so warm and quiet. It's such a treat to have the day to yourself to just relax and take it easy. Think about the warm, beautiful day.

You walk toward the water, feeling the soft, lush grass under your feet. You reach the beach and start across it. It is very warm and very nice. Now visualize yourself wading into the water slowly up to your ankles, up to your knees. The water is so warm, it's almost like a bath. The water is so warm, so comfortable, as the breeze continues to blow. You look around you, and you are still alone. You still have this lovely spot all to yourself.

Far across the lake you can see a sailboat, tiny in the distance. It is so far away you can just make out the white sail jutting up from the blue water. You take another look around and decide to return to your spot to lie down and enjoy the sun. You head across that warm sand to the grass. You can feel the hot sun warming your skin. It must be 90 degrees, but it is clear and dry. The heat isn't too much to take, it's just nice and warm and comfortable.

You sit down and look around at the peaceful scene. You lift the can of lemonade to your mouth and smell the pungent citrus aroma. You take a drink from the can and taste the cool tangy liquid. It is very refreshing. You lie down on the blanket partly in the sun and partly in the shade and feel the deep, soft grass under you head. You're looking up at the sky, seeing those great billowy clouds floating by, far, far above. In the distance you can hear the rustle of the water on the beach. You can hear the sound of a bird singing in a tree nearby. You can even smell the sweet grass around you. You can feel the gentle breeze in your hair and on your skin. You are very comfortable, quite at ease, and totally relaxed. Take a minute or two to sit back and continue the image on your own, enjoying the positive feelings you have been able to bring forth.

From Turk, Meichenbaum, and Genest (1993). *Pain and Behavioral Medicine: A Cognitive-Behavioral Perspective.* Guilford Press. Adapted with permission.

Assertiveness and communication skills

Assertiveness training enables patients to reestablish their roles, particularly within the family, and thus to regain a sense of self-esteem and potency. By role playing existing tension-producing interpersonal transactions, patients and therapists can identify and modify maladaptive thoughts, feelings, and communication deficiencies that underlie nonassertiveness and practice adaptive alternatives. Patients may find assertiveness training useful in addressing reactions from family members and health care providers that oppose patients' self-management objectives.

Exercise and activity pacing

Physical exercise and activities are important not only in building muscle strength, flexibility, and endurance, but also in bolstering a sense of personal control over physical functioning. In addition, some evidence suggests that physical exercise can facilitate the release of endorphins, the body's own natural painkiller.

Patients should begin physical exercises at reasonably comfortable levels and gradually increase the activity levels. For example, at first it may be possible for a person with back pain to walk only half a block before experiencing pain. He or she may start by walking only one-quarter of a block and then over several days or weeks increase the distance walked. This permits early success and enhances confidence as successive goals are accomplished.

Patients with chronic pain need to learn that pain onset or exacerbation does not necessarily mean that harm is being done. Pain may simply be the result of using muscles that have been weakened from disuse. Chronic pain patients need to set an activity goal for each day and record progress toward that goal. They need to learn to pace their activities and rest only after completing the specified activity, rather than at the experience of pain. To record progress in meeting activity goals, patients can construct simple graphs with the days of the week on the horizontal axis and the amount of activity, for example, distance walked, on the vertical axis. In time, the benefits of exercise will be evident not only on the paper record, but also in feelings of improved physical and emotional health.

Skills consolidation

During the skills-consolidation phase of cognitive-behavioral treatment, patients practice and rehearse the skills gained during the skills-acquisition phase and apply them outside the clinic. This treatment phase employs mental rehearsal in which the patient imagines using the skills in different situations, role playing, and role reversal. An important goal of rehabilitation is development of the patient's ability to use newly learned skills in his or her own environment. Thus, home practice of all skills learned during the skills acquisition phase is critical. As patients practice skills at home, they should record their experiences, including difficulties that arise. Problems that arise in practice become subjects for discussion between therapist and patient.

Role playing and role reversal

Role playing is useful not only in the rehearsal of new skills but also in the identification of potential problem areas that may require special attention. Typically, patients are asked to identify and role play with therapists in situations that dramatize particular problems.

In role reversal, a variation of role playing, patients and therapists reverse roles. The patient is instructed to act as a therapist who is teaching specific pain-management skills to a patient with physical diagnoses similar to his or her own. The therapist acts as a patient. This exercise employs principles derived from research on attitude change, namely, that when people must improvise their responses, as in role playing or role reversal, they generate exactly the kinds of arguments, illustrations, and motivating appeals that they regard as most salient and convincing. In such situations, they not only emphasize those aspects of the skills training that are most convincing to them, but they also focus less on conflicting thoughts, doubts, and unfavorable consequences. In short, these exercises contribute to self-persuasion as well as permitting therapists to determine areas of confusion and potential difficulties.

Preparation for generalization and maintenance

To maximize the likelihood of maintenance and generalization of treatment gains, cognitive-behavioral therapists focus upon the cognitive activity of patients as they confront problems throughout treatment, for example, failure to achieve specified exercise goals or recurrent stresses. These events become opportunities to help patients learn how to handle such inevitable setbacks, lapses, and pain flare-ups because they will certainly occur once treatment is terminated.

Relapse prevention

In the final phase of treatment, discussion focuses on possible ways of predicting and avoiding or dealing with symptoms and symptom-related problems following treatment termination (see *Relapse prevention following therapy*). Patients are helped to identify high-risk situations such as a nonsupportive spouse or conflict with a child and to note the types of responses that may be necessary for successful coping.

Discussion of relapse must unfold delicately. On the one hand, therapists do not wish to convey an expectancy of treatment failure, but on the other hand, they wish to anticipate the potential for relapse by assisting patients to identify stressors that may precipitate an abandonment of newly acquired coping skills or an exacerbation of symptoms.

During this treatment stage, therapists should encourage patients to anticipate specific, symptom-exacerbating events, such as stress,

PAIN MANAGEMENT PRACTICE

Relapse prevention following therapy

- Discuss the importance of adherence to home practice throughout treatment, not just at termination.
- Address the patient's understanding of recommendations and why they are necessary. Be specific.
- Be proactive. Help the patient to anticipate problems; for example, identify high-risk situations that may undermine coping efforts.

- Teach patient how to deal with problems, setbacks, side-effects, and lapses in effort.
- Encourage self-reinforcement and the use of charts to self-monitor behavior and progress.
- Explain to significant others the necessity and importance of treatment recommendations and home practice.
- Enlist the assistance of significant others.

exercise, and conflicts, and to plan how they will deal with them. For example, one patient was anticipating his daughter's wedding soon after therapy termination. Using a future-oriented, problem-solving approach, the patient could identify both expected and potential problems, for example, dancing at the wedding reception, and poor service by the caterer. He was able to develop a plan to cope with such situations and with general, unanticipated problems and thereby decrease the likelihood of relapse and exacerbation of symptoms.

It is important to note that all possible problematic circumstances cannot be anticipated. Rather, the goal of this treatment phase, as of the entire treatment strategy, is to enable patients to develop the belief that they have the skills to respond appropriately to problems. In this phase of treatment patients learn to anticipate future difficulties, plan adaptive responses, and adjust behavior accordingly. Successful responses to problems further enhance patients' sense of self-efficacy and help to form a "virtuous circle" in contrast to the "vicious circle" created by inactivity, passivity, physical deconditioning, helplessness, and hopelessness.

The generalization and maintenance phase serves at least two purposes: It encourages patients to anticipate and plan for the post-treatment period and it focuses on the necessary conditions for long-term success. More specifically, relapse prevention helps patients understand that minor setbacks are inevitable and do not signal total failure. Rather, these setbacks should be viewed as cues to use the coping skills mastered during treatment. Most importantly, patients must accept ongoing personal responsibility for adherence to treatment recommendations.

During the final sessions, all aspects of the treatment should be reviewed. Therapists should focus discussions on what patients have learned, how they have changed during treatment, and how their own efforts have contributed to the positive changes. At this time, review of patients' self-monitoring charts fosters self-reinforcement of accomplishments. The goal is to help patients realize that they have skills and abilities within their repertoires to cope with their circumstances without contacting their therapists and without becoming dependent on others. Patients should no longer view themselves as patients but as competent people who happen to have some physical symptoms and discomfort.

Concluding comments

For patients, pain complaints connote distress and are pleas for assistance. The subjective experience of pain includes an urge to escape from the cause or, if that is not possible, to obtain relief. The overwhelming desire to terminate pain gives it power. It can produce fear and depression and, ultimately, a diminished will to live.

It has become abundantly clear that no isomorphic relationship exists between tissue damage and pain report. This chapter has discussed the view of pain as a perceptual process not directly proportional to nociceptive input but rather the result of nociceptive modulation at a number of different levels in the central nervous system.

Current knowledge suggests that pain must be viewed as a complex phenomenon that incorporates physical, psychosocial, and behavioral factors. The range of centrally important psychological variables along with current understanding of the physiological basis of pain were reviewed. Also described were the gate control and cognitive-behavioral models, both of which incorporate much available research and clinical information. The latter section of the chapter focused on comprehensive assessment techniques and cognitive-behavioral treatment modalities designed to reduce maladaptive thoughts, feelings, and behaviors associated with the pain experience.

Pain has become an area of vigorous research, and the virtual explosion of information will surely lead to refinements in understanding and advances in clinical management.

REFERENCES

American Psychiatric Association. *Diagnostic and Statistical Manual*, 4th ed. Washington, D.C.: American Psychiatric Association, 1994.

Bandura, A., et al. "Perceived Self-Efficacy and Pain Control: Opioid and Nonopioid Mechanisms," *Journal of Personality and Social Psychology* 53(3):563-71, September 1987.

Bergner, M., et al. "The Sickness Impact Profile: Development and Final Revision of a Health Status Measure," *Medical Care* 19(8):787-805, August 1981.

Bernstein, D.A., & Borkovec, T.D. *Progressive Relaxation Training.* Champaign, Ill.: Research Press, 1973.

Beutler, L.E., et al. "Inability to Express Intense Affect: A Common Link Between Depression and Pain?" *Journal of Consulting and Clinical Psychology* 54:752-59, 1986.

Blumer, D., & Heilbronn, M. "Chronic Pain as a Variant of Depressive Disease: the Pain-Prone Disorder," *Journal of Nervous and Mental Disease* 170:381-406, 1982.

Bonica, J.J. "Cancer Pain: Importance of the Problem," in *Advances in Pain Research and Therapy*, vol 2. Edited by J.J. Bonica and V. Ventafridda. New York: Raven Press, 1979.

Council, J.R., et al. "Expectancies and Functional Impairment in Chronic Low Back Pain," *Pain* 33(3):323-31, June 1988.

Engel, G.L. "Psychogenic Pain and the Pain-Prone Patient," *American Journal of Medicine* 26:899-918, 1959.

Fairbank, J.C.T., et al. "The Oswestry Low Back Pain Disability Questionnaire," *Physiotherapy* 66(8):271-73, August 1980.

Fernandez, E., and Turk, D.C. "The Utility of Cognitive Coping Strategies for Altering Pain Perception: A Meta-Analysis," *Pain* 38(2):123-35, August 1989.

Flor, H., et al. "Assessment of Stress-Related Psychophysiological Responses in Chronic Back Pain Patients," *Journal of Consulting and Clinical Psychology* 53(3):354-64, June 1985.

Fordyce, W.E. *Behavioral Methods for Chronic Pain and Illness.* St. Louis: Mosby–Year Book, Inc., 1976.

Holbrook, T.L., et al. *The Frequency of Occurrence, Impact and Cost of Selected Musculoskeletal Conditions in the United States.* Park Ridge, Ill.: American Academy of Orthopaedic Surgeons, 1984.

Jamner, L.D., and Tursky, B. "Syndrome-Specific Descriptor Profiling: A Psychophysiological and Psychophysical Approach," *Health Psychology* 6(5):417-30, 1987.

Jensen, M.P., et al. "Correlates of Improvement in Multidisciplinary Treatment of Chronic Pain," *Journal of Consulting and Clinical Psychology* 62(1):172-79, February 1994.

Kanfer, F.H. *Helping People Change: A Textbook of Methods*, 4th ed. Needham Heights, Mass.: Allyn & Bacon, 1992.

Kerns, R.D., et al. "The West Haven-Yale Multidimensional Pain Inventory (WHYMPI)," *Pain* 23(4):345-56, December 1985.

Lawrence, R.C., et al. "Estimates of the Prevalence of Selected Arthritic and Musculoskeletal Diseases in the U.S.," *Journal of Rheumatology* 16(4):427-41, April 1989.

Manning, M.M., and Wright, T.L. "Self-Efficacy Expectancies, Outcome Expectancies, and the Persistence of Pain Control in Childbirth," *Journal of Personality and Social Psychology* 45(2):421-31, August 1983.

Melzack, R. "The McGill Pain Questionnaire: Major Properties and Scoring Methods," *Pain* 1(3):277-99, September 1975.

Melzack, R., and Wall, P.D. "Pain Mechanisms: A New Theory," *Science* 50:971-79, 1965.

Merskey, H. "Classification of Chronic Pain: Descriptions of Chronic Pain Syndromes and Definitions of Pain Terms," *Pain* Suppl.3, S1-S225, 1986.

National Center for Health Statistics. Koch, H. "The Management of Chronic Pain in Office-Based Ambulatory Care: National Ambulatory Care Survey," *Advanced Data from Vital and Health Statistics.* No. 123, DHHS Pub No (PHS) 86-1250. Hyattsville, Md.: Public Health Service, 1986.

O'Leary, A., et al. "A Cognitive-Behavioral Treatment for Rheumatoid Arthritis," *Health Psychology* 7(6):527-44, 1988.

Osterweis, M., et al. *Pain and Disability: Clinical, Behavioral, and Public Policy Perspectives.* Washington, D.C.: National Academy Press, 1987.

Peebles, R.J., and Schneidman, D.S. *Socioeconomic Factbook for Surgery, 1991-1992.* Chicago: American College of Surgeons, 1991.

Raj, P.P. "Pain Relief: Fact or Fancy?" *Regional Anesthesia* 15(4):157-69, 1990.

Rickard, K. "The Occurrence of Maladaptive Health-related Behaviors and Teacher-rated Conduct Problems in Children of Chronic Low Back Pain Patients," *Journal of Behavioral Medicine* 11(2):107-16, 1988.

Roland, M., and Morris, R. "A Study of the Natural History of Back Pain. Part I: Development of a Reliable and Sensitive Measure of Disability in Low Back Pain," *Spine* 8(2):141-44, March 1983.

Schmidt, A.J.M. "Cognitive Factors in the Performance Level of Chronic Low Back Pain Patients," *Journal of Psychosomatic Research* 29(2):183-89, 1985.

Spiegel, D., and Bloom, J.R. "Pain in Metastatic Breast Cancer," *Cancer* 52(2):341-45, July 15, 1983.

Stewart, W.F., et al. "Prevalence of Migraine Headache in the United States: Relation to Age, Income, Race, and Other Sociodemographic Factors," *Journal of the American Medical Association* 267(1):64-69, January 1, 1991.

Tota-Faucette, M.E., et al. "Predictors of Response to Pain Management Treatment: The Role of Family Environmental Changes in Cognitive Processes," *Clinical Journal of Pain* 9(2):115-23, June 1993.

Turk, D.C., and Meichenbaum, D. "Cognitive-Behavioral Approach to the Management of Chronic Pain," in *Textbook of Pain*, 3rd ed. Edited by Wall, P.D. and Melzack, R. New York: Churchill Livingstone, 1994.

Turk, D.C., et al. *Pain and Behavioral Medicine: A Cognitive-Behavioral Perspective.* NY: Guilford Press, 1993.

Turk, D.C. and Melzack, R. *Handbook of Pain Assessment.* New York: Guilford Press, 1992.

Turk, D.C., and Nash, J.M. "Psychological Issues in Chronic Pain," in *Contemporary Neurology.* Edited by Portenoy, R.K., et al. Philadelphia: F.A. Davis, in press.

Turk, D.C., and Salovey, P. "Chronic Pain as a Variant of Depressive Disease: A Critical Reappraisal," *Journal of Nervous and Mental Disease* 172(7):398–404, July 1984.

Turk, D.C., and Salovey, P. "Illness Behavior: Normal and Abnormal," in *Psychosocial Management of Chronic Illness.* Edited by Nicassio, P. and Smith, T.W. Washington, D.C.: American Psychological Association, in press.

CHAPTER 6

Noninvasive techniques for managing pain

Mary F. Bezkor, MD
Mathew H. M. Lee, MD, MPH, FACP

Many types of pain can be managed by the use of noninvasive or conservative techniques that do not pierce the skin or disturb the integrity of the body. Invasive procedures often require a recovery phase that necessitates intensive monitoring or even hospitalization. Noninvasive measures provide symptom relief without adding the problems of wound healing or postprocedure recovery. Noninvasive techniques frequently incorporate readily available objects or methods. Other advantages include a generally lower risk of infection and complications.

The cooperation of patients is often a key factor in the use of noninvasive pain relief measures. The use of exercise, bracing, and physical means such as heat or cold application, all common elements of noninvasive pain management, require the participation and consent of patients. The recovery process may often be slow, occurring gradually and subtly over time. Patients who have experienced a dramatic change in pain status as a result of invasive measures may lose motivation during a slower course of conservative therapy. With proper supervision and guidance these patients can often maintain steady and gradual gains if educated about what to expect in this type of recovery.

Many common pain syndromes, such as low back pain, arthritis, and ligament strain, are managed in the early phase of recovery through immobilization, temporary bracing, and physical modalities such as heat and cold treatments. They address the acute situation and help to contain severe pain. Selection of appropriate treatment is essential to success, and assessment, physical exam, and diagnostic testing are always the first steps in the process. After initiation of primary measures, caregivers should develop a progressive treatment plan that includes follow-up and maintenance in order to insure optimal recovery.

Later recovery involves mobilization, exercise, and a return to a more fully functional lifestyle. Progression during this phase frequently requires clinical skill and insightful supervision. Therapists must maintain patient motivation while remaining attentive to changing patterns of pain. At times a physical condition can change or become more complex and then require different treatment, which may include invasive measures.

Some types of pain, for example cancer pain or diabetic neuropathy, require special consideration. The use of the physical techniques described in this chapter must be very selective for any disease that results in impaired sensation or compromised skin integrity. The origin of the pain, whether from skin, muscle, joint, or bone, will often determine the correct choice of noninvasive treatment. Proper assessment and diagnosis always come into play. To reach these various levels, different types of penetration or intensity are required. Choice of technique or physical modality will vary according to the anatomical origin of the pain. Superficial pain, for example, may respond well to modalities with minimal penetration, such as hot packs. Deep pain may require the use of ultrasound or deep massage. Muscular spasticity, another element complicating the spectrum of pain, can also be addressed through noninvasive techniques. Understanding of the anatomy involved and the physical principles of the chosen technique remains essential to safe and effective treatment. Attentiveness to all aspects of the pain cycle is a necessary element to choosing proper treatment.

Therapeutic heat and cold

Therapeutic heat and cold have long been tools in effective pain management through noninvasive measures. They have the advantages of easy application and ready availability, and in many cases, they offer a safe, effective alternative to medication (see *How heat and cold affect pain*).

Regional heating—heat therapy of selected body areas within a certain temperature range—can offer immediate temporary pain relief. The sedated area can then tolerate mobilization to a greater degree than when untreated. Heat is often applied in preparation for a therapeutic exercise routine. Regional heating can have a systemic effect resulting from the autonomic reflex responses to localized heat application. These reflex-mediated responses may cause elevated temperature, increased blood flow, or other physiologic changes in areas distant

PAIN MANAGEMENT PRINCIPLES

How heat and cold affect pain

Both heat and cold can produce analgesia for various types of pain. The mechanisms for analgesia produced by the different temperature extremes are not completely known, but it is possible to point out the general physiologic effects of heat and cold and to speculate on how they affect the pain response.

Heat

The effects of heat therapy include increased blood flow, increased tissue metabolism, and decreased vasomotor tone. Heat also increases the viscoelasticity of connective tissue, an effect that produces temporary relief of joint stiffness. The overall effects of local heat application include analgesia, sedation, relief of muscle spasticity and vascular congestion, and elevation of the pain threshold.

Unwanted side effects of heat include increased inflammation and accumulation of edema. Increased metabolic demands of the tissue exposed may result in vascular insufficiency and subsequent ischemia. Patients with sensory impairment of the area may experience burning or skin damage. Metal implants and bony prominences are particularly vulnerable to the undesirable side effects of heat.

Cold

Cold therapy tends to reduce vascular flow and as a result is often helpful in reducing or controlling the effects of edema. Cold therapy counteracts inflammation and fever and also diminishes muscle spasticity. In addition, cold application to free nerve endings reduces nerve conduction velocity, an effect that may elevate the pain threshold. Cold analgesia fits into the gate control theory of pain, or regulation of pain perception through a gating mechanism at the dorsal horn of the spinal cord. Vasoconstriction and decreased nerve conduction velocity result in reduced transmission of noxious stimuli to the "gate."

Cold therapy is not suitable for patients with vascular insufficiency, cold intolerance, and conditions directly aggravated by cold, such as Raynaud's phenomenon (cold-induced arterial spasm and subsequent numbness in the fingers), cryoglobulinemia (the presence of abnormal blood proteins that crystalize upon exposure to cold), and paroxysmal cold hemoglobinuria (a condition in which exposure to cold leads to passage of hemoglobin into the urine).

from the heated site. Regional heating may sometimes result in total body temperature elevation. This response is called reflex heating.

Contraindications to heat exposure include active infection, active bleeding, vascular insufficiency, skin desensitization, and neoplasm. Exposure to heat may sometimes accelerate an undesirable process. The body, when compromised, may be unable to meet the additional metabolic demands associated with heat exposure.

Therapeutic heat is delivered to the body by three means:

- conduction, the direct transmission of heat from a thermal energy source
- convection, the delivery of heat via warmed liquid or gas
- conversion, the delivery of heat through the partial transformation of nonthermal energy such as soundwaves into thermal energy.

Therapeutic cold within a certain temperature range also has pain-reducing qualities and can be additionally helpful in the control of spasticity. Cold can reduce swelling and inflammation in the acute stage; however, extreme cold exposure can lead to vascular incompetence and subsequent tissue necrosis.

Thermotherapy

Hot packs, or hydrocollator packs, the most common heat conduction device used in therapy, are composed of a cloth-covered silica gel core, which is chosen for its ability to retain heat. The pack is heated in a hot water bath, then dried and wrapped in insulating terry cloth to protect the skin from burns. The unit is then placed on the body for 20 to 30 minutes, during which time heat is conducted to the skin from the pack. Hot packs provide regional heating to the trunk, spine, or limbs and are effective in the treatment of muscle spasm, tendinitis, and bursitis. The heat penetration is superficial, only a few millimeters into the skin. Paraffin bath, another heat conduction method, is frequently effective in treatment of the arthritic hand. The paraffin is mixed with mineral oil to improve skin tolerance and avoid burning. Progressive dips are performed in the bath to produce a paraffin "glove" that delivers safe and penetrating heat.

Ultrasound is a commonly used form of conversion heat. The energy generated from a quartz crystal passes from an applicator through a transmission gel covering the patient's skin and into the targeted area of the patient's body. The energy is ultimately converted to heat wherever it is reflected, especially at interfaces of soft tissue and bone. Some ultrasound is converted to heat at the level of skin, subcutaneous tissue, and muscle, but most of the heating effect is deep. Ultrasound treatment results in increased blood flow, pain threshold elevation, and increased tissue metabolism. Since superficial heating may be minimal, some types of pain are treated with a combination of a hot pack for superficial penetration and ultrasound for treatment of deep tissues.

Undesirable side effects of ultrasound include cavitation, damage that results when a sound wave pattern induces formation of gas bubbles in tissue. Cavitation is avoided through use of a stroking technique in applying the treatment or by using pulsed sound waves. Ultrasound cannot be used over the eye or over fluid-filled sacs. It should not be used near the site of an abscess or neoplasm and must be avoided or used with caution in patients who have had previous spinal surgery. It can cause periosteal superheating if used over bony surfaces.

Infrared and ultraviolet light, both forms of radiant energy that convert to produce superficial heating, are less commonly used in a therapeutic setting. Skin carcinoma is a serious side effect associated with exposure to ultraviolet light. Radiant heat is less desirable as a therapeutic choice because it is not applied to the body directly and therefore may spread to areas not intended for treatment.

Microwave diathermy is an electromagnetic wave that produces conversion heating. Microwaves are selectively absorbed by tissues with high water content. Microwave treatment is effective in relieving pain associated with rotator cuff tears, sprains, strains, herniated disks, and arthritis. The use of microwave diathermy is contraindicated in persons with implanted cardiac pacemakers. Shortwave diathermy, yet another form of electromagnetic conversion heat, assists in recovery from low back pain and tenosynovitis (inflammation of a tendon sheath).

Hot packs and ultrasound are the most common heat modalities used in the therapeutic setting. However, emergency and home use alternatives are also necessary to manage pain. Electric heating pads are a safe alternative method if people are properly instructed. Attention to product intactness, package instructions, and limitation of time exposure can usually eliminate the chance of injury. Children, elderly or frail patients, and patients who lack normal temperature or pain sensations should use these products only under close supervision.

Cryotherapy

Cool and cold modalities provide immediate pain relief and are additionally helpful in reducing or preventing edema and swelling. Spasticity can also be effectively controlled by the use of therapeutic cold.

Cold therapy is often appropriate for acute pain, especially the pain of sports-related injuries, such as muscle sprains and ligament sprains of a joint. Also, postfracture pain and swelling can frequently be reduced through the use of cold modalities.

Ice is often used for pain relief but can be too harsh if applied directly to the skin. An ice bag, a waterproof pack covered with insulating material, provides effective protection from skin chafing, but the irregular shapes of the individual ice pieces often cause uneven temperature exposure. The flexible pack filled with an ice and water slurry effectively delivers cold to uneven surfaces, allowing the treatment to be adapted to different body parts.

The cool pack, another common, useful item, consists of a cold-retaining gel enclosed in a soft plastic pouch. The gel maintains a cool temperature when refrigerated for a relatively brief period of time. These packs are inexpensive, reusable, and quite effective for both clinical and home use. Patients with pain that is responsive to cold should have several cool packs on hand so that at least one pack can remain refrigerated while the other is in use.

Regional cooling has also been used to affect body temperature and produce mild or relative hypothermia. Most people are familiar with the use of cooling compresses to reduce a fever. Cooling can provide pain relief for patients whose disease symptoms would be worsened by the application of heat. For example, heat application to a joint with acute synovial inflammation from rheumatoid arthritis increases the inflammatory response and aggravates symptoms. In multiple sclerosis elevation of body core temperatuure can worsen disease symptoms. The proposed mechanism of this effect is a thermally induced block in nerve conduction. Thermal cooling suits have been used in this disorder to produce beneficial effects.

Application of cold by aerosol sprays is also used as part of a muscle-stretching treatment for painful trigger points in myofascial pain syndromes (see "Medication combined with physical modalities" later in this chapter).

Hydrotherapy

Water, a classic and extremely versatile therapeutic modality, can deliver convection heat or it can cool. It offers total body immersion or regional exposure of a selected body part. Many people who resist medication or technical machinery easily adapt to the familiarity of water in a therapeutic setting.

Pool therapy (total body immersion in a pool) is used in pain management. The buoyancy of the water provides an antigravity effect that unloads painful joints and muscles and allows patients to move more freely than on land. Patients may also move their limbs against the resistance of the water to receive a beneficial exercise effect. Pool therapy is effective for relief of low back pain as well as pain associated with arthritis and osteoporosis. It is also used to reduce painful spasticity associated with spinal cord injury and multiple sclerosis.

Immersion of the body in water also produces a systemic effect. If the pool is warm, there may be a resultant decrease in blood pressure and increase in vascular dilation. Cool temperature settings may produce an initial increase in heart rate and vasoconstriction. The therapist must be attentive to temperature tolerance in various pain-associated conditions. Arthritic persons may have a relatively high tolerance for heat. Those who are cardiac- and pulmonary-impaired are usually heat-intolerant. Cooler settings are more appropriate for intensive exercise or sports.

There are other concerns to be addressed prior to initiating pool therapy. Open wounds are contraindicated since the lesion may either become infected or infected material may drain from it. Bowel and bladder incontinence is another contraindication to pool therapy. Chlorine or chemical sensitivity is also an issue. Inability to swim need not interfere with pool therapy, but a life vest should be used for these patients.

Individual immersion systems

A Hubbard tank is a smaller total body immersion system used for individual treatment. For patients who are at risk for infection this device allows immersion along with isolation and protection. The Hubbard tank is useful in the control of pain associated with burns because the small volume of water permits close temperature regulation and the addition of electrolytes, both of which are necessary for safety in treating burn pain.

Whirlpool therapy adds gentle agitation of the water for a therapeutic effect. It is useful in pain management of muscle sprains and chronic spinal conditions. Smaller whirlpool tanks can also be used to treat a painful extremity. The pain of skin debridement from wounds such as burns can be greatly reduced with whirlpool therapy. The skin-moistening effects of the water help alleviate the pain of debridement, and the agitation of the water helps loosen the necrotic skin. Mobilization of a contracted or spastic extremity can be achieved in a less painful manner with whirlpool therapy.

Water is also used as a regional soak that allows wound cleansing and then debridement with less pain. Selective use of regional soaks encourages drainage of painful fluid accumulation. In addition, regional soaks are effective in cooling a body affected by fever or exertion.

Electrical modalities

Electricity is an effective pain management tool. Both direct (galvanic) and alternating (faradic) currents can be applied. Muscle activity is, in fact, based on electrochemical activity at the interface between nerve and muscle and within the muscle fibers themselves. Therefore, electric current can affect muscular response and assist in pain reduction.

Electricity must, of course, be used with understanding and an appropriate level of caution. Electric modalities are contraindicated in persons with artificial cardiac pacemakers or defibrillators. Other implanted devices that function to pump insulin or antispasticity medication would also be adversely affected by exposure to a second electrical device. Good candidates for some types of electrical treatments may be those who are intolerant of heat modalities. When performed in therapeutic settings, electrical stimulation alone does not expose the patient to a heating effect.

Galvanic current is a direct, continuous, and unidirectional flow of current between the positive, or acid, anode and the negative, or alkaline, cathode. It can cause a contraction in denervated muscle and is used for patients with paralysis to retard muscle atrophy. For true clinical success in maintaining muscle bulk, the length of exposure and intensity of contracture is still an area that encourages further research. Direct current also causes an increase in blood and lymph flow, an increase in tissue metabolism, and a pain-reducing effect. Direct current is also used in iontophoresis, or ion transfer, to drive acidoid or alkaloid materials into the skin. Ionotophoresis with salicylates and lidocaine combined with active exercise are used to treat musculoskeletal pain and pain of neuromuscular origin, including low back pain, sprains, bursitis, sciatica, and shoulder muscle spasm.

Alternating current changes direction constantly. Both faradic and sinusoidal currents are examples of alternating current. The application of alternating current to innervated muscle may produce muscle relaxation, alleviation of spasticity, and pain reduction. It is used in spinal cord trauma in those cases where the cord has not been severed. Localized pain problems, such as frozen shoulder and tendinitis, also respond to stimulation with alternating current.

Transcutaneous electrical nerve stimulation (TENS) is commonly used for pain management in the therapeutic setting (see *Some current uses of TENS*). It is a form of alternating current delivered through a small, compact battery. TENS units possess two channels and up to four lead placements. The settings allow adjustment of wave frequency, duration, and intensity. Waves can be delivered in a continuous mode for a low-level numbing effect or in a burst mode, which simulates the sensation of an "electrical massage." Therapists often preset some of the unit options, but patients usually control the intensity. With practice and careful instruction, patients can achieve a fair tolerance for electrical stimulation.

TENS seems to affect trigger points. Perpendicular placement of the leads can have an effect similar to trigger-point massage, acupuncture, or injection. It also seems to affect the pain threshold and may have other autonomic effects as well. Controlled studies of TENS seem to produce conflicting results. Distraction and the placebo effect have been cited by those who doubt the efficacy of TENS for pain management. TENS units are often used by patients for home treatments. Proper instruction in the use of the device is essential. Careful clinical assessment and case selection eliminate the problem of overprescribing this modality.

PAIN MANAGEMENT PRACTICE

Some current uses of TENS

Transcutaneous electrical nerve stimulation (TENS) must be prescribed by a physician and is most successful if it is administered and taught to the patient by a therapist skilled in its application. TENS has been used for temporary relief of acute pain such as postoperative pain and for ongoing relief of chronic pain such as sciatica. Pain problems that responded to TENS include:

• Arthritis
• Bone fracture pain

• Bursitis
• Cancer-related pain
• Low back pain
• Myofascial pain
• Musculoskeletal pain
• Neurogenic pain (neuralgias, neuropathies)
• Phantom limb pain
• Postoperative incision pain
• Sciatica
• Whiplash

Traction

Traction is an effective and sometimes powerful technique when used with appropriate clinical assessment and precautions. It employs weights and a pulley system to apply a distracting force to the spine or extremity. The application of this force separates normally contingent bony surfaces or enlarges the space within a joint without rupturing or displacing the associated ligaments. It is often used in the hospital setting for stabilizing limb fractures. Traction is applied to the spinal column in the treatment of vertebral fracture and dislocation with associated spinal cord injury.

Traction of reduced intensity is used to apply a gentle pulling force appropriate for pain management, particularly for cervical and lumbar spine pain. In these cases traction produces soft-tissue stretching and relief of muscle spasms. Spinal traction is often applied through the familiar suspended weight and pulley system. Sometimes, though, the body itself can be suspended to produce its own traction effect. Inversion or suspension of patients in traction frames use the weight of the body as a distraction force on the spine. This type of traction requires very careful attention to individual tolerance as patients may experience intense vascular congestion below the level of suspension, an effect that can sometimes cause loss of consciousness.

The weights used in low-intensity traction systems may be simple metal plates or flexible containers filled with water. The water-filled containers offer certain advantages that improve the safety of home units, namely the ability to make small additions of weight to the system and the ability to unload the system quickly if necessary.

Traction can also be applied by an electrically driven distracting force. These units are used in therapeutic settings and require proper clinical assessment and skill for safe use. The traction force may be applied through continuous or intermittent exposure. Tolerance to these two techniques may vary widely. Patient selection tends to be a key factor.

Certain precautions must always be observed in patient selection and technique application. Special attention must be taken to avoid injury or excessive pressure to the area where the force is applied. Dental injuries, nerve entrapment, and skin damage are usually preventable when safety measures are followed and protective padding is used. Traction cannot be applied to an artificial joint. Traction for pain control may be unsafe in patients with certain underlying skeletal abnormalities, such as metastatic disease or multiple myeloma.

Cervical spine traction, commonly seen in a clinical setting, is helpful in reducing the pain associated with cervical arthritis and muscle tension. It should not be applied to patients with an acutely herniated disk or spinal instability; therefore, proper clinical assessment is essential. Diagnostic testing, including X-ray, MRI, or CT scan of the spine, is usually required prior to traction application.

Lumbar spine traction for acute low back pain was once a common cause for hospitalization but now is not as commonly used. Strict bed rest may, in fact, be as effective as lumbar traction. However, traction is often used to help improve patient compliance for bed rest. It serves as a continuous reminder to patients to maintain immobilization yet can be removed easily for safety, hygiene, and bathroom privileges.

Massage and manipulation

Massage, a hands-on approach to pain management, means rubbing, kneading, or manipulating various soft tissues (skin, muscles, ligaments, tendons, or fascia) to produce a pain-relieving and muscle-relaxing effect. Increased blood and lymph flow to the massaged area plays a role in the therapeutic response.

Therapists employ a range of massage methods. Techniques can be very light or deep and penetrating. Massage is traditionally a manual technique, but many different types of electrically powered massage units are now commonly available, and they enable therapists to deliver treatment without experiencing manual fatigue. Electrical units also enable massage to be applied in the home setting. Some models offer effective self-administration of massage.

Massage induces a range of physiologic changes associated with analgesia, including relief of muscle spasms as well as arteriole dilation and constriction, effects that improve blood and lymph flow. Massage also loosens soft tissue adhesions, enhances muscle flexibility, and stimulates peripheral nerves through the repetitive movement of the therapist's hands or massage device. These known physiologic effects reveal why many people experience overall feelings of wellness following treatment.

Massage is also one of several techniques employed to deactivate trigger points. These tender muscle foci may be painful on direct palpation, but they also may refer pain to other anatomical sites. In addition to massage, TENS, spray-and-stretch techniques, and acupuncture have been shown to be effective in treating trigger-point pain. Injection of trigger points with either 5% lidocaine or normal saline also provides relief. Myofascial pain and fibromyalgia are two pain syndromes characterized by trigger points.

Massage should not be performed over bony prominences, exposed nerves, or compromised tissue. It also should be avoided in regions of active phlebitis or over arterial vascular structures. Knowledge of anatomy is essential to ensure safe technique.

Due to the pain-relieving and muscle-relaxing effects, many people with chronic pain request massage. As with all treatments, massage cannot be provided indefinitely. To achieve full recovery, people in pain must acquire a repertoire of self-management techniques such as an active exercise program. Massage is a passive experience. The later addition of an active exercise program enables patients to recondition and strengthen the muscles involved.

Manual manipulation

Manual manipulation is the delivery of forceful movement that articulates a joint in a manner not possible for patients to achieve independently. It brings about the passive stretching of adhesions in periarticular or intra-articular areas and results in restored ranges of motion. Therapists perform the movement in a quick manner, and a noticeable "click" or "snap" is often heard. Many times, the maneuver is combined with a sustained stretch. Effects of manipulation can be appreciated immediately in many cases. At times, slight discomfort may be experienced after the treatment.

Manipulation remains controversial in conventional allopathic medicine. Its mode of action and effectiveness for pain relief have still not been firmly established by the medical literature, yet it is a traditional form of treatment delivered to large numbers of patients, especially by osteopaths and chiropractors. Manipulation should be done only by trained professionals who are skilled in this particular technique. Proper clinical assessment and evaluation, including diagnostic testing, are required prior to treatment.

Manipulation is contraindicated in fractures, metastatic or neoplastic processes, and osteoporosis. Instability of the spine and large vertebral disk herniation are conditions in which manual manipulation should be avoided. Active infection or bleeding also endangers the patient. Although manipulation is a noninvasive technique, it has significant risks if used without proper assessment. The subject must be reevaluated between maneuvers. Local heat treatments prior to manipulation facilitate relaxation.

Medication combined with physical modalities

Both prescription and nonprescription medication can be used to enhance the benefits of physical modalities.

Spray-and-stretch treatment combines the use of cooling, medicated aerosol sprays (usually methyl fluoride or ethyl chloride) with the technique of passive or active stretching. The spray, chosen for its mild muscle-relaxing or anesthetizing properties, is directed at both the muscle origin and the point of insertion. The muscle is then exercised actively or passively to enhance the analgesic and antispasticity effects of the spray. Improved range of motion is achieved in this manner. A trained clinician or therapist is required for this technique. Spray-and-stretch is effective for persons who cannot tolerate heat modalities, but it is not suitable in the presence of skin infection or open lesions. Some patients may develop an allergy or skin sensitivity to the vapocoolant chemicals.

Iontophoresis is a technique that involves the use of direct electrical current to facilitate the introduction of charged acidoid or alkaloid substances into the skin. Lidocaine, a drug commonly applied in this technique, provides local analgesia so that the therapist can perform full range-of-motion movements necessary to relieve spasticity and reduce soft-tissue adhesions.

Phonophoresis employs ultrasound to deliver medication through the skin. Steroid preparations are applied in this manner to help reduce local musculoskeletal inflammation. The ultrasound reportedly improves drug diffusion.

Therapists must use caution when exposing patients who take prescription medications to a physical modality. For example, patients taking sulfa-based antibiotics are especially susceptible to burns produced by ultraviolet light. Transdermal medicine patches can dramatically change absorption rates if exposed to local heat treatments. The important point to remember is that physical modalities have the potential to affect the absorption and efficacy of various medications. Realizing this, the treating clinician can either use the effect therapeutically or take steps to avoid unwanted interactions.

Immobilization and bracing

For the intense pain related to trauma, acute illness, or injury, immobilization may be the best choice. A new injury, trauma, or surgical procedure may leave an individual unable to cope with the swelling, bruising, and fluid accumulation that often occur.

Immobilization of the body is achieved through simple bed rest. This is frequently a first-line management choice in acute lumbar pain. Bed rest offers a beneficial antigravity effect and is usually indicated for pain that is exacerbated by weight-bearing, such as fractures, ligament sprains, or muscle strains. Horizontal positioning also assists in reducing edema.

Immobilization permits scar formation between tissue interfaces, such as occurs following the suturing of a laceration or the casting of a fracture. It fosters an important step in the healing process, and pain reduction accompanies it. Immobilization is also appropriate for the acute pain associated with repetitive motion. The acute stages of carpal tunnel syndrome and degenerative arthritis are examples of disorders in which pain is exacerbated by repetitive motion.

However, immobilization cannot be used indefinitely. Undesirable complications of immobilization include muscle atrophy and dysfunction, skin breakdown, bone loss (osteoporosis), and venous stasis and inflammation (phlebitis). In venous complications involving deep veins, vascular stasis can result in life-threatening clots that travel to the lungs (pulmonary embolisms). Muscle dysfunction resulting from immobilization may be temporary, but it also sometimes requires significant active intervention to reverse.

A recuperative stage usually follows periods of prolonged immobilization. For pain that has been treated with initial immobilization, early mobilization (early reversal of the stasis period) through passive or active exercise techniques is frequently the key to successful management of the overall problem.

It may not be desirable to restrict people to bed rest after many types of injuries. Through the desirable alternatives of bracing or splinting, the trunk or affected extremity can be selectively immobilized. This strategy preserves the freedom of the person experiencing pain.

Bracing and orthotics

Bracing and orthotic devices have traditionally been used to achieve selective immobilization and alignment during treatment of soft-tissue and joint injuries as well as of fractures. In addition to partial and, in some cases, almost complete immobilization of a body part, bracing and orthotics can reduce pain and improve function. The devices, which originated with the primitive use of wood to make simple splints, can range from soft fabric garments to complex implements of metal and plastic. The selection of the appropriate brace requires proper clinical assessment of the problem being treated.

Orthotic devices and braces can be used on a temporary or long-term basis. Patients with acute injuries usually require temporary bracing and splinting. Patients who need assistance with function or ambulation may use braces over a long period of time. Chronic pain conditions that are aggravated by repetitive motion are often treated by the use of splints that are worn only during the pain-exacerbating activities.

Rigid versus soft orthotics

For strict alignment or positioning, such as treatment of long-bone fractures of the extremities, rigid bracing using metal and molded plastic orthotics is appropriate. Metal or custom-molded plastic is also used in the fabrication of braces that assist ambulation. The rigid structure helps position and unload painful weight-bearing joints. Although rigid bracing systems allow for some pain relief, they are coupled with the risk of skin breakdown. Careful skin monitoring is required in rigid bracing systems.

Soft bracing is the treatment of choice when pain management is the primary focus and strict alignment is a lower priority. Soft bracing usually permits significant degrees of movement within the device, a feature that increases patients' tolerance of bracing. The soft devices can be used for long periods of time with reduced risk of skin breakdown. Most soft bracing systems are designed for intermittent use and can be put on and removed with little effort.

Bracing side effects

Brace dependency is an unwanted side effect of orthotics. Even short-term immobilization of a body part can result in muscle atrophy and dysfunction. Early mobilization after bracing is one way of avoiding this problem. Selective active exercise can sometimes be done within the brace in order to help preserve muscle function. Isometric exercise is frequently chosen for this purpose since it does not involve joint movement. Active exercise without the brace or with intermittent selective bracing may also be permitted when the chosen activity presents little danger of reinjuring the affected part.

Bracing for common pain problems

Hand injuries are frequently managed by using splints. Finger splints are simple items that greatly reduce the pain and swelling associated with tendon ruptures. Splints for carpal tunnel syndrome support the wrist, relieve pain, and prevent repetitive stress to the median nerve. Custom-molded hand splints relieve the pain associated with rheumatoid arthritis.

Braces are often used in treating pain associated with various conditions of the cervical and lumbar spine. Soft cervical collars allow the neck to maintain a restful position and avoid further nerve outlet impingement. Lumbar supports may be fabricated of cloth or synthetic material and are worn like a garment. Usually, they are constructed for easy self-application.

Braces for painful extremities and joints can be rigid or soft, depending on the intended use. Soft joint splints are commonly used for protection and pain relief in sports injuries. Such splints can continue to be worn for protection when the person returns to the sport.

For painful feet, a common problem that leads to limited mobility for many people, shoe orthotics and inserts can provide relief and contribute to improved function. Heel wedges, arch supports, and other shoe modifications are commonly used to ensure proper positioning of the foot and ankle, which sometimes results in relief of lumbar spine discomfort.

Equipment and ADL items

Long-term pain due to injuries or chronic conditions can be disabling, but proper selection of equipment for home, work, and recreation can greatly enhance the functioning of people in pain.

Activities of daily living (ADLs) are the necessary functions people normally perform in a day: dressing, eating, grooming, and personal hygiene. When people perform these activities independently and without pain, they experience greater personal freedom and improved self-esteem. ADL items are assistive devices that permit people with pain-related disabilities to perform these ordinary self-care routines independently (see *Assistive devices for people in pain*, page 194). Recovery from pain in a rheumatoid hand, for example, can be enhanced through the use of such simple ADL items as a reacher, a jar opener, or an adapted pen. These items unload unnecessary stress and perform functional tasks while minimizing further pain.

Chronic pain due to repetitive activities is usually managed by choosing an appropriate adaptive device to mechanically unload or cushion the body part being stressed. Examples of adaptive devices that offer musculoskeletal cushioning during repetitive activity include

Assistive devices for people in pain

Specialty catalogues offer many devices to help patients with pain-related disabilities maintain independence in daily activities. The ADL items shown here assist patients whose pain affects hand and fin- ger function. For example, patients with pain, muscle weakness, or paralysis of the hand can write by just dragging the finger pen across the paper.

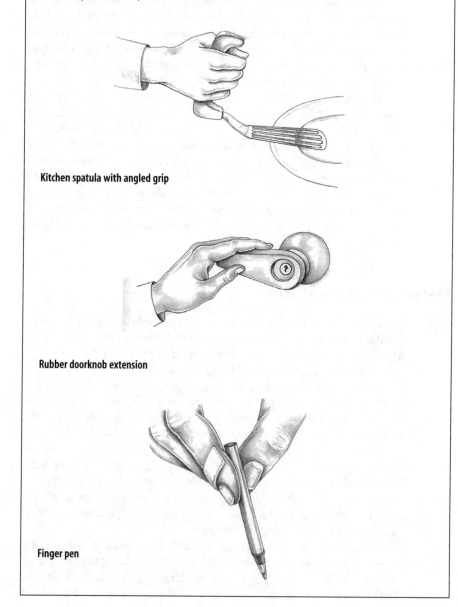

Kitchen spatula with angled grip

Rubber doorknob extension

Finger pen

padded gloves, padded doorknob covers, and easy-open pill contain-ers. Tools used in the work setting can also be adapted for improved performance and reduced stress on muscles and joints. Examples of tools adapted to reduce musculoskeletal stress include hammers with padded handles, scissors with properly contoured handles to improve grip, and power tools with improved shock absorption.

The proper selection of chairs and bedding is often an essential component of the treatment plan for persons with chronic spinal pain. Cushions, pillows, and pads are widely available for cervical and lumbar conditions.

Patients with arthritis or osteoporosis may experience painful ambulation. Assistive devices for ambulation, such as canes, walkers, or crutches, can relieve painful legs or feet and improve mobility.

To select appropriate assistive devices for home or work, thera-pists need an understanding of body mechanics, an assessment of which functions require assistance, and if possible, an on-site inspec-tion of the patient's actual environment. Home equipment, such as tub seats, grab bars, and raised toilet seats, can relieve pain and improve safety by enhancing function, especially for many geriatric patients. For patients with pain-related functional impairments, thoughtful use of these home devices contributes to independent community-based living.

Adaptive equipment and ADL items are hidden resources and valuable tools for therapists involved in pain management.

Acupuncture

Acupuncture, an ancient Chinese healing art, probably dates to the times of prehistory. Now practiced in a modern form, acupuncture is the subject of research in the United States, China, Sweden, and Canada. In the United States it is considered an experimental proce-dure by the U.S. Food and Drug Administration, but acceptance and availability have been growing since the 1970s. The National Institutes of Health has been a vital force in sponsoring research projects. Acupuncture is best considered a complementary form of pain man-agement that can enhance other treatments or therapies. It does not claim to be a cure-all.

Thin, sterile stainless steel needles are inserted into the body at precisely mapped acupuncture points. The needles are approximately half the diameter of the finest needles used in more common medical procedures. Skin penetration is minimal. Needle placement is select-ed according to the particular problem being treated. The needles are often twirled to increase the therapeutic effect. No chemicals are injected and there is usually no bleeding.

Pain relief varies. Subjects may have an immediate response of relaxation, drowsiness, or even euphoria. The pain-relieving effect is probably mediated through the release of endorphins, the natural morphine-like substances in the body. The technique has been successful in the relief of back, neck, arthritis, neuralgia, and myofascial pain as well as other conditions.

Acupuncture is somewhat invasive in that a sterile needle enters the body, but no substances or chemicals are injected. The needles must be sterile. Many practitioners use disposable acupuncture needles, which are readily available. The risk of hepatitis B or HIV transmission through the use of nonsterile needles is very real. Proper training and strict attention to sterile technique is essential. Some serious complications of acupuncture have been cited, including reports of hemothorax and pneumothorax (blood or air in the lung cavity) in some types of needle placements.

Acupuncture principles have contributed to the development of other pain management techniques, particularly for musculoskeletal pain. Trigger points, localized painful areas within muscles, often occur in the same anatomical locations as traditional acupuncture points. Treatment for certain types of musculoskeletal pain involves injection of the trigger points with saline or local anesthetic, localized massage, called acupressure, or other stimulation, including application of intense cold or TENS at the trigger points. Shiatsu or acupoint massage involves finger pressure treatment of these tender pain loci.

Exercise

Mobilization through exercise is an important component of most successful pain management programs. Immobilization is usually required during the acute stages of injuries, but early mobilization is the key to completing the recovery course. Certain painful disease processes, such as rheumatoid and infectious arthritis, may respond to rest during the inflammatory phase, but early mobilization during the remission and recovery phase is necessary to prevent muscle atrophy and dysfunction.

Active exercise, muscle contraction entirely through the patient's own efforts, is the best means of achieving early mobilization and normal function. Also essential for mobilization is range of motion, a simple yet encompassing exercise technique that involves the movement of a body part throughout all the motions permitted by the joint. Range of motion can be done passively, actively, or in an active-assistive manner.

Range of motion

Passive range of motion is movement of a joint through its entire range without active contraction of the muscle. The limb or body part is moved by another person. In many cases, patients can be trained to self-apply this technique. Passive range of motion can also be achieved by the use of electrically powered continuous passive motion (CPM) devices. Passive range of motion is commonly applied to paralyzed extremities to help mobilize the limb and prevent contractures (the loss of flexibility and normal range of motion in muscles, ligaments, tendons, fascia, and joint capsules). Pain is inevitably a feature in immobilized paretic muscles and joints. Passive range of motion helps control pain by promoting release of the reversible elements of contracture. Fixed contractures are reversible only through surgery or other invasive measures.

Active range of motion is performed with active contraction of the muscle through patients' own efforts. Active exercise more effectively returns the body to functioning, but in early healing stages patients may not be able to move the body part actively through the complete range of motion. In that case, patients benefit from an active-assistive routine.

Active-assistive range of motion incorporates an additional passive force, applied by therapist or patient, along with the patient's own active efforts in order to complete the range of motion. The end degrees of a joint's range of motion are the most vulnerable and the first to become contracted. If these areas are not addressed, contracture inevitably develops.

Active and active-assistive range of motion are used in the recovery of function in partially paralyzed limbs as well as in the treatment of arthritis. These two approaches are also used in recovery from fracture, ligament sprain, and muscle tendon strain.

Three types of exercise

Different types of exercise achieve different results. Isotonic, isometric and isokinetic exercise are three methods that produce varying beneficial effects.

Isotonic exercise is active muscle contraction. Patients simply move a joint without assistance partially or completely through its range of motion. Simple examples of isotonic exercise are flexing and extending the knee while seated as part of recovery from knee arthritis or bringing the knees to the chest while lying down as part of recovery from low back pain. Isotonic exercise is frequently a component of mobilization because it is easy to perform and requires no specialized instruction or equipment. It can be performed with or without resistance. If with resistance it is usually a free weight, which patients move or lift as part of the exercise. Resistance applied during isotonic exercise increases its strengthening effect. In general, isotonic exercise increases strength and muscle size or bulk.

Isometric exercise is also an active exercise except that during the active muscle contraction, the joint remains static. This form of exercise may be preferred when joint mobility is restricted. Isometric exercise is frequently performed by persons confined in a cast. It is also employed in recovery from disorders that are exacerbated by excessive joint mobility such as the early healing phases of septic or inflammatory arthritis. Isometric exercise increases strength with a less significant bulk effect on the muscle.

Isokinetic exercise, another form of active exercise, is always performed against variable resistance. The resistance is applied in a manner that forces the muscle to exert maximal force throughout the entire range of motion. This type of exercise requires specialized equipment. It can achieve positive effects throughout the entire range of motion of the joint. Both strength and muscle size are increased in isokinetic exercise.

Exercise in pain management

Therapists have special roles in relation to people in pain. Most people are not familiar with the principles of therapeutic exercise, which is the use of specific exercise activities to promote healing, release contractures, enhance range of motion, develop correct function, and relieve pain. Often injury occurs when those in pain try to develop their own recovery programs because they lack anatomical knowledge of the injured or symptomatic body parts. Therapists may take the role of a very specialized "personal trainer" during the process of recovery. Supervision, attention to exercise performance, and sensitivity to clinical response are essential elements in a successful therapeutic exercise program.

In pain management, the decision-making process is very important and requires experience and clinical skill. The therapist is responsible for a number of different treatment parameters and effects. These should include the timing of the rest or immobilization period and its coordination with the early mobilization phase, the selection of the style of exercise, the progression of intensity in an active exercise program, the number of repetitions of a given exercise, and the prevention of muscle strain from overly vigorous activity.

Patients require the attention and assistance of therapists in order to tolerate the discomfort of the early mobilization phase. Often, initial weight-bearing and movement may be difficult and patients must be encouraged to perform the exercises correctly and safely. Therapists must exercise judgment to guide patients through simple and then progressively more complex physical activity.

When a specific anatomical area is the origin of pain, the recovery plan employs site-specific exercise protocols to address this pain. This practice is quite common in recovery from orthopedic surgery such as knee and hip replacement. Therapeutic exercise programs that address the predictable pain and immobility associated with these surgeries help to ease postoperative pain. The addition of active exercise helps to complete the physical and functional recovery following surgery.

Exercise is typically part of the recovery plan for cervical, thoracic, and lumbar spine pain. Exercise programs may vary in style and theory but they are based on common principles. For example, precautions taken to avoid spinal impact and repeated spinal flexion in osteoporosis or to avoid early vigorous exercise and spinal impact in acute disk herniation may be quite similar in the various exercise techniques. Either spinal flexion or extension may be emphasized within one protocol, while another protocol may combine the two activities. Use of correct body mechanics, an issue that is usually covered in "back school" programs, is usually reviewed in all therapuetic back exercise protocols. Efforts to return patients with back pain to the work environment in a timely manner are usually addressed in "work hardening" programs.

Solutions to exercise problems

One-to-one exercise with a therapist is a traditional and effective pain management method, but cost-containment measures may place this option out of reach for many people. Patients also face the concern of how to manage active exercise for long-term pain problems. Therapeutic exercise classes are a solution to both considerations. Although a group setting lacks the personal nature of individual treatment, it offers other advantages, such as the opportunity for patients to share insights and ideas and the capacity to treat a large number of patients effectively and efficiently. Group classes also offer additional motivation and supervision to patients with long-term pain management problems.

Another creative solution is the use of instructional video tapes or film. Patients are able to view the proper exercise technique and hear the instructions. Repeated viewing aids in further understanding and comprehension. Video tapes, of course, cannot answer questions or correct misunderstandings, and written instructions sheets have the same drawbacks. There is no substitute for individual counseling; therefore, videos and written instructions are most effective when combined with personal instruction.

Maintenance of achieved goals is a difficult accomplishment. Patients are often advised to perform active exercise programs on an ongoing basis. At first, motivation may be strong, but with time, boredom, forgetfulness, and distractions lead to failure to continue active exercise programs. Sometimes refresher sessions are helpful when people experience relapses or fall into periods of inactivity.

Active exercise remains an essential element in achieving complete recovery and function. Maintenance of this effect is achievable with ongoing activity. When reversal of pain is not possible, active exercise plays an important role in optimizing function and thereby the quality of life.

Long-term pain management

Many pain-associated conditions are not completely reversible. People may experience low-level pain over a period of months or even years. Some conditions fluctuate between pain exacerbation and remission in a cyclical fashion. Immobility and dysfunction, both hazards of long-term pain, cause changes in muscle, bone, skin, and vascular structures. Muscle weakness and atrophy lead to debility. Bone loss, or osteoporosis, increases fracture risk and pain. Skin breakdown or decubitus ulcers are caused by lack of activity. Immobility is also associated with deep venous clots, which in turn can lead to life-threatening emboli in the lung.

Avoiding the long-term physical hazards of pain is clearly desirable, but people faced with chronic pain also need care that addresses the overall quality of life, in addition to physical and therapeutic management. Patients may benefit from psychological counseling to assist them in dealing with issues provoked by chronic pain, such as changes in function and self-image, depression, reduced self-esteem, and sexual dysfunction. The last case can be an important issue that people find difficult to discuss. Sensitivity to the problem, proper recognition of the symptoms, and referral for appropriate evaluation and counseling are essential for successful management of pain-related sexual dysfunction.

Balanced nutrition assists in recovery and is a helpful addition to any overall treatment plan. For patients with chronic pain problems, attentiveness to the nutritional risks associated with long-term illness is essential.

Conditions associated with long-term pain can lead to periods of unemployment. Vocational counseling, including exploration of educational options, is often required. Many occupations involve manual tasks that are too stressful for people in pain. Alternative jobs or even careers may have to be considered. Returning to the job market can often be a difficult process that requires counseling.

Appropriate options and alternatives help persons dealing with chronic pain to reorganize their lives and thereby increase function, quality of life, and self-esteem.

Alternative noninvasive techniques

Many noninvasive techniques have been reviewed here, but it is important to remember that there are many alternative noninvasive techniques, too. Many of these techniques alter patients' cognitive habits to help them manage symptoms in a different way. They are useful complements to other forms of pain management.

Therapies that affect patients' thought patterns include hypnosis, distraction, and mental imagery. In hypnosis, people's cognitive functions, motivation, and susceptibility to hypnotic suggestion all play a role. Hypnosis may also help to deal with unconscious issues in persons who are resistant to health. Self-hypnosis, a technique that allows people to treat themselves, provides better personal control of pain and better outcome. Distraction is a technique in which people focus their attention on other activities or stimuli. Mental imagery involves using pleasant or functional images or mental associations to reshape or control the pain experience.

Natural body functions can also be used to alter pain perception. Progressive relaxation training and diaphragmatic breathing instruction help to reduce pain and provide an important component in self-regulation of autonomic arousal. Both of these activities promote self-control, which is an important factor in avoiding learned helplessness as a reaction to pain.

Biofeedback uses the electrical signals generated by biological activity to provide information to patients, who, in turn, use the information to self-regulate biological functions. Electromyography (EMG) (signals elicited from muscles) and electroencephalography (EEG) (brain signals) are commonly used to provide information to patients concerning their levels of tension or arousal. Learning to control arousal by this method can produce relaxation, pain reduction, and decreased anxiety. Follow-up sessions seem to be essential to sustain positive effects.

Environmental alteration

Environment and the arts can have effects on pain perception. Temporary alteration in normal brain hemisphere dominance may play a role in this effect. The right hemisphere of the brain dominates in musical and artistic skills. The left hemisphere deals with math, logic, language, and symbolic interpretation.

Music therapy involves playing, singing, or listening to music for therapeutic results. Pain reduction, elevation of pain threshold, relaxation, changes in respiration, and reduced anxiety are reported effects of this form of therapy. Listening to music may assist in reducing the anxiety involved in tolerating certain medical procedures or diagnostic tests. Music therapy to alleviate pain may involve distraction, changes in affect, or alterations in cognitive and sensory processes to achieve the therapeutic effect. Music therapy's pain-alleviating effects may also result from an increased sense of control and self-esteem.

Pet therapy is an interactive treatment approach that brings people into contact with live, domestic animals. Of course, this treatment can present certain problems, but when carried out in a caring and professional manner it can produce great success. Geriatric patients, in particular, have experienced positive outcomes from encounters with pet therapy. Improved self-image has been reported. This technique may benefit people experiencing chronic or disabling pain.

Horticultural therapy is a treatment that includes viewing, touching, and cultivating plants. The potential benefits include pain reduction, relaxation, reduced fatigue, and relief of tension. When gardens are available in hospital settings, great benefits to patients and families can result. The garden provides a separate atmosphere of peace and tranquillity. Light, window views, and perceived space can influence patients' perceptions of pain and levels of anxiety. Horticultural therapy may also be interactive. Active participation in gardening can provide patients with distraction from pain and chronic illness. Further research is required to explore possible benefits of this therapy, including issues of improved self-esteem and self-image.

Pain management through noninvasive techniques offers many innovative and creative alternatives. The multidisciplinary approach of combining different noninvasive techniques and expertise seems to result in optimum pain control and sustained positive outcome.

REFERENCES

Albright, G.L., and Fischer, A.A. "Effects of Warming Imagery Aimed at Trigger-point. Sites on Tissue Compliance, Skin Temperature and Pain Sensitivity in Biofeedback-trained Patients with Chronic Pain: A Preliminary Study," Part 2. *Perceptual & Motor Skills* 71(3):1163–70, December 1990.

Appel, P.R. "The Use of Hypnosis in Physical Medicine and Rehabilitation (Review)," *Psychiatric Medicine* 10(1):133-48, 1992.

Beckham, J.C., et al. "Biofeedback as a Means to Alter Electromyographic Activity in a Total Knee Replacement Patient," *Biofeedback & Self Regulation* 16(1):23-35, March 1991.

Dean, B.Z., et al. "Pain Rehabilitation: 4. Therapeutic Options in Pain Management," *Archives of Physical Medicine & Rehabilitation* 75(5-S):S21-S30, May 1994.

Flor, H., and Birbaumer, N. "Comparison of the Efficacy of Electromyographic Biofeedback, Cognitive-Behavioral Therapy, and Conservative Medical Interventions in the Treatment of Chronic Musculoskeletal Pain," *Journal of Consulting & Clinical Psychology* 61(4):653-58, August 1993.

Goddard, M.J., et al. "Pain Rehabilitation 1. Basic Science, Acute Pain, and Neuropathic Pain," *Archives of Physical Medicine & Rehabilitation* 75(5-S):S4-S8, May 1994.

Goldberg, R.T., and Maciewicz, R.J. "Prediction of Pain Rehabilitation Outcomes by Motivation Measures," *Disability & Rehabilitation* 16(1):21-25, January-March 1994.

Herring, S.A. "Rehabilitation of Muscle Injuries," *Medicine & Science in Sports & Exercise* 22(4):453-56, August 1990.

Ilacqua, G.E. "Migraine Headaches: Coping Efficacy of Guided Imagery Training," *Headache* 34(2):99-102, February 1994.

Jones, D., and Churchill, J.E. "Archetypal Healing," *American Journal of Hospice & Palliative Care* 11(1):26-33, January-February 1994.

Karlstrom, E., and Abel, G.G. "Biofeedback for Musculoskeletal Pain," *JAMA* 270(22):2736, December 8, 1993.

King, J.C., and Goddard, M.J. "Pain Rehabilitation: 2. Chronic Pain Syndrome and Myofascial Pain," *Archives of Physical Medicine & Rehabilitation* 75(5-S):S9-S14, May 1994.

Kleinhauz, M., and Eli, I. "When Pharmacologic Anesthesia is Precluded: The Value of Hypnosis as a Sole Anesthetic Agent in Dentistry," *Special Care in Dentistry* 13(1):15-18, January-February 1993.

Kottke, F.J., and Lehmann, J.F. *Krusen's Handbook of Physical Medicine and Rehabilitation,* 4th ed. Philadelphia: W.B. Saunders Co., 1982.

Lee, Mathew H.M. *Rehabilitation, Music and Human Well-Being.* Saint Louis: MMB Music Inc., 1989.

Lee, Mathew H.M., and Itoh, M. "Rehabilitation," in *The Merck Manual of Geriatrics.* Edited by Abrams, W.B., and Berkow, R., 16th ed. Rahway, NJ: Merck & Co., Inc, 1995.

Lee, Mathew H.M., et al. "Physical Therapy and Rehabilitation Medicine," in *The Management of Pain,* 2nd ed. Edited by Bonica, J.J. Baltimore: Williams & Wilkins, 1990.

Levitan, A.A. "The Use of Hypnosis with Cancer Patients (Review)," *Psychiatric Medicine* 10(1):119-31, 1992.

Liao, Sung J., et al. *Principles and Practice of Contemporary Acupuncture.* New York: Marcel Dekker Inc., 1994.

Magill-Levreault, L. "Music Therapy in Pain and Symptom Management," *Journal of Palliative Care* 9(4):42-8, Winter 1993.

Mather, C.M., and Ready, L.B. "Management of Acute Pain (Review)," *British Journal of Hospital Medicine* 51(3):85-88, February 2–15, 1994.

McCracken, L.M., and Gross, R.T. "Does Anxiety Affect Coping with Chronic Pain?" *Clinical Journal of Pain* 9(4):253-59, December 1993.

Menegazzi, J.J., et al. "A Randomized, Controlled Trial of the Use of Music During Laceration Repair," *Annals of Emergency Medicine* 20(4):348-50, April 1991.

Middaugh, S.J., et al. "Biofeedback-Assisted Relaxation Training for the Aging Chronic Pain Patient," *Biofeedback & Self Regulation* 16(4):361-77, December 1991.

Miller, A.C., et al. "A Distraction Technique for Control of Burn Pain," *Journal of Burn Care & Rehabilitation* 13(5):576-80, 1992.

Miller, M.E., and Bowers, K.S. "Hypnotic Analgesia: Dissociated Experience or Dissociated Control?" *Journal of Abnormal Psychology* 102(1):29-38, February 1993.

Nanneman, D. "Thermal Modalities: Heat and Cold. A Review of Physiologic Effects with Clinical Applications," *AAOHN Journal* 39(2):70-75, February 1991.

Reigler, F.X. "Update on Perioperative Pain Management (Review)," *Clinical Orthopaedics & Related Research* 305:283-92, August 1994.

Rhiner, M., et al. "A Structured Nondrug Intervention Program for Cancer Pain," *Cancer Practice* 1(2):137-43, July-August 1993.

Rivenburgh, D.W. "Physical Modalities in the Treatment of Tendon Injuries (Review)," *Clinics in Sports Medicine* 11(3):645-59, July 1992.

Roberts, A.H., et al. "Behavioral Management of Chronic Pain and Excess Disability: Long-Term Follow-up of an Outpatient Program," *Clinical Journal of Pain* 9(1):41-8, March 1993.

Rosenfeld, J.P. "Applied Psychophysiology and Biofeedback of Event-Related Potentials (Brain Waves): Historical Perspective, Review, Future Directions," *Biofeedback & Self Regulation* 15(2):99-119, June 1990.

Rosomoff, H.L., and Rosomoff, R.S. "Comprehensive Multidisciplinary Pain Center Approach to the Treatment of Low Back Pain (Review)," *Neurosurgery Clinics of North America* 2(4):877-90, October 1991.

Schoen, M. "Resistance to Health: When the Mind Interferes With the Desire to Become Well," *American Journal of Clinical Hypnosis* 36(1):47-54, July 1993.

Singh, J., and Miabach, H.I. "Topical Iontophoretic Drug Delivery in Vivo: Historical Development, Devices and Future Perspectives (Review)," *Dermatology* 187(4):235-38, 1993.

Spira, J.L., and Spiegel, D. "Hypnosis and Related Techniques in Pain Management," *Hospice Journal* 8(1-2):89-119, 1992.

Theorell, T., et al. "Pain Thresholds during Standardized Psychological Stress in Relation to Perceived Psychosocial Work Situation. Stockholm Music I Study Group," *Journal of Psychosomatic Research* 37(3):299-305, April 1993.

Turk, D.C., and Rudy, T.E. "Neglected Topics in the Treatment of Chronic Pain: Patients—Relapse, Noncompliance, and Adherence Enhancement (Review)," *Pain* 44(1):5-28, January 1991.

Van Dalfsen, P.J., and Syrjala, K.L. "Psychological Strategies in Acute Pain Management," *Anesthesiology Clinics of North America* 7(1): 171-81, 1989.

Von Korff, M., et al. "Effects of Practice Style in Managing Back Pain," *Annals of Internal Medicine* 121(3):187-95, August 1, 1994.

Warner, S.B. Jr., and Baron, J.H. "Restorative Gardens: Green Thoughts in a Green Shade," *British Medical Journal* 306(6885):1080-1081, April 24, 1993.

Williams, A.C., et al. "Evaluation of a Cognitive Behavioral Programme for Rehabilitating Patients with Chronic Pain," *British Journal of General Practice* 43(377):513-18, December 1993.

Williams, F.H., and Maly, B.J. "Pain Rehabilitation: 3. Cancer Pain, Pelvic Pain and Age-related Considerations," *Archives of Physical Medicine & Rehabilitation* 75(5-S):S15-S20, May 1994.

CHAPTER 7

Medical and surgical pain management techniques

Richard V. Gregg, MD
Ann Tuttle, MD

Pain management as a medical focus and discipline is relatively new in the United States. The first text on the subject was *The Management of Pain*, published by John Bonica in 1953, but the idea of pain management as a separate discipline did not catch on significantly until the late 1970s. Within the past five years, federal guidelines have been published for the management of acute pain and cancer pain, thus establishing a place for those disciplines as well as reasonable guidelines for performance and documentation of services.

Pain management assumes or requires that adequate or reasonable medical management of underlying disease processes is completed or ongoing, and the focus of the pain management team is on the pain itself. As an example, an attack of acute cholecystitis (gallbladder disease) would reasonably be treated with removal of the patient's gallbladder, which would normally result in resolution of the pain of cholecystitis, but rather than discussing that treatment per se, the information here covers the control of the patient's pain before and after gallbladder surgery (acute pain), medical methods for controlling pain from the surgical scar (chronic benign pain), and, if disseminated cancer were discovered at the time of surgery, controlling the pain associated with the tumor (cancer pain) as a task separate from trying to control the tumor itself.

The hypothetical patient with gallbladder disease illustrates three major divisions and concepts in pain management: acute pain, chronic benign pain, and cancer, or malignant, pain. Approaches to managing each of these pain problems vary according to expectations regarding the pain problem and the patient's expected longevity. Acute pain from trauma, surgery, or acute medical disease is expected to last for a fairly well-defined period of time during which medical management will adequately treat the problem and stop the pain. It is possible therefore to use medications and invasive treatments that are effective for short time periods but perhaps not reasonable for extended time periods.

A classic example of chronic benign pain is low back pain. In many cases, this disorder does not have a reasonable end point, and even with medical management, the pain may persist with the expectation that to some extent it will last for the rest of the patient's life. Under these circumstances, treatments that have significant risks or reduced likelihood of prolonged effectiveness may not be a reasonable choice. Psychosocial and physical disability issues become equally important in the management of low back pain, and short-term relief may offer only false hope and ultimately be psychologically devastating, rather than helpful. Although medical management plays a role in the treatment of such a patient, it should focus on a rehabilitation approach in which management of the problem rather than cure is the expectation. This form of pain rehabilitation is generally performed by a team of providers, usually including a physical therapist, a psychologist, and a physician whose efforts are aimed at helping the patient return to work or maximizing his ability to function in day-to-day living.

Malignant, or cancer, pain is managed in the context of the assumption that the patient has an undefined but probably shortened life expectancy, and treatment often focuses on pain relief at any cost. Just as in the case of managing acute pain, in this circumstance, pain alleviation treatments that may fail with prolonged use become reasonable, although quality of life and ability to function are extremely important issues as well.

In keeping with the categorization of pain as acute, chronic benign, or malignant, this chapter includes the principles of managing these three different types of pain. Subsequently, the chapter provides specific information about medications, techniques, and procedures used in pain management.

Acute pain

Acute pain is expected to heal or go away. The pain may be constant such as a burn, intermittent such as a muscle strain that hurts with activity only, or both such as an abdominal incision that has some pain at rest but hurts significantly more when the patient is moving, breathing deeply, or coughing. Acute pain management must consider the varying levels of pain during the patient's course of treatment.

Pain management has benefits beyond relief of pain alone. If acute pain is severe, the patient is inactive. A patient who has pain with breathing, such as with a rib fractures or an abdominal incision, does not take deep breaths and risks pulmonary complications. Pain, the stress response, and other features associated with surgery or acute illness also pose potential risks to the cardiovascular system, particularly in a patient who already has preexisting cardiovascular abnormalities. Almost any other system in the body can be affected by special circumstances surrounding acute pain; therefore, caregivers must consider the possibility of other medical complications when choosing the means of pain management.

Treatment of acute pain

Just as there is a World Health Organization "ladder" for the management of increasing severity of cancer pain (see page 297), it is reasonable to establish a ladder of treatment options related to severity of acute pain, preexisting illness, and the likelihood of complications. At the bottom of that ladder, for minor pain problems, acetaminophen and nonsteroidal anti-inflammatory drugs (NSAIDS) are common choices (see *Characteristics of some common NSAIDs*, pages 208 and 209). The anti-inflammatory effects of these drugs may actually be helpful in rapid healing and restoration of normal function.

The next step up the ladder is oral opioids. At this time, there is a large variety to choose from (see *Opioid analgesics*, page 240). A distinction exists between those opioids that give long-lasting relief and those that last for only 2 to 4 hours. Most of the familiar medications fall into the second category of short-duration opioids. These are reasonable analgesics for moderate pain, particularly if it is activity-related. More severe levels of activity-related pain would be controllable by reducing activity as well as by using the opioid. For pain that is fairly severe and is expected to be consistent for several days or more, consideration should be given to the long-acting opioids, either slow-release forms or those with a long half-life. Although at this time slow-release morphine and methadone are the only commonly used long-acting opioids available, it appears that in the future there will be a number of slow-release formulations for opioids that will probably work equally well. With the increasing focus of medicine on the cost-benefit ratio, the use of oral medications, even for a patient in the hospital, should be the first choice if the patient is tolerating oral intake.

Characteristics of some common NSAIDs

Generic name	Trade names (U.S.A.)	Analgesia	Anti-inflammatory effects	Comments
acetaminophen	Tylenol, many others	+	0	No clotting or ulcer effects.
salicylates				
aspirin (acetylsalicylic acid)	Bayer, many others	+	++	Clotting effect lasts for life of platelet, about 10 days (others 24 to 48 hrs.).
diflunisal	Dolobid	+	+/−	Minimal clotting effects.
magnesium or choline trisalicylate	Trilisate, Salflex, Magsal, Mono-Gesic	+	+	Minimal clotting effects.
propionic acids				
ibuprofen	Motrin, many others	++	++	
naproxen	Naprosyn, Anaprox, Aleve	++	++	
fenoprofen	Nalfon	+	+	
flurbiprofen	Ansaid	++	+	
ketoprofen	Orudis	++	++	
oxaprozin	Daypro	++	++	
acetic acids				
indomethacin	Indocin	++	+++	High incidence of ulcers.
diclofenac	Voltaren, Cataflam	++	++	Concentrated in joints.
ketorolac	Toradol	+++	++	Available IM/IV. High incidence of ulcers.

Characteristics of some common NSAIDs *(continued)*

Generic name	Trade names (U.S.A.)	Analgesic	Anti-inflammatory effects	Comments
acetic acids, *continued*				
etodolac	Lodine	++	+	
sulindac	Clinoril	+	++	Reduced kidney problems.
others				
piroxicam	Feldene	++	++	High incidence of ulcers.
mefenamic acid	Ponstel	++	++	One week maximum use due to side effects.
meclofenamate	Meclomen	++	++	Increased diarrhea.
nabumetone	Relafen	++	++	Minimal clotting effects. Possible reduced ulcers.

0 = no measurable effect; + = a measurable effect; ++ = a greater measurable effect; +++ = greatest measurable effect; +/- = equivocal evidence of a measurable effect

A number of medications are considered adjuncts to pain management. These include sleeping pills, muscle relaxants to decrease muscle spasm, and antihistamines to reduce side effects such as itching and to give some mild sedation. Although they do not provide analgesia, they do help to reduce some side effects.

Parenteral opioids for acute pain

The next step up the ladder for managing acute pain is parenteral opioids. The old standard for this was intramuscular administration of opioids such as morphine or meperidine (Demerol) on an intermittent basis. Parenteral drug administration has changed significantly over the past 10 or 15 years to include transdermal administration (a patch soaked with medication that penetrates the skin, allowing slow, consistent systemic absorption), subcutaneous infusions, and intravenous bolus or infusion.

Pain relief varies with different parenteral methods. Medication delivered via a standard intramuscular (I.M.) injection is not absorbed immediately but takes from 15 to 30 minutes to be significantly absorbed and, therefore, that same length of time to initiate pain relief. Pain relief can last from 2 to occasionally as long as 6 hours after I.M. administration of the commonly used opioids. I.M. medications are often prescribed every 4 to 6 hours. Consequently, those patients who get relief for only 2 hours endure a significant amount of time during which pain is inadequately controlled. That is in addition to the pain of the I.M. injection and the 15- to 30-minute wait for relief after the injection.

The only transdermal opioid available at this time is fentanyl. It comes as a variably sized patch designed to release a particular dose of fentanyl into the bloodstream over a set period of time. The patches last for 3 days and should be considered long-acting opioids. After a patch is first applied, approximately 12 hours must pass before the drug reaches a consistent level in the blood stream. Because of the delay in onset of analgesia, transdermal fentanyl is essentially useless for acute increases in pain or management of activity-related pain. Since it also takes 12 hours for the medication to stop being effective after patch removal, if the patient develops side effects, such as oversedation or nausea and vomiting, it will take 12 hours for those side effects to cease. However, for constant, fairly severe pain the transdermal fentanyl patch can be reasonably effective in providing steady relief over time without large variations in plasma concentrations of drug.

Subcutaneous or intravenous infusions can also provide a consistent plasma level of opioid and thus a consistent level of relief of relatively constant pain. Intravenous boluses with or without the intravenous infusion can deliver rapid increases in the opioid level and, therefore, rapid relief of breakthrough pain. The capacity to deliver an I.V. bolus of opioid is very important for relieving intermittent increases in pain. Relief generally occurs within 3 to 10 minutes, much less time than is required for relief from an I.M. injection.

These methods of delivering opioids are chosen for patients who cannot have anything by mouth (NPO) or for patients who cannot achieve adequate pain control with oral medications.

Patient-controlled analgesia for acute pain

The last step of the ladder for acute pain management involves the use of drug delivery technology and regional analgesia techniques in an attempt to maximize pain relief and minimize side effects or potential complications. The most common system at this time is a patient-controlled analgesia (PCA) machine for administering I.V. opioids. This computer-controlled device holds a syringe of medication that is attached directly to the patient's I.V. line. The patient can push a button and receive a dose of the opioid through the I.V. Safety features in the PCA device will not allow administration of an overdose, and most of the devices are capable of delivering a constant infusion along with the on-demand bolus feature.

Although PCA may seem like a more expensive way to supply what an I.V. infusion and routine nursing care could accomplish, it actually offers significant benefits. Small boluses of opioid on demand allow the patient to titrate the medication to his own needs. One patient might have greater pain than another and one patient might be remarkably less sensitive than another to a given opioid. The amount of medication required by patients with similar acute pain problems may vary as much as fourfold or fivefold. PCA allows the patient to determine those needs rather than having to rely on a nurse's assessment of the patient's pain level. The device also markedly reduces or eliminates the time lapse between the desired pain relief and administration of the medication into the I.V. Also, by allowing a number of small but frequent doses, it reduces the side effects caused by high systemic levels of opioid relative to the level of analgesia achieved. One other benefit is that the patient can have control over something at a time when other aspects of necessary care may make the patient feel passive or even victimized. This experience in self-control should not be underestimated when assessing a patient's satisfaction with the use of these devices.

Regional analgesia for acute pain

Another remarkably effective means of relieving pain, particularly in postoperative or post-trauma patients, is to place a catheter in the epidural space (see *Catheterization of the epidural space*, page 249) and administer opioids and local anesthetics through that catheter to provide "regional analgesia." In the United States the pain of labor and childbirth is often relieved by the use of an epidural catheter. By placing the catheter at various levels within the epidural space of the spine, it is possible to relieve not only labor pain but also pain from abdominal or thoracic incisions and even pain caused by broken ribs.

When local anesthetics are infused through catheters, they reduce all sensation in the nerves near the tip of the catheter. The number of nerves affected can be changed by varying the flow rate of the infusion. Since opioid receptors for reducing pain perception are in the spinal cord, opioids given through the epidural catheter are regionally effective in a manner similar to local anesthetics. Epidural administration of opioids allows a higher concentration of opioid at the spinal pain receptors without exposing other receptors that cause nausea, vomiting, sedation, or constipation to high levels of opioid. The availability of both local anesthetics and opioids for use through an epidural catheter allows a pain management physician to tailor the analgesia of a patient specifically to the pain problem as well as to the medical condition.

Although this epidural technique sounds like a panacea for pain, there are some drawbacks. Pain around the head and neck often cannot be treated in this fashion because the nerves supplying pain sensitivity to those areas do not travel through the epidural space. Local anesthetics not only change sensation, they can also cause the blood vessels in the areas they numb to open up significantly, sometimes causing the blood pressure to fall below acceptable levels. Higher concentrations of local anesthetics also block the motor nerve fibers, causing muscle weakness. In the chest and abdomen, this is often not much of an issue. When it affects the legs, it stops ambulation and, in fact, can slow the patient's recovery if allowed to continue.

In the case of the opioids, even though the epidural catheter allows regionally placed pain relief, the possibilities of sedation, nausea and vomiting, and even respiratory depression are still present. If the patient expects or demands absolutely no pain, these side effects can result from efforts to achieve it, even when the opioid is placed into the epidural space. One side effect is, in fact, increased when using opioids through epidural catheters as compared to the other systemic applications; that is itching. At times it can be sufficiently severe for the patient to request no further epidural administration, although generally it is merely a nuisance. These side effects and potential problems must be considered when tailoring a patient's epidural pain relief.

Peripheral nerve blocks by single injection or placement of a catheter near the nerve can be performed for pain after surgery or injury. Anesthesiologists are trained to perform nerve blocks to anesthetize various regions of the body so that surgery can be performed without a general anesthetic. In fact, these same techniques can be used after surgery to relieve pain, and a single injection can last as long as 8 to 12 hours. If pain relief is needed for a longer time, a catheter can sometimes be placed to allow repeat administration or a continuous infusion. In general, only local anesthetics are used through these catheters because delivering opioids by this method has not consistently been shown to be of help.

Integration of pain management with acute care
Sometimes a patient needs extremely complex management that requires the integration of pain services with care provided by other physicians. A common example is a car accident victim with fractures in legs, arms, and ribs, with contusion to the chest and subsequent

abdominal surgery for bleeding. That patient may have a history of heart disease and be at risk for further heart problems under the present stressful conditions. The management of a patient in these circumstances is critical. In fact, pain management techniques such as epidural analgesia, along with careful medical management, can markedly reduce the complications associated with these injuries and help keep the patient off mechanical ventilation for breathing difficulties associated with the broken ribs and abdominal incision.

To insure that the pain of the broken bones and other injuries is adequately addressed, it is necessary to examine the patient frequently, discuss progress, and adjust medications as needed. Multiple-trauma patients gain the most from this kind of careful attention to pain management. Along with better pain relief, these patients will have fewer pulmonary complications, including pneumonia and the need for mechanical ventilation, as well as less cardiac stress and fewer complications. In addition, the total cost of such a patient's care has been demonstrated to be lower because of the integration of attentive pain management with the overall medical care.

This brings up one last issue associated with acute pain management. Although the trauma patient discussed here will probably get better, it is certainly not going to occur in one to four weeks. After extensive injuries, a patient commonly takes as much as a year or more to fully recover. It then becomes important to make sure that pain management is carried on as the patient transfers from the acute care setting into the rehabilitation setting, where he or she regains normal breathing function, use of extremities and, ultimately, activities of daily living. Addressing pain issues early in the patient's care can help to reduce the long-term pain problems that the patient suffers while getting back to normal functioning. It can also help to reduce or avoid the development of chronic pain, which is discussed in the next section.

Chronic benign pain

In this chapter, the term *benign* indicates the absence of a malignant disease process and therefore the presence of a normal life expectancy. *Chronic benign pain* is used to describe recurring pain that is not associated with a malignant (neoplastic) process. It does not indicate that the pain described is less severe; indeed, some physicians object to the use of the term to describe pain.

Chronic benign pain is poorly defined because the change from an acute pain problem to a chronic pain problem occurs gradually. Most textbooks choose a point somewhere between 3 and 6 months as a normal time frame for development of chronic pain, but actually the exact time period for development of chronic pain is irrelevant. Chronic benign pain problems develop when changes occur in a patient's body that may be secondary to the pain itself but that cause secondary disability by themselves. These problems are often broken down into physical and psychological categories, although these two areas cannot truly be separated any more than the mind can be separated from the body. See *A patient with chronic benign pain* for an illustration of the development of chronic benign pain in a patient with a previously normal medical history.

The classic issues of chronic benign pain are fairly obvious in the patient described in this history. The patient does continue to have ongoing pain organically based in degenerative disk disease and a herniated disk. On top of that, the patient has severe physical deconditioning because of a fairly inactive lifestyle, previous obesity, and an inability to maintain any significant physical function during the past 4 to 6 months. A number of psychological or behavioral issues apply to this person's pain problem as well. Preexisting difficulties at work make him pessimistic about a reasonable return to work even if he has no pain or back problems at all. These issues, along with back pain, may make him significantly depressed and reduce his self-image to that of an invalid, unable to escape pain or perform significant physical activity, with nowhere to turn.

Patients with these difficulties learn significant illness behavior among friends and family, including the avoidance of social interaction, which may have become difficult. Such patients may often obtain secondary gains in the form of help from family and friends, who by their overly solicitous behavior contribute to the patient's physical debility. Finally, the patient is dependent on medications that provide reduced relief over time, that cloud mental clarity, and that expose him to periods of partial relief alternating with no relief at all. This patient may have become labeled as drug-seeking or even addicted, even though the medications have been prescribed by the physicians who have been caring for him.

Rehabilitation approach to chronic benign pain

The patient described above exemplifies the issues of pain, physical deconditioning, behavioral change, and medication dependence. The presence of these problems does not indicate that the patient is malingering or has psychogenic pain problems, although they too may occur in a psychologically disturbed patient. Since all of the issues become problems to some extent for many chronic pain patients, a number of health care professionals must be involved in such a patient's care in order to treat all of the identified problems. A

PATIENT HISTORY

A patient with chronic benign pain

John G., a loading dock employee, is a labor union member with a poor education and few other job skills. He has had three or four episodes of significant back pain during eight years of employment without requiring significant time off or medical treatment. Other factors of concern are his moderate obesity, a lack of exercise outside the job, a poor relationship with the loading dock foreman, and information that a number of layoffs are about to occur at the loading dock. One day, while lifting a heavy load, John G. suddenly has severe back pain with pain radiating down into one leg. He is placed off work and prescribed bed rest for a few weeks, a program that does not significantly reduce his pain. His attempts to return to work cause immediate increase in his pain, making him unable to be physically active. Various medications and other treatments do not help consistently, and ultimately surgery is performed to remove a disk herniation in his lower back. Unfortunately, pain continues after this surgery and attempts to return to work markedly worsen his pain complaints. This course of events leading to the patient's chronic pain occurred over a period of about 6 months.

---

rehabilitation approach is necessary. Such an approach has a number of clear goals:

- to maximize the patient's functional abilities, both physical and psychological
- to minimize the pain the patient experiences during rehabilitation and for the rest of his life
- to teach the patient how to manage whatever pain remains as well as how to handle pain exacerbations that arise due to increased activity or for unexplained reasons.

The rehabilitation approach requires the patient's motivation and active participation as well as input from physicians, physical therapists, psychologists, and vocational rehabilitation workers to assess the patient's maximum functional capacity, the possibility of job placement, or the potential need for retraining. These same issues are important for all patients, including those not covered by the Workers' Compensation Act.

Pain rehabilitation programs focus on outcomes quite different from those expected of normal medical care. Some of the outcome measures examine benefits to the patient and some examine benefits to society. Patient outcome measures include reduced pain, reduced need for pain medication, increased activities of daily living, demonstrably improved physical flexibility, strength and endurance, reduced depression and illness behavior, improved self-image, demonstrated use of and benefit from pain management techniques, and the ability to return to gainful employment. The last outcome measure would also be one of society's benefits along with others, such as reduced use of the health care system resulting in reduced cost to society, the employer, and the insurance company.

With all of these considerations, a pain management physician can be only one member of a large team of care providers. To maximize the patient's improvement, care must be integrated among all providers, and the information the patient receives from the various professionals must be consistent and correct. It is not uncommon for a medical treatment to be reasonable in an isolated circumstance but unreasonable for a particular patient with unique physical and psychological needs. Medical treatment for chronic benign pain should always be determined in the context of the patient's long-term benefit rather than on the narrow basis of today's pain complaint.

Medical treatment of chronic benign pain

Medical management for chronic benign pain focuses on long-term safety and efficacy. There are almost no well-designed scientific studies documenting the effectiveness of any of these treatments alone in managing long-term pain because of the difficulty of conducting long-term scientific studies, the lack of a consistent patient population, and the use of the presence or absence of pain as a relatively inexact outcome measure. It is also true, however, that medical management alone is almost never effective for long-term, chronic benign pain problems. Many medical treatments either make a small impact on a patient's pain complaints for a prolonged period of time or reduce pain complaints significantly for a short period of time to help the patient perform in a physical rehabilitation program, which will ultimately improve function and will probably reduce pain. Treatment generally consists of medication and temporary or permanent invasive therapies such as nerve blocks or surgery.

Most pain management physicians attempt to categorize a patient's pain source(s) by the type of tissue or the part of the body. Although this may sound obvious, it is often a fairly difficult process, and "unknown etiology" is not an uncommon categorization. The three general categories of pain are somatic, visceral, and neuralgic. Somatic pain includes pain arising from the skeleton, muscles, ligaments, skin, and bones. Visceral pain originates in the contents of the chest and abdomen and perhaps all blood vessels. Neuralgic pain generally comes from either the peripheral nervous system or the central nervous system, with the brain and spinal cord making up the central nervous system.

These categories are important in guiding the choice of treatment plans, particularly medications and physical therapy regimens as well as for establishing reasonable expectations for pain alleviation. Somatic pain is generally increased by activity, although it can often be markedly reduced by a well-designed physical therapy program. Visceral pain is often unrelated to activity and unpredictable. It is frequently unresponsive to activity programs. Neuralgic pain may or may not be responsive to activity. It is felt to be one of the more difficult pain problems to treat, and it requires specific kinds of medications.

Medications for chronic benign pain

A few groups of medications can be helpful for all types of pain. The most commonly used is the NSAID group. NSAIDs are generally more effective for inflammation-based pain, but they are direct analgesics and can, therefore, also reduce pain from noninflammatory origins. The other group of medications commonly used for chronic pain on a long-term basis is antidepressants. There are a number of such drugs, each with quite different side-effect profiles (see *Antidepressants available in the United States*, page 218), but their basic mechanism increases the activity of one or more of the central nervous system pathways that inhibit pain perception. The response rate to antidepressants is significantly less than 100%, and many patients seem not to benefit from them.

The use of opioids for chronic benign pain has been a source of great controversy ever since tolerance, dependence, and addiction have been understood. Although there are great social and political pressures against the use of opioids or any other medication with abuse potential, there has been a recent increase in the use of opioids for chronic benign pain. There are pain management physicians who stand vehemently in each camp, some proposing the use of opioids consistently and some condemning it consistently. The issue is yet to be resolved. When considering opioids for chronic benign pain, the authors of this chapter employ some uniform guidelines. The first guideline is to try to get satisfactory pain management without the use of opioids. The second guideline involves placing the patient in a rehabilitation program that includes a behavioral approach to pain management prior to committing to long-term opioid use with the attendant issues of dependence, tolerance, and medical or social ostracization. Beyond that, there are a number of predominantly behavioral issues that determine whether the chronic use of opioids is appropriate.

One important job of pain management physicians is to provide a humane weaning program to reduce use of opioids already prescribed while avoiding withdrawal symptoms and minimizing pain exacerbation caused by opioid tolerance coupled with the decreasing dosage. There is generally significant iatrogenic cause for opioid dependence under these circumstances, and labeling the patient as a medication abuser or addict is inappropriate. Other medications

Antidepressants available in the United States

Tricyclics	Quaternary cyclics	Serotonin-specific	Specific, multiple receptor	Other
• amitryptyline *Elavil, Endep, Emitrip*	• trazodone *Desyrel*	• fluoxetine *Prozac*	• venlafaxine *Effexor*	• bupropion *Wellbutrin*
• amoxapine *Asendin*		• paroxetine *Paxil*	• nefazodone *Serzone*	
• desipramine *Norpramin, Pertofrane*		• sertraline *Zoloft*		
• doxepin *Adapin, Sinequan*				
• imipramine *Tofranil, Janimine, Tipramine*				
• maprotiline *Ludiomil*				
• nortriptyline *Aventyl, Pamelor*				
• protriptyline *Vivactil*				
• trimipramine *Surmontil*				

prescribed for pain, such as benzodiazepines, barbiturates, and the like should also be humanely reduced and eliminated if possible.

Medications for neuralgic pain are generally not classic analgesic medications (see *Medications used for neuralgic pain*) and are generally ineffective for pain from other tissue sources. Frequently, combinations of these medications are far more effective than any one of them alone, but unfortunately a significant number of patients have minimal apparent benefit after an extensive trial of these drugs. As the mechanisms of nerve pain are becoming better understood and newer medications become available, the response rate continues to improve. Neuralgic pain is currently the primary focus of research for pain management.

Medications used for neuralgic pain

Medications	Examples	Comments	Side effects
antidepressants	amitriptyline, imipramine, nortriptyline, desipramine, doxepin, fluoxetine[1], paroxetine, venlafaxine	Documentation shows these are the most effective in relieving neuralgic pain. They produce analgesia at doses less than required to treat depression.	Sedation/confusion, constipation, dry mouth, urine retention, tachycardia, weight gain/fluid retention
neuroleptics	fluphenazine, perphenazine, haloperidol, chlorpromazine, methotrimeprazine[2]	Usually used in combination with antidepressants.	Alpha blockade/orthostatic hypotension, sedation/confusion, acute extrapyramidal reaction, tardive dyskinesia
anticonvulsants	carbamazepine, valproic acid/sodium valproate, phenytoin, gabapentin	Best for intermittent, sharp, "shooting" neuralgia but can be effective for constant pain.	Sedation/confusion, GI distress, bone marrow suppression, hepatic toxicity, gingival hyperplasia (phenytoin)
baclofen		Combination with carbamazepine optimal for tic douloureux; usually used in combination with other neuralgic medications.	Sedation /confusion, GI distress/ intolerance, CNS withdrawal symptoms with abrupt discontinuation
mexiletine		Perhaps more useful for diffuse neuralgia such as in diabetes	Sedation/confusion/ "lightheaded," GI intolerance, tremor
clonazepam		May work best in combination with baclofen.	Dependence, sedation/ confusion, withdrawal symptoms with abrupt discontinuation

[1] Different side effect profile; see text.

[2] I.M. preparation only, has been used S.L..

Adapted from *Seminars in Spine Surgery*, Vol. 6, No. 2, June 1994, p. 158. Used with permission.

Nerve blocks for chronic benign pain

Nerve blocks, or injection therapy, for chronic pain management generally fall into three basic categories: diagnostic blocks, short-term therapeutic blocks, and destructive, or "neurolytic," blocks.

Diagnostic blocks consist of a local anesthetic injection into an area thought to be a pain source or around the nerves supplying an area thought to be a pain source in order to determine the relative significance of that particular source in the patient's complaints.

The results of blocks must be interpreted with great care. A placebo response occurs in approximately 30% of the normal population, giving significant false-positive responses. Pain is a very difficult thing to quantify, so percentages of relief or changes in pain scales can be interpreted only as a trend rather than as a hard and fast number. The practitioner also must consider that a number of behavioral and psychosocial issues make it difficult for some patients to report significant pain relief, even under the circumstances of a diagnostic block. All of these issues make a diagnostic block difficult to interpret when performed perfectly. Add to these uncertainties the technical difficulties of performing the blocks, and the use of diagnostic blocks is revealed to be less precise than most people would imagine possible in the field of medicine.

Short-term therapeutic blocks can be injected at the site of a pain source or along the path of the nervous system to the spinal cord. The various blocks are described later in this chapter, but for chronic benign pain some important points must be considered:

- The ability to temporarily block a chronic pain is not a sufficient reason to perform a therapeutic block. In fact, for some patients it is detrimental to demonstrate a remarkable relief in pain for only a short period of time, only to have the pain return in full force.
- Some objective measure of improvement must be chosen (improvement in physical activity, improved ability to focus on behavioral techniques, and so forth) as a measure of the block's effectiveness.
- A patient will *occasionally* have an extremely long-term or apparently permanent relief of pain from a short-term block. This response cannot be explained medically except by invoking the patient's return to normal activity or the rather unscientific principle of "breaking the pain cycle" as the probable cause of relief. These long-term positive responses are fairly rare and should not be presented to patients as any reasonable expectation.
- Nerve blocks *can* be remarkably effective for some patients by helping them to complete a rehabilitation program faster and with reduced pain.

Neurolytic blocks (permanent destruction of nerve tissue) are generally inappropriate for patients with chronic benign pain problems. Technical failures and inappropriately placed medication become far more important when permanent damage can be the result. Also, a remarkable phenomenon occurs in patients who have had permanent neurolysis. After a while, generally six to twelve months, the perception of pain in the treated area often reoccurs. A number of theories explain this phenomenon, including regeneration of nerves and changes in afferent processing mechanisms in the central nervous system. The recurring pain is frequently somewhat different from the initial pain but, unfortunately, often far more severe. The new pain is usually neuralgic and frequently very difficult to treat or to help at all. The problem of recurring pain also appears when a neurosurgical procedure instead of a neurolytic injection interrupts the nerve; therefore, neurosurgical nerve-interruption procedures should also be viewed skeptically for most chronic benign pain problems.

Spinal cord stimulators and catheters for chronic benign pain

Recently, the technology of pain management has advanced to include two new treatment options: spinal cord stimulators and spinal catheters. Technical information about these devices appears later in this chapter. Spinal cord stimulators are most useful for neuralgic pain in an area on one side of the body that is not adequately controlled by less invasive treatment. For a select group of patients with these complaints, insertion of a spinal cord stimulator can produce remarkable pain relief that allows those patients to return to more normal function. This procedure is not a panacea, however, and like any other treatment option, it has its problems and failures.

The cord stimulation system involves very specific placement of stimulating electrodes close to the spinal cord. The electrodes can move or break, making them no longer functional. Even with continued appropriate stimulation, some patients lose pain relief over time, and some patients, even with neuralgic pain as described, do not get any benefit or even may have worse pain symptoms with the stimulation. Obviously, in those patients who get no relief, the system would not be permanently placed, but spinal cord stimulators are intended to be a life-long implantation requiring only occasional battery changes.

Analgesia via spinal catheters involves an infusion or sometimes a bolus injection of medications, usually opioids or local anesthetics, into the epidural space in a manner similar to the epidural catheter infusions described in the acute pain section. There is a great deal of controversy about the appropriate use of such catheters in chronic benign pain patients. The same tolerance and dependence issues occur with this technologically advanced system as with simple oral administration of opioids. There is a fairly high cost for the placement of the catheter and continued refilling of the pump. There also exists the potential for complications or infection involving the spinal cord or brain. For these reasons, spinal catheters are generally reserved for cancer pain. As the safety record of these devices improves and as data on long-term use is gathered, it is possible that in the future they will serve a greater role in chronic benign pain management.

Cancer pain

Cancer is diagnosed in more than one million Americans annually and causes one in every five deaths in the United States. Several studies document that pain in cancer patients is frequently undertreated (Bonica 1990). The incidence of pain depends on the type and stage of disease with 30% to 50% of patients complaining of moderate to severe pain in early stages and nearly 75% in late stages (Bonica 1990). The National Cancer Institute 1990 consensus statement said that "the undertreatment of pain and other symptoms of cancer is a serious and neglected public health problem" and concluded that "every patient with cancer should have the expectation of pain control as an integral aspect of his or her care throughout the course of the disease." (National Cancer Institute 1990).

A number of other diseases, although they are not classified as cancer, are consistently progressive and fatal, such as AIDS and some other autoimmune diseases, and pain problems in populations with these diseases should be handled in the same way as pain problems in cancer patients. Even the most common disease processes may ultimately reach the state of severe, unrelieved pain. There are certainly patients with severe heart disease whom surgery will not benefit, and yet these patients have constant anginal pain and might be termed "cardiac cripples." Similarly, the pain of severe lung disease requiring home oxygen and limitation to almost no physical activity should be considered as compelling as malignant pain. Pain management in these cases may take on the role of pain relief at any cost. Since other activities that affect quality of life are so restricted, constant pain simply removes comfort as one of the last remaining values available to give the patient a reasonable quality of life.

Rationale for treatment of cancer pain

The physical and psychological effects of chronic pain can be devastating in patients who are already debilitated. The treatment of cancer pain should be a high priority to avoid unnecessary suffering and to allow increased function. Unrelieved pain diminishes activity, appetite, and sleep. It prevents patients from working productively, enjoying recreation, or taking pleasure in their usual role in the family and society. The psychological effect of cancer pain can also be devastating. Whether the pain is due to the cancer or the treatment, it can often cause the patient to lose hope, believing that the pain heralds the progress of a fatal, painful disease. Pain can exacerbate individual suffering by worsening helplessness, anxiety, and depression. The suffering of a patient with terminal cancer can often be relieved by demonstrating to the patient that his or her pain truly can be controlled (Cassel 1982).

Causes of undertreatment of cancer pain

One possible factor contributing to the undertreatment of cancer pain is the complexity of the pain problem. Pain may originate from several different sources, including bone, muscle, nerves, or visceral structures. These patients may have pain from several etiologies including these:

- tumor progression and related pathology
- invasive diagnostic or therapeutic procedures
- toxicity of chemotherapy and radiation therapy
- infection
- muscle aches associated with limitations in physical activity.

Another cause for undertreatment of pain is fear of addiction, a common dread of both patients and care providers. Use of opioids for pain control does not lead to addiction. For the few patients with a history of addiction or with other social concerns such as drug diversion, these issues in and of themselves should not lead to undertreatment of pain. A clear outline of the care provider's expectations of the patient and close follow-up is often sufficient to allow pain treatment of individuals with a history of drug-related problems. Inadequate knowledge of the pharmacology of opioids leading to fear of respiratory depression can also lead to undertreatment of pain.

Medications for cancer pain

Pharmacologic management as the primary means of cancer pain relief is effective in greater than 80% of patients. Medications are titratable and suitable for pain that is multifocal or progressive. Effects and side effects are reversible, and widespread implementation does not depend on sophisticated technology or scarce resources. Treatment with opioids is the mainstay of pharmacologic management. A simple, well-validated, and effective method for chosing the appropriate titration of therapy for cancer pain is to follow the analgesic ladder developed by the World Health Organization (WHO 1990) on page 297.

NSAIDs or acetaminophen are used alone as initial therapy in mild pain and combined with opioids and adjuvant analgesics if pain intensity increases. A combination of NSAIDs and opioids can provide more analgesia than either of the two classes of drug can provide alone. NSAIDs also exhibit a "dose-sparing" effect on opioids, such that using acetaminophen or an NSAID with an opioid provides effective analgesia at a lower-than-usual dose of the opioid. NSAIDs do not produce tolerance or physical or psychological dependence, but there is a ceiling on their analgesic potential.

The next step on the analgesic ladder employs opioids, usually taken by mouth. Full agonists are generally used for cancer pain because they offer analgesia without a ceiling effect. Agonist-antagonists should not be given to patients who are regularly taking agonists, as they can precipitate withdrawal symptoms.

Opioids for cancer pain

Opioid tolerance and physical dependence are expected with long-term opioid treatment and should not be confused with psychological dependence or addiction. For most cancer patients, the first indication of tolerance is a decrease in the duration of analgesia for a given dose. Increasing dose requirements are consistently correlated with progressive disease, which produces increased pain intensity (Foley 1985).

Effective pain relief is best accomplished by the anticipation and prevention of pain. In patients with persistent or daily pain, opioids should be given on a regular schedule rather than only as needed. As the scheduled medication is being titrated to effect, patients can then take additional doses as needed to cover breakthrough pain. The optimal dose is that which controls pain with the fewest side effects, such as sedation, mental clouding, nausea, or constipation. If a particular side effect is not well tolerated, switching to another opioid can help manage the problem. The oral route is the preferred route because it is the most convenient and cost-effective.

Generally, opioid analgesics with longer durations of action, such as controlled-release morphine, methadone, levorphanol, and the fentanyl patch are preferable because they provide sustained analgesia and require administration at less frequent intervals. Mild and incident pain can be relieved by codeine, oxycodone, hydromorphone, or immediate-release morphine, depending on the severity of the pain and the side effects of the medication.

Even though chronic opioids are administered orally whenever possible, alternate routes are necessary in up to 70% of patients at some time. Though I.M. or I.V. routes are most commonly used, the subcutaneous route should also be considered. Studies have shown that subcutaneous dosing produces stable blood levels that correlate closely with continuous intravenous infusion. Subcutaneous PCA has been shown to be as effective as intravenous PCA. A weekly change of the infusion site to avoid local toxicity or infection can easily be performed by a home health nurse using a butterfly needle.

Other routes to consider for administration of opioids include rectal, nasal, sublingual or buccal, and transdermal. These routes can be considered on an individual basis in those patients unable to take medications by mouth.

Adjuvant analgesics for cancer pain

Though opioids are rightfully recognized for their analgesic value, other pharmacologic therapy is often undervalued in treating cancer pain. For example, NSAIDs can be beneficial in the management of osseous metastases, and analgesic adjuvants, such as antidepressants, anticonvulsants, sodium channel blockers, amphetamines, and corticosteroids, can be helpful in controlling neuropathic and other pain syndromes while limiting opioid side effects.

Tricyclic antidepressants can be especially useful for patients complaining of neuropathic pain such as dysesthetic or burning pain. Limited studies have been performed in cancer patients, including one placebo-controlled study, in which imipramine was found to decrease morphine requirements (Walsh 1986). Potentially beneficial side effects of tricyclics, including restoration of a normal nighttime sleep pattern and improved mood, can also be used to the patient's advantage.

Corticosteroids have been shown to decrease pain and increase appetite and activity, but some studies demonstrate an effect of only 2 to 4 weeks' duration. There are also risks associated with these medications, including immunosuppression and infection, proximal myopathy, psychiatric symptoms, and possibly a higher incidence of gastrointestinal and cardiovascular side effects. Thus, the relative risk versus the benefit of using these medications should be considered on an individual basis.

Phenothiazines (a class of antipsychotic agents sometimes used for sedation or as antiemetics) and benzodiazepines (a class of sedative agents often used as anxiolytics) do not have good evidence supporting their use for adjuvant analgesia. However, they may be used for their beneficial effect on anxiety, sleep disturbance, or muscle spasm. Their use is appropriate if they do not take the place of opioids or psychosocial intervention when indicated. The one exception is methotrimeprazine (a phenothiazine derivative), which provides analgesia comparable to morphine plus a potent antiemetic effect and thus can be invaluable in the acute setting when opioid side effects are not well tolerated. Its use is limited by the fact that it can be administered only parenterally and by its common side effects of sedation and orthostatic hypotension.

Amphetamines (a class of stimulants) have been shown to increase significantly the analgesic effect of morphine, while decreasing sleepiness and increasing activity, appetite, and intellectual performance. However, in certain patients they may decrease appetite, increase anxiety, increase delirium, and cause a paranoid reaction. These reactions may be less common with methylphenidate, which has a shorter half-life than dextroamphetamine, but must always be watched for, especially in the elderly. When opioid-related sedation becomes a limiting factor despite continued pain, the amphetamines can significantly decrease pain and increase function.

Palliative radiation therapy for cancer pain

Radiation therapy is complementary to analgesic drug therapies and may enhance their effectiveness because it can be used to eradicate or substantially depopulate the tumor cells; therefore, it directly targets the cause of pain. A balance is required between the killing of tumor cells and the adverse effects of radiation on normal tissue. The toxicity of radiation is determined by the structures included within the radiation portal, the dose per fraction, the total dose, and the radiation sensitivity of the tissues involved.

Greater than one-third of radiation therapy is palliative. Most retrospective and prospective studies report that 75% or more of patients obtain relief from pain and that about one-half of those who achieve relief become pain-free (Nielsen et al. 1991).

Palliative radiotherapy should be administered with the minimum number of hospital visits and length of overall treatment time so that precious remaining time with friends and family can be maximized.

Indications for the radiation of bone metastases include pain relief and the prevention or promotion of healing of pathologic fractures. Spinal cord compression associated with vertebral collapse due to bony or epidural metastases requires emergency radiation therapy, sometimes in coordination with surgical intervention to preserve neurologic integrity. Painful nerve compression or infiltration by a malignant tumor can sometimes be alleviated by radiation therapy. Dosage is limited by the proximity of the tumor to radiosensitive structures such as the spinal cord. Peripheral nerves, however, can tolerate higher doses.

ß-emitting radiopharmaceuticals are used to relieve the pain of widespread osteoblastic skeletal metastases and require only one intravenous injection. Iodine-131, phosphorus-32-orthophosphate, strontium-89, rhenium-186, and samarium-153 phosphorate chelates have demonstrated 50% to 80% efficacy in clinical trials.

Brachytherapy involves the placement of a radioactive source within the tissue to deliver localized radiation and is frequently applied to treat recurrent disease in an area previously treated by external beam radiation. Advantages include the sparing of critical structures close to the tumor and brevity of treatment (hours to days). Difficulties involve primarily anatomic constraints on implant placement.

A radiation oncologist should be consulted to determine if radiation is appropriate. For palliative purposes, even the "radioresistant" tumors frequently respond favorably.

Palliative chemotherapy for cancer pain

Although many cancers today remain incurable, few cancers are untreatable. With properly applied antineoplastic therapy, symptomatic palliation can be achieved. When treating a patient's cancer pain, one must not forget to treat the underlying disease. When considering palliative treatment, toxicity and the ability of a particular patient to tolerate that toxicity are particularly important. Tumor histology is also an important factor in this decision tree. The chance a malignancy will respond to therapy and the ability of the patient to tolerate therapy decreases with each successive treatment.

A thorough discussion of the types of chemotherapy for each type of cancer is beyond the scope of this chapter. Refer to recent texts for further information (Kurman 1993; DeVita et al. 1985; Hellmann and Carter 1987). In general, the clinician needs a broad knowledge of the natural history of the patient's disease, a thorough understanding of the physiologic effects and pharmacology of systemic treatment, and an intimate knowledge of the patient's medical and psychological state.

Local anesthetic nerve blockade for cancer pain

Anesthetic nerve blockade is a procedure in which a local anesthetic is injected around various nerves or ganglia or into the epidural or intrathecal spaces of the spinal cord. Any pain-relieving effects that result from a local anesthetic nerve blockade are usually temporary. For the cancer patient, local anesthetic nerve blocks may fulfill diagnostic, prognostic, and therapeutic roles in the management of pain. Although this technique does not generally provide long-term relief, it does provide immediate relief of regional pain and can be invaluable in guiding future treatment. Diagnostic nerve blocks can identify the anatomic source of the pain and determine whether it is visceral or sympathetic in origin, as opposed to somatic. For example, a patient's response to a celiac plexus blockade versus an intercostal nerve blockade would help direct the next step in therapy by identifying how much of the patient's abdominal pain originates from visceral structures (relieved by celiac plexus block) and how much from the abdominal wall (relieved by intercostal block).

Local anesthetic blocks may also be used to predict the efficacy of permanent, ablative procedures such as celiac plexus neurolysis (permanent destruction of the celiac ganglion), rhizotomy (permanent interruption of the dorsal root of a spinal nerve), or sympathectomy (permanent interruption of some portion of the sympathetic nerve pathways). They allow the patient to experience the neurologic changes that are likely to accompany a more definitive procedure such as a neurolysis. Even if the patient experiences temporary relief from a local anesthetic nerve block, however, the response does not guarantee that the patient will gain long-term pain relief from a surgical or neurolytic block. The pain-relieving results of any neurodestructive procedure can be thwarted by postsurgical nerve regeneration, chronic deafferentation syndrome, and dysesthesias, among other complications. However, since a lack of response to local anesthetic blocks reliably predicts failure of the more permanent surgical or neurolytic procedure, it is still worthwhile to perform predictive blocks when a more permanent procedure is being considered.

Neurolysis for cancer pain

Neurolysis is the permanent destruction of nerve tissue using various ablative techniques, including the injection of a neurolytic substance such as phenol. Neurolysis should be considered only after more conservative modalities have first been exhausted. It should be performed only by an experienced clinician. Though newer nondestructive analgesic infusion techniques may have decreased the need for neurolysis, it is still appropriate in many cases. Neurolytic blockade in general can be considered in a patient who meets all of these criteria: limited life expectancy, localized or regional pain, adequate response to local anesthetic block, pain that is not relieved by less invasive modalities.

Intrathecal neurolysis (destruction of nerve roots or the spinal cord within the spinal fluid) is limited by a high-risk profile and only fair long-term results. It is indicated only for cancer patients with pain that is unresponsive to more conservative therapy and only when all possible measures are instituted to ensure that the injection is made at the intended site. The pain should be localized to two to three dermatomes (spinal nerve levels), should be somatic in origin, and should respond favorably to a prognostic block. Risks include inadequate pain relief, limb paresis, spinal cord damage, and bowel and bladder dysfunction. The patient is positioned so that the neurolytic agent contacts posterior (sensory) roots and, it is hoped, avoids anterior motor roots, though increased spread can cause complications. Because the cell bodies are not destroyed, axon regeneration may eventually occur. The average duration of relief is 2 to 4 months.

Epidural neurolysis (destruction of nerve roots within the epidural space) has the advantage of less risk of spread of the neurolytic agent and no meningeal irritation; however, results from this procedure have been disappointing. Recent reports using repeated administration of a neurolytic substance through an indwelling catheter claim 70% of patients achieve appreciable relief lasting for an average duration of 5 to 8 months (Korevaar et al. 1987). Though perhaps less common, the same risks apply as with intrathecal neurolysis.

Nerve blocks for sympathetically mediated pain

Sympathetically mediated pain is often more responsive to neurolysis than somatic pain. When performed properly, destruction of sympathetic nerves is not accompanied by numbness or weakness, and the development of neuritis or deafferentation pain are not significant risks. Sympathetic pain may be neuropathic in origin, such as Pancoast's syndrome, lumbosacral plexopathy, causalgia, or reflex sympathetic dystrophy (RSD); or of visceral origin such as pancreatic cancer. Patients may develop RSD due to tumor invasion or anti-tumor therapy and will present with classic symptoms that usually appear solely in the affected body part, often an extremity. RSD-associated symptoms include allodynia, hyperesthesia, hyperpathia, and atrophy of the involved extremity, as well as vasomotor and sudomotor changes, such as intermittent cyanosis, rubor or pallor, edema, abnormally diminished or increased perspiration, and increase or decrease in skin temperature. In RSD, a series of local anesthetic blocks (see above) to sympathetic nerves can result in complete resolution of symptoms in addition to providing the diagnosis. However, visceral pain caused by tumor progression into sympathetic nerves will likely require neurolysis for resolution of symptoms after a diagnostic block confirms the etiology of pain. The sympathetic blocks performed most commonly for cancer pain are the celiac plexus block, the lumbar sympathetic block, and the hypogastric plexus block.

Celiac plexus block is most commonly used for pancreatic cancer but can be used for pain arising from other sites, such as the distal esophagus, stomach, or liver. Significant relief is reported by 70% to 94% of patients, with most studies reporting successful results in the higher ranges (Cousins and Bridenbaugh 1988). Duration of relief varies between weeks and a year or more, though the majority of treated patients experience relatively pain-free deaths. Efficacy and duration are presumed to relate to the completeness of celiac ablation and the relative presence of concomitant pain of somatic origin. In the hands of a skilled clinician, serious complications such as paraplegia or urinary and sexual function abnormalities are extremely rare, although they are possible. Hypotension and diarrhea are fairly common side effects of this procedure and should be anticipated or treated prophylactically.

Lumbar sympathetic neurolysis may be used for intractable RSD or nonoperable ischemic pain of the lower extremities. Cancer involving the lower extremities is usually somatically mediated as well and thus would require other therapy.

Recently, superior hypogastric plexus block has been frequently used for visceral pelvic pain. The procedure is minimally hazardous and provides significant pain relief. It may be used for pain emanating from the descending colon and rectum, vaginal fundus and bladder, prostate and prostatic urethra, testes, seminal vesicles, uterus, and ovary. In a study of 28 patients, this procedure produced a mean decrease of 70% in pain scores with only two having some return of symptoms before death. There were no serious complications (Plancarte et al. 1990).

Orthopedic procedures for cancer pain

Maintenance of maximal functional activity can prevent numerous complications from tumor involvement in bone, including muscle weakness, decreased ambulation, joint stiffness or contractures, spinal deformities, osteopenia from inactivity, thromboembolism, and hypercalcemia. Surgical fixation of impending or completed pathologic fractures, maintained ambulatory status, and rehabilitative programs such as physical therapy and occupational therapy can reduce or avoid these problems.

A patient with bone pain may have a normal X-ray because nearly 50% of trabecular bone must be destroyed before a lytic lesion (an area of cell destruction) becomes evident on a plain X-ray. A bone scan is a much more sensitive indicator of bone involvement, and an MRI will demonstrate early marrow involvement but is generally not necessary as a screening tool.

Bone pain that is not likely to cause a fracture can be treated with local radiation therapy, which is the mainstay of pain control with metastatic lesions and multiple myeloma (malignant neoplasm of plasma cells, usually arising in the bone marrow). However, surgical stabilization followed by radiation therapy to permit healing is indicated with an impending fracture in a weight-bearing extremity. Radiation therapy alone may be sufficient for lesions in the axial skeleton, which heal more readily. Lesions of the spine are often dectected early because patients usually present with back pain before there is significant bone destruction; however, following radiation therapy, if pain recurs, if the spine is unstable, or if a neurological deficit progresses, surgery may be necessary.

Neurosurgical procedures for cancer pain

As with neurolytic procedures, before neurosurgery is considered, more conservative methods of pain management must be exhausted, and an experienced clinician must be available to evaluate the patient. Procedures to ablate nervous tissue are generally avoided unless the patient is known to have a life-shortening malignancy. If the patient's life expectancy is less than 60 to 90 days, pain is usually managed through appropriate administration of opioids or through a percutaneous procedure such as neurolytic injection or nonincisional neurosurgery. Neurodestructive surgery would be more appropriate in a cancer patient with a life expectancy of 6 months or greater. The following discussion addresses only the more commonly used procedures. A more thorough discussion can be found in recent textbooks (Bonica 1990; Wall and Melzack 1994).

Percutaneous radiofrequency coagulation is a neurodestructive procedure that involves inserting a probe through the skin and into the target ganglion or nerve. By passing a radiofrequency electrical current through the inserted probe, the surgeon creates a heat lesion in the targeted nervous tissue. This technique has been refined in recent years and is recommended when possible over an open neurosurgical technique. The extent of the lesion can be controlled by monitoring the current applied and the temperature achieved at the probe tip. As opposed to the application of chemical neurolysis, radiofrequency can confirm that the intended lesion site will reduce the patient's pain. This is done by electrical stimulation of the intended lesion site to mimic the pain as well as recording possible increased nerve electrical activity at the intended site if that is present. Recording of electrical impedance after the thermocoagulation can determine if the nerve or ganglion has been adequately destroyed.

Though attractive due to its simplicity, peripheral neurectomy is less likely to be used because it causes both motor and sensory loss and can cause new pain syndromes with nerve regeneration. Examples of this procedure include multilevel intercostal neurectomy for chest wall pain and cranial neurectomy for head and neck cancer. Motor loss is less problematic in these examples, but there is still significant risk of anesthesia dolorosa (denervation hypersensitivity) and recurrence of or increase in pain with nerve regeneration.

Dorsal rhizotomy (cutting sensory nerve roots just outside the spinal cord) is preferable to peripheral neurectomy as it selectively destroys the dorsal nerve root. This spares motor function while reducing nociceptive perception in the affected area. However, multilevel dorsal rhizotomy of all roots supplying an extremity renders it functionally useless due to loss of proprioception and a propensity for charcot joints (disintegration of joints, even major joints such as knees or hips, after loss of sensory innervation). The likelihood of this impairment is lessened by sparing at least one dorsal root. However, in practice this procedure is considered only for localized pain in the trunk or abdomen or, rarely, for an extremity that is functionless preoperatively. As with peripheral neurectomy, its use is limited by potential anesthesia dolorosa and late loss of efficacy.

Cordotomy for cancer pain

Anterolateral cordotomy (spinal tractotomy) destroys the fibers of the spinothalamic tract in the anterolateral quadrant of the spinal cord. Cordotomy provides selective loss of pain and temperature sensation in a variable number of segments below and contralateral to the segment at which the lesion is placed. Anterolateral cordotomy is indicated for unilateral, mainly somatic pain below the midcervical dermatomes. The percutaneous approach with radiofrequency ablation has provided excellent results with decreased complications compared to the open technique. However, with improved conservative management of cancer pain, there may be fewer neurosurgeons with experience in this approach, and an open procedure would then be indicated. Potential complications include Ondine's curse (sleep apnea), ataxia, paresis, bowel and bladder and sexual dysfunction, and unmasking of dysesthetic pain. Studies report greater than 90% of patients are pain-free immediately after cordotomy, 84% at 3 months due to dysesthesias and incomplete analgesia, and 60% at 2 years (Bonica 1990). This procedure is a reasonable option, especially for unilateral pain in the cancer patient with a limited life expectancy.

Commissural myelotomy interrupts the spinothalamic tract bilaterally as it crosses in the midline of the spinal cord. Indications for myelotomy include bilateral and midline pelvic or perineal pain. Potential complications include dysesthesias and limb apraxia (inability to carry out purposeful movements) in addition to variable duration of pain relief. There is great variability in sensory loss and pain relief.

Intracranial procedures for cancer pain

Stereotaxy is a precise method of applying lesions to brain structures after they have been located within a system of three-dimensional coordinates. Using stereotaxy, both radiofrequency and chemical hypophysectomy (removal of the pituitary gland) offer a 40% to 85% likelihood of cancer pain relief in all areas of the body. This procedure has its greatest success for hormonally dependent tumors such as prostate and breast malignancies and is almost as successful with hormonally independent tumors. It is also successful for bilateral or diffuse bone pain from metastatic disease that has failed to respond to all other hormonal, radiation, or medical therapies. Complications include anterior hypopituitarism in 80% to 90% of patients, visual and oculomotor disturbances, and the recurrence of pain in 3 to 4 months. Hormone replacement therapy may be needed to replace pituitary secretions.

Thalamic lesions applied via stereotactic techniques can be useful with widespread metastases, midline, bilateral, or head and neck cancer pain. Nonfatal complications, usually consisting of transient confusion or other cognitive disorders, are experienced by 10% to 20% of patients. As with to other destructive procedures, the long-term failure rate limits its usefulness. The initial reported success of 80% for this procedure can drop to about 30% by the end of 1 year.

Psychosurgical procedures, although rarely used, aim at destroying or stimulating brain integrative pathways involved in assignment of meaning to peripheral stimuli. Pain continues, but the emotional response and reactivity to pain are reduced, especially with respect to the patient's anticipation and memory of pain. The most favored procedure, bilateral cingulumotomy, either alone or in conjuction with lesions elsewhere, is considered effective in patients with significant depression or anxiety. A recent review of this procedure concluded that one-half to three-quarters of pain patients so treated derived short-term relief from cingulumotomy, but that long-term relief was "equivocal" (Bouckoms 1994).

Cancer pain can be relieved not only by intracranial neurolytic procedures but also by modulation of electrical activity in certain parts of the brain. Electrical stimulation of the periventricular-periaqueductal gray area of the brain via implanted electrodes, a process that is thought to activate descending inhibition of nociceptive impulses traveling through the spinothalmic tract, has a reported 60% to 80% chance of relieving pain. This technique offers the great advantage of reversibility and therefore lowered risk but is limited by the costly equipment. Risks include neural trauma (up to 11%), infection (4% to 5%), device failure (3% to 9%), lead breakage (11%), and lead migration (7%) (Wall and Melzack 1994).

Intraspinal opioids for cancer pain

Intraspinal opioid therapy probably represents the most significant advancement in contemporary cancer pain management. In contrast to neurolytic blocks and neurosurgery, intraspinal opioid therapy produces reversible analgesia that is more likely to be effective for multiple pains or for pain that is bilateral or crosses the midline. Intraspinal opioid therapy works best for somatic and visceral pain, both of which are common in cancer. A trial application using the less invasive percutaneous catheters can easily help to predict the patient's response to this type of opioid therapy. Development of opioid tolerance and other complications of chronic opioid use are less of an issue in the cancer pain patient due to limited life expectancy.

By means of a catheter the opioid is introduced into either the epidural (peridural) space or the subarachnoid (intrathecal) space. Intraspinal analgesia classically refers to the administration of opioids only, which leaves the motor, sensory, and sympathetic systems unaffected. However, combinations of opioids and dilute concentrations of local anesthetics, which potentially can cause motor weakness, sensory anesthesia, and interference with sympathetic function at higher doses, are becoming more common. Studies have confirmed the additive effects, or synergism, between local anesthetics and opioids.

Physical and chemical properties of drugs influence onset, duration of action, and migration away from the primary site of delivery. Morphine is the most commonly used narcotic and the most hydrophilic (water-soluble), reaching peak effect in 30 to 60 minutes and having a duration of analgesia of 6 to 24 hours. The lipophilic (fat-soluble) agents such as sufentanil and fentanyl peak in about 10 minutes and last 2 to 5 hours. The lipophilic agents do not spread as readily in the epidural space; therefore, when using these agents with an epidural catheter, they must be placed near the site of pain.

The side effects of intraspinal opioids include respiratory depression and loss of normal gastrointestinal motility. The risk of respiratory depression generates the most clinical concern and can occur early (less than 2 hours after a dose) or late (4 to 24 hours after a dose). Lipophilic agents are more likely to cause early respiratory depression; morphine poses the potential for late respiratory depression. Fortunately, such depression occurs relatively rarely if at all in the opioid-tolerant cancer patient.

Other dose-limiting side effects are also rare in cancer patients who have been chronically exposed to systemic opioids. Systemic opioids decrease gastrointestinal motility, presumably by their action on opioid receptors in the gut. Clinically, gastrointestinal motility seems to be much less affected by intraspinal opioids, but adverse effects may appear as dosage is increased. Nausea and vomiting are infrequent if the patient has had prior chronic exposure to opioids and generally resolve with continued administration. A more lipophilic opioid or antiemetic therapy may be necessary to control nausea in certain patients. Urinary retention is rarely observed in opioid-tolerant cancer patients but can be treated with intermittent bladder catheterization if necessary. Pruritus is also uncommon in cancer patients, though it is very common in opioid-naive patients. It generally responds to antihistamines or an opioid antagonist given systemically.

Complications of intraspinal opioids

Probably the most serious, though uncommon, complication of intraspinal opioid therapy is infection at the catheter exit site, along the superficial or deep catheter track, or within the epidural or intrathecal space. Infection at the catheter exit site may occur in up to 6% of patients and is one rationale for the use of tunneled catheters. The DuPen Epidural Catheter with VitaCuff (Davol, Inc., Salt Lake City, Utah) incorporates a silver-impregnated cuff near the exit site to further impede infection. Epidural space infection is associated with constant, nonspecific back pain, pain on injection, fluid collection near the proximal incision, and reduced analgesia. Untreated, an epidural abscess may lead to serious neurologic deficits, including hemiparesis. Good local skin care, filtered and aseptic administration of the opioid, and vigilant assessment for signs of infection are mandatory. Immediate neurosurgical consultation is also critical if infection is suspected.

Another serious and unfortunately all too common complication is misinjection. A wide variety of substances have been inadvertently injected into intraspinal catheters with complications ranging from severe permanent neurologic injury to self-limited back pain and spasm. Distinct labeling of any external lines or pumps and no availability of accessory ports are critical.

As with neurolysis and neurosurgery, the most widely accepted indication for chronic therapy with intraspinal opioids is intractable pain that is unresponsive to aggressive systemic pharmacologic management. Some would argue for earlier administration of intraspinal opioids due to the reversibility and low risk of the procedure, but the cost of the equipment and follow-up care may be a limiting factor.

Delivery techniques for intraspinal opioids

Intraspinal opioids can be administered by continuous infusion or by bolus techniques. Continuous infusion provides the advantage of a stable spinal level which can decrease both pain and complications and thus is often preferred if resources are available. PCA by spinal catheter returns some control to the patient and addresses one of the patient's greatest fears: uncontrolled pain. However, PCA is not suitable for patients who are uncomfortable with it, who have a significant history of drug-seeking behavior, or who have cognitive deficits. Lipophilic agents are especially suited to PCA use due to their quick onset, but morphine boluses can also be effective as rescue doses.

Depending on life expectancy and medical resources, two general types of intraspinal opioid delivery systems can be used. The oldest type has the drug reservoir and pump outside the body, requiring a catheter or needle through the skin. This is less expensive initially and requires less technology but has increased risk of infection. This device cannot be used with an intrathecal catheter since defense against infection is poor in the intrathecal space; these systems use epidural catheters. The other system is entirely implanted, including the pump and reservoir. The reservoir requires refilling every 1 to 4 weeks, but no other direct access is needed. Since an implanted reservoir must be small, these devices must be used to deliver intrathecal opioids because intrathecal dose requirements are approximately one-tenth the dose requirements for epidural administration.

The implanted pumps can now be programmed externally to change the infusion rate, give boluses at specific times consistently, and vary the rate for specified hours of the day, making them as adjustable as external pumps. The maintenance costs of internal pumps is lower, even though initial costs are much higher. This makes them cost-effective after 3 to 6 months of use.

Intraspinal opioid therapy is contraindicated if the patient has a bleeding diathesis, is on anticoagulation therapy, or has infection at the insertion site. Systemic sepsis, localized tumor invasion that prevents safe access to the spinal canal, or inability to care for the catheter are additional contraindications. Installation by an anesthesiologist or neurosurgeon trained in these techniques is mandatory.

Descriptions of pain management techniques

This section provides further information about some of the medications, techniques, and procedures mentioned earlier. For greater detail, refer to the resource list at the end of this chapter for textbooks and journals with in-depth information on the medical and surgical management of pain.

Use of NSAIDs

NSAIDs have analgesic properties in peripheral tissues and in the central nervous system. Most of their analgesic and other properties are due to their capacity to inhibit production of prostaglandins or related substances. In peripheral tissue prostaglandin inhibition decreases the inflammatory response and the generation of pain transmitters and potentiators. In the spinal cord and probably in the brain, it reduces the perception of pain and reduces certain causes of increased pain perception over time.

In the stomach and small intestine, the inhibition of prostaglandin production partially breaks down the protective coating of the mucosa and makes patients taking NSAIDs more susceptible to gastritis or ulcers. In the blood stream, NSAIDs cause reduced platelet function and therefore, inhibition of the normal clotting mechanism of the blood. In the case of an injury or an ulcer, this can lead to increased loss of blood, but the effects on platelet function can also be used to advantage in patients with blood vessel disease around the heart or brain; merely taking one aspirin a day can reduce the chances of having a blood vessel suddenly occlude and cause a stroke or heart attack. In the hypothalamus, prostaglandin inhibition reduces the fever response.

Certain NSAIDs have statistically greater or lesser effect on any one of these systems, and acetaminophen has essentially no effect on the gastric lining, blood clotting, or inflammation. Another key issue is idiosyncratic response. A given patient may have tremendous pain relief with few side effects with one NSAID and not with others, and the response does not necessarily coincide with the statistical norms.

Use of antidepressants

Several classes of medications have antidepressant properties (see the table on page 218). They share a common function thought to relieve depression: blocking reuptake of the neurotransmitters norepinephrine and serotonin after they have been released into the synaptic cleft. This increases the effects of the neurotransmitters. These same two neurotransmitters function in the central nervous system to decrease the perception of pain. By blocking the reuptake of these neurotransmitters, it is possible to increase their availability in the central nervous system and therefore, decrease the perception of pain. The pain-relieving effects of antidepressants are not related to relief from depression; the doses of antidepressant that provide pain relief usually are subtherapeutic for depression.

The tricyclic antidepressants and trazodone all share some common side effects, although each one may vary in the intensities of these effects. For the most part, these effects are sedation, constipation, dry mouth, blurred vision, increased heart rate, and increased sweating. Some patients, particularly elderly males, also have difficulty voiding urine. Frequently, these side effects are sufficiently disturbing that the patient discontinues the treatment. Sedation may be a beneficial side effect if the patient is having trouble sleeping, but if the sedation carries over into normal waking hours, it is often unacceptable.

A newer group of antidepressants, the selective serotonin reuptake inhibitors (SSRIs), affect only serotonin reuptake and have a significantly different side-effect profile. The effects on sleep are variable and often nonexistent, although some patients note some sedation or insomnia. Gastrointestinal upset is a little more common with these drugs, but the other side effects such as dry mouth, constipation, and difficulty urinating are fairly infrequent. In men, however, there is a significant side effect of impotence, which may prove intolerable.

Currently, new receptor-specific antidepressants with slight variations in side effects or in the receptors affected are being developed and marketed. Although the effect of SSRIs on pain has not been tested, their mechanism of action would indicate that, in fact, they should also give pain relief in the same manner as the other antidepressants.

Antidepressants for pain relief can be chosen according to which side effects the patient desires or can tolerate. Even patients who have great difficulty with side effects can generally tolerate at least one of these medications. It frequently takes 1 to 3 weeks to notice a significant effect on pain levels, and in order to maintain the pain-relieving effect, the medications must be taken consistently, rather than as needed. Most of these drugs require only once-a-day dosage.

Use of medications for neuralgic pain

Medications for neuralgic pain are a diverse group of drugs that frequently have no value for pain from tissue other than the nervous system (see the table on page 219). It is thought that most of these medications reduce excessive firing of pain nerve fibers or act within the central nervous system to decrease the perception of nerve pain. Most have the potential to cause sedation or mental side effects that some patients find intolerable. Some also have potentially significant side effects, actually causing long-term damage to certain tissue or organ systems, so trials with these medications can be difficult and may require significant time and medical monitoring. Also, they require consistent, rather than as-needed administration in order to be effective.

Use of opioids

Opioids are a large class of medications named for the opium poppy. There are specific opioid receptors within the body that, when activated, have both beneficial and detrimental effects. There are several different classes of opioid receptors, and most of them have pain relief as one of their effects. Analgesia originating at opioid receptors occurs not only in the brain and spinal cord but also out in the peripheral tissues, particularly if inflammation is present. The body actually produces opioid receptors at the site of inflammation, and when those receptors are activated, they reduce pain and inflammation.

The side effects of consuming opioids are commonly known: nausea and vomiting, itching, constipation, and sedation. Along with the sedation, opioids cause an inhibition in the brain stem respiratory center, which normally produces the drive to breathe. In high enough doses, this inhibition will actually cause complete apnea or no drive to breathe at all. Opioids that are either partial agonists or agonists/antagonists have a ceiling effect on respiratory depression, which perhaps makes them slightly safer. However, in a patient who has consistently been taking complete agonist opioids for a significant period of time, swiching to an agonist/antagonist or a partial agonist may cause abrupt withdrawal symptoms, which range from uncomfortable to life-threatening. The opioids also have the potential to cause a euphoria or a dysphoria, depending on the patient. Certain opioids produce an increased incidence, statistically, of dysphoria or a decreased incidence of euphoria, but in any given patient, either one may occur.

Whenever a patient is started on chronic opioid therapy, consideration should be given to starting a stool softener or laxative. Though not all patients will require such therapy with the initiation of opioids, oversight of this issue may cause increased pain and decreased appetite as well as intestinal pseudo-obstruction and even colonic perforation.

Tolerance, dependence, and addiction

Three definitions are important regarding opioids: tolerance, dependence, and addiction. Tolerance is defined as the decreased effect of a medication when taken over a prolonged period of time, with other conditions remaining constant. This is one of the features of the opioids, although there has been some debate about it, and it means that over time, a given dose of opioid that has been effective in relieving pain may no longer be effective. The patient's need for a higher dose of opioid to obtain pain relief does not necessarily imply dependence or addiction.

Dependence is generally broken down into physical dependence and psychological dependence. Physical dependence means that if the medication is abruptly discontinued, the patient will demonstrate the withdrawal symptoms of increased activity in the sympathetic nervous system and the central nervous system. The nervous system changes may cause a general flu-like syndrome with malaise and achiness, marked diarrhea or nausea and vomiting, increased heart rate and blood pressure, profuse sweating, and perhaps confusion, seizures, or even death. It should be noted that if the opioid withdrawal is gradual rather than sudden, withdrawal symptoms are markedly reduced or eliminated.

Psychological dependence involves the patient's belief that he or she must take the medication to cause or to stop a particular effect. The desired effect of opioids is to reduce pain, although many patients state that taking an opioid allows them to function. Psychological dependence has some similarities to addiction.

Addiction is a complex of behaviors associated with drug-seeking or manipulative behavior and involves taking a medication for reasons other than pain relief, frequently for the euphoria or sedation that is a side effect of the chosen drug. Understanding the difference between dependence and addiction is important. When the informa-

Opioid analgesics

The first group are agonists/antagonists. When used alone, they work as agonists. They bind to the opiate receptors and provide analgesia. When used in combination with an agonist, such as the opioids listed in the other columns, they block the agonist effect and produce withdrawal symptoms.

Agonists/antagonists or partial agonists
buprenorphine
butorphanol
dezocine
levallorphan
nalbuphine
nalorphine
pentazocine
tramadol

Less potent opioids, short duration of analgesia
codeine
dihydrocodeine
hydrocodone
propoxyphene
- dezocine*
- evallorphan
- nalbuphine
- nalorphine
- pentazocine
- tramadol

More potent opioids, short duration of analgesia
fentanyl
hydromorphone
meperidine
morphine
oxycodone
oxymorphone
sufentanil
- buprenorphine
- butorphanol

More potent opioids, long duration of analgesia
methadone
levorphanol
slow-release morphine
fentanyl patch (slow release through the skin)

* Medications offset with (•) are agonists/antagonists or partial agonists.

tion intended to be conveyed is that the patient has physical dependence or tolerance, caregivers should avoid describing the patient in terms that imply addiction because addiction has very negative social and medical/legal implications.

Short-duration opioid analgesics are divided into two categories: less potent and more potent agonists (see *Opioid analgesics*). This division is arbitrary, but it conforms to many other tables available in medical literature.

Use of nerve blocks

The term "nerve block" has become a catch-all term for the injection of a large variety of substances into an equally diverse variety of anatomical sites. Here, descriptions of the substances injected as nerve blocks are followed by descriptions of the more common sites for injection.

Local anesthetic blocks

Local anesthetics are the classic nerve-block medications and probably the best understood. There are several local anesthetics with slightly different properties, usually varying in their effective duration. Local anesthetics are relatively nontoxic when used appropriately. As a single injection, none of the local anesthetics will last longer than 6 hours consistently, and many of them last only 1 hour. Occasionally other medications are added to them to try to increase their duration, but these are usually effective only for the short-acting local anesthetics.

The exact mechanism of action of local anesthetics is still being defined, but the basic function is to block nerve excitation and transmission by deactivating sodium and calcium channels in the nerve cell membrane. The block is concentration-dependent, so that lower concentrations of drug produce only a partial block.

In general, small-diameter nerve fibers are more easily blocked than larger ones. Pain nerve fibers are among the smallest diameter nerve fibers in the body; thus, pain can be relieved without blocking all sensory nerve function or motor nerve function necessary for movement. Unfortunately, there is no single consistent concentration of any local anesthetic that always blocks pain without blocking some sensations or motor functions. Each patient requires a slightly different concentration or amount of local anesthetic for pain relief. Local anesthetics relieve pain by blocking electrical activity at the local nerve endings. Local anesthetics also work at some distance from the pain site if the nerve fibers carrying the pain information stay together in a nerve bundle, or plexus. The most central place local anesthetics are injected is the area where the spinal nerves enter the spinal cord.

Glucocorticoid injection

"Steroids" is a term often used to describe glucocorticoids. A number of other medications fall into the category of steroids, but they have dissimilar effects. Only the glucocorticoids are used for nerve blocks. Another common term for glucocorticoids is "cortisone," which was the most commonly used glucocorticoid in the past.

Glucocorticoids have a number of local and systemic actions, both beneficial and detrimental. They reduce inflammation and probably stabilize hyperexcitable nerve membranes. As both inflammation and nerve hyperexcitability can cause prolonged pain, steroids can be effective in reducing that pain.

A large number of glucocorticoids are available. Some of them are effective for 1 to 3 days; others last for 2 to 3 weeks after the injection.

The duration of reduced inflammation or pain may not correspond with the expected duration of the medication and may last shorter or longer than the period during which the medication actually remains at the injection site. At times, even when inflammation is the cause of significant pain, steroid injections can be ineffective in reducing the inflammation and its associated pain. Nonetheless, they are the most effective medication for reducing inflammation.

Glucocorticoids are associated with a number of potential side effects, but by injecting them at a focused site, many of the side effects associated with systemic dosing can be markedly reduced or eliminated. Specifically, these medications reduce the immune response and, therefore, increase the risk of infection. They also slow healing as well as reduce scarring. In systemic doses, they change the entire metabolic system, usually resulting in elevated blood sugar at the expense of protein and fat metabolism. There can also be fluid retention resulting in increased blood pressure or even heart failure in susceptible individuals. Beyond that, a large number of diverse and sometimes severe potential complications are associated with glucocorticoids, but these complications are usually associated with extremely high doses or prolonged administration.

The reduction in inflammation associated with glucocorticoids is due to inhibition of the inflammation chemical cascade, including prostaglandin inhibition. In this sense, they have properties similar to NSAIDs, although they are more effective than NSAIDs and do inhibit a significant number of other inflammatory functions beyond prostaglandin production. Recent research indicates that some extreme neuralgic pain problems have prostaglandin as one of the pain pathway transmitters at the spinal cord. It is possible that steroids in the region may produce relief by inhibiting of prostaglandin production.

Opioid injection

Although opioids have been injected into many sites, only two currently have scientific basis or demonstrated benefit. The best proven location for opioid injection is near the spinal cord, either in the epidural or intrathecal (subarachnoid) space. Opioids thus delivered are thought, although poorly proven, to diffuse or be transported to opioid receptors in the spinal cord area where the sensory nerve roots enter. In that area they reduce transmission of pain messages by inhibiting both neurotransmitter release and subsequent excitation of secondary neurons. Although opioids can be very effective under these circumstances, they generally cannot block 100% of pain messages, particularly upon such strong stimulation as surgery itself.

The other potential use for opioids by injection is at the site of inflammation. Since opioid receptors are produced by the body at those sites, an injection in the area of inflammation, such as an inflamed knee after surgery, may reduce pain transmission as well as inflammation. The injection of opioids on nerves between the site of inflammation and the spinal cord is generally ineffective and inappropriate.

Neurolytics

The term "neurolytic" means lysis, or destruction, of nerves. A fair amount of research has gone into finding medications that safely destroy nerves in a consistent fashion. Unfortunately, science has found no substance that will consistently destroy nerves without destroying other tissue. Of the many substances that have been investigated, only two are in significant current use for neurolysis: ethyl alcohol and phenol.

Ethyl alcohol is used in concentrations of 50% to 100%, with 100% being extremely damaging to any tissue near the injection site. Ethyl alcohol is not particularly toxic systemically; it is the same alcohol as that found in alcoholic beverages. The concentration of phenol that will produce neurolysis is strongly dependent upon the carrier solution used for the phenol. The carrier solution can be glycerin, water, saline, or radiopaque dye.

Phenol has some local anesthetic properties at the time of injection; therefore, a phenol injection is not particularly painful. It may actually give better immediate pain relief as a local anesthetic than it will provide in its neurolytic function. This can make dosage of phenol somewhat difficult to determine at the time of injection. Alcohol, on the other hand, is often painful as an injection but its neurolytic properties will give pain relief at least equal to the relief achieved immediately after an injection and perhaps even better relief over 1 to 2 weeks. Alcohol tends to be more completely tissue-destructive than phenol and therefore may offer a more permanent block in areas where nerves can regenerate. Note that the sympathetic nervous system is extremely good at regenerating, peripheral nerves are fairly good at regenerating, and the spinal cord and brain are essentially incapable of regeneration.

Peripheral blocks

Nerve blocks at the periphery are generally intended to block pain signals at a site of injury or inflammation, while any blocks more proximal than the injury site are usually intended to block nerve transmission of pain signals from those sites. Occasionally, the nerves themselves are the site of injury, so a block at that position may block both the transmission and the site.

The most common "nerve block" is not a nerve block at all but a muscle block. The common terms are trigger-point injection or myoneural block. The location of the injection is determined by palpating a muscle that the patient indicates is sore until a point of maximum tenderness is determined. Frequently, the examiner will feel a

Injecting a trigger point

To inject a painful muscle trigger point with saline or a local anesthetic, the examiner first palpates for a taut band of muscle (marked with an oval), then positions the band between two fingers and injects the maximally tender point (dark spot within the oval).

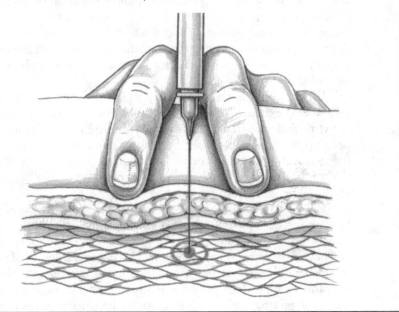

hard "knot" at the tender site. Dry needling or injection of saline, local anesthetic, or a steroid may provide acute and occasionally long-term relief from the pain at that site (see *Injecting a trigger point*). A similar injection site is at a scar from previous surgery or injury. Nerve and other tissue can get entrapped in a scar and become quite painful. Injections such as this are frequently much more effective when combined with physical manipulations of the scar after the injection to help reduce entrapment.

Nerve fibers from a given muscle or region frequently join to form peripheral nerves. As those nerves approach the central nervous system, they often group together into a plexus such as the brachial (arm) plexus or lumbosacral (leg) plexus. From there, they regroup into spinal nerves before entering the spinal cord. *Injection of a local anesthetic* illustrates a block of the suprascapular nerve, a peripheral nerve that supplies the scapula and several muscles associated with the scapula. This nerve could be blocked to relieve acute pain from scapular fracture, chronic pain from nerve entrapment, or pain from a tumor in this region, to give examples of nerve block for acute, chronic, and cancer pains.

Injection of a local anesthetic

Injection of a local anesthetic near a peripheral sensory nerve (shown here, the suprascapular nerve) temporarily relieves pain to areas served by that nerve. Injection of a neurolytic agent, such as alcohol or phenol, produces a disruption of neural tissue and long-term analgesia, which remains effective until the nerve tissues regenerate.

Sympathetic blocks

A portion of the sympathetic nervous system: The paravertebral ganglia, page 246, demonstrates the sympathetic ganglia located next to the spine. Although this chain of ganglia can be blocked anywhere along its course, the two most common sites are at the stellate ganglia (near the top ribs) for arm or facial pain and at the lumbar ganglia (between the lowest ribs and the pelvis) for leg pain. It is important to remember that not all pain transmission from legs, arms, and face passes through these ganglia. However, when an accurate blockade of one of these ganglia is performed, pain from the affected area is reduced without loss of strength or other normal sensations. A number of other functions may also be affected as a result of such a block:

- increased heart rate, contractility, and blood vessel tone (and blood pressure elevation as a result of these)
- increased peristalsis of the gastrointestinal tract
- various effects on other organs.

Occasionally, more often with permanent blocks, loss of normal sympathetic functions can cause a problem.

Anatomy of celiac and hypogastric plexuses, page 247, shows the
(Text continues on page 248.)

A portion of the sympathetic nervous system: The paravertebral ganglia

The sympathetic nervous system contains three types of ganglia: terminal ganglia (lying near the innervated organ), prevertebral ganglia (located in the abdomen and pelvis near the vertebral column), and paravertebral ganglia (lying on each side of the vertebral column as shown here). A nerve blockade of particular sympathetic ganglia alleviates certain types of pain without the loss of motor or sensory functions; for example, blockade of a stellate ganglion (one of the paravertebral ganglia) relieves some types of arm or facial pain.

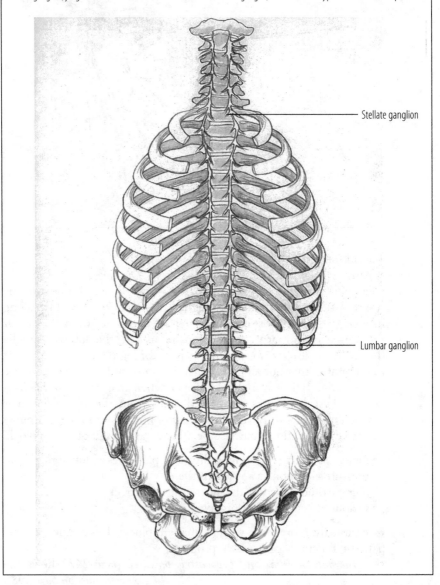

Stellate ganglion

Lumbar ganglion

Anatomy of celiac and hypogastric plexuses

The celiac and hypogastric plexuses are part of the sympathetic innervation of the abdomen and pelvis, respectively. Celiac plexus blockade relieves cancer pain originating in the upper abdominal viscera. Blockade of a hypogastric plexus relieves cancer pain originating in the pelvic viscera.

Greater splanchnic nerve

Lesser splanchnic nerve

Least splanchnic nerve

Celiac ganglion and plexus

Common hepatic artery and hepatic plexus

Gastroduodenal artery

Left gastric artery and plexus

Splenic artery and plexus

Superior mesenteric ganglion, artery and plexus

Aorticorenal ganglion and renal artery with plexus

Abdominal aortic plexus

Inferior mesenteric ganglion, artery and plexus

Superior hypogastric plexus

Inferior hypogastric plexus

Pelvic plexus

Pelvic splanchnic nerve (nervus erigens)

Pudendal nerve

A cross section of the spinal cord

This illustration shows a cross section of the spinal cord within the vertebral foramen. Note the epidural space located between the outer and inner layers of dura mater as well as the subarachnoid space located beneath the arachnoid mater. As a means of analgesia, a variety of drugs (opioids, local anesthetics, or corticosteroids) may be injected into either one of these spaces.

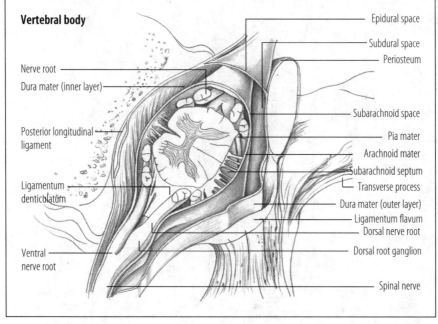

Vertebral body

Nerve root

Dura mater (inner layer)

Posterior longitudinal ligament

Ligamentum denticulatum

Ventral nerve root

Epidural space

Subdural space

Periosteum

Subarachnoid space

Pia mater

Arachnoid mater

Subarachnoid septum

Transverse process

Dura mater (outer layer)

Ligamentum flavum

Dorsal nerve root

Dorsal root ganglion

Spinal nerve

sympathetic innervation to the abdomen and pelvis, respectively. Cancer pain from the liver, pancreas, stomach, small intestine, or first part of the large intestine can be reduced on a long-term basis by a neurolytic celiac plexus block. Chronic benign pain from these organs usually is not relieved long-term by this same block; currently we are unable to explain this difference in response. In this context, "long-term" means 6 months to 2 years of pain relief.

Central blocks

A cross section of the spinal cord illustrates the relationship between the vertebrae and the spinal cord along with the intrathecal and epidural spaces. The intrathecal space (also called the subarachnoid space) around the spinal cord is filled with cerebrospinal fluid. The epidural

Catheterization of the epidural space

As shown here, a needle may be used to introduce a catheter into the epidural space of the spinal cord. A similar technique allows placement of a catheter in the subarachnoid space. Epidural or subarachnoid catheters allow delivery of a constant infusion or of intermittent boluses of analgesic drugs to the spinal cord.

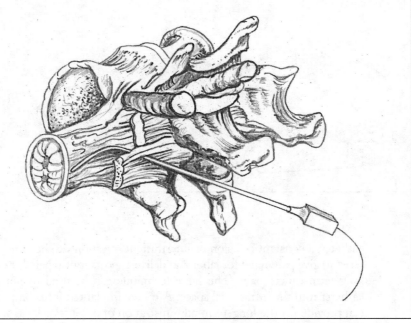

space is an essentially empty space extending from the base of the skull to the tip of the sacrum and coccyx. It easily allows injection of medications. This space can be disturbed or interrupted by previous surgeries or space-occupying problems such as tumors. Spinal nerves travel through both the epidural and subarachnoid spaces as they approach the spinal cord. Local anesthetics can block the spinal nerves in the epidural or intrathecal spaces. Opioids injected into the epidural space must travel through the dura and cerebrospinal fluid to reach the spinal cord where the opioid receptors are located. This does not necessarily take a long time, and the time between injection and pain relief is generally quite similar for intrathecal and epidural injections.

Catheterization of the epidural space demonstrates threading a catheter through a needle and into the epidural space. Through this

An implanted pump for delivery of spinal analgesia

One delivery system for continuous spinal analgesia uses a drug reservoir and pump outside the body, requiring a catheter or needle through the skin. An alternate system, shown here, is totally implanted, including the pump and reservoir, and can be programmed externally to vary the rate of drug delivery or deliver a bolus dose at specific times.

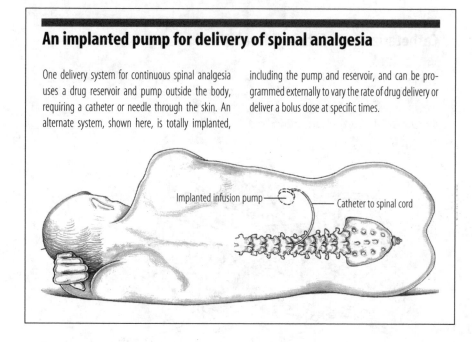

Implanted infusion pump

Catheter to spinal cord

catheter, a constant infusion or intermittent injection can be administered to give pain relief for labor and delivery, postsurgical pain, or even long-term cancer pain. The same technique can be used to put the catheter into the intrathecal space. A totally implanted infusion pump can provide for the long-term administration of opioids or local anesthetics (see *An implanted pump for delivery of spinal analgesia*).

Electrical stimulation of the spinal cord provides pain relief for selected patients. Using a technique similar to threading a catheter through a needle, an electrode for stimulation of the spinal cord can be inserted through an epidural needle for trial or permanent placement of a spinal cord stimulator system. Since precise positioning of the spinal cord stimulator is necessary, an optional and more stable system can be placed during laminectomy surgery (see *An implanted electrode for electrical stimulation of the spinal cord*). The inset demonstrates the placement of the stimulator. The space where the stimulator enters the spine is made by removal of vertebral bone on the dorsal surface of the spine. This can be done without any destabilization of the spine and usually does not result in any long-term pain problem.

An implanted electrode for electrical stimulation of the spinal cord

The implantation of a strip electrode for spinal cord stimulation requires a laminectomy to allow insertion of the electrode. Alternatively, wire electrodes can be implanted percutaneously by insertion through a nee- dle. If trial electrical stimulation alleviates the patient's pain, a second surgery is performed to internalize the electrical pulse generator.

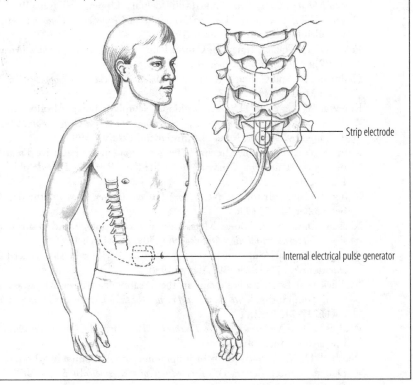

Strip electrode

Internal electrical pulse generator

REFERENCES

Bonica, J.J. *The Management of Pain*, Philadelphia: Lea & Febiger, 1953.

Bonica, J.J. *The Management of Pain*, 2nd ed. Baltimore: William & Wilkins, 1990.

Bouckoms, A.S. "Limbic Surgery for Pain," in *Textbook of Pain*, 3rd ed. Edited by Wall, P.D. and Melzack, R. New York: Churchill Livingstone, Inc., 1994.

Cassel, E.J. "The Nature of Suffering and the Goals of Medicine," *New England Journal of Medicine* 306(11):639-45, March 18, 1982.

Cousins, M.J., and Bridenbaugh, P.O., eds. *Neural Blockade in Clinical Anesthesia and Management of Pain*, 2nd ed. Philadelphia: Lippincott-Raven, 1988.

DeVita, V.T., et al., eds. *Cancer: Principles and Practice of Oncology*, 4th ed. Philadelphia: Lippincott-Raven, 1993.

Foley, K.M. "The Treatment of Cancer Pain," *New England Journal of Medicine* 313(2):84-95, July 11, 1985.

Hellmann, K., and Carter, S.K. eds. *Fundamentals of Cancer Chemotherapy*. New York: McGraw-Hill, 1987.

Korevaar, W.C., et al. "Thoracic Epidural Neurolysis Using Alcohol," in *Pain Research & Clinical Management, Proceedings 5th World Congress on Pain*, vol. 3. Edited by Dubner, R., et al. Amsterdam: Elsevier, 1987.

Kurman, M.R. "Systemic Therapy (Chemotherapy) in the Palliative Treatment of Cancer Pain," in *Cancer Pain*. Edited by Patt, R. Philadelphia: J.B. Lippincott Co., 1993.

National Cancer Institute. *NCI Workshop on Cancer Pain*. Bethesda, Md. September 14-15, 1990.

Nielsen, O.S., et al. "Bone Metastases: Pathophysiology and Management Policy," *Journal of Clinical Oncology* 9(3):509-24, March 1991.

Plancarte, R., et al. "Superior Hypogastric Plexus Block for Pelvic Cancer Pain," *Anesthesiology* 73(2):236-39, August 1990.

"A Review of Local Radiotherapy in the Treatment of Bone Metastases and Cord Compression," *International Journal Radiation Oncology, Biology, Physics* 23(1):217-21, 1992.

Wall, P.D., and Melzack, R. eds. *Textbook of Pain*, 3rd ed. New York: Churchill Livingstone, Inc., 1994.

Walsh, T.D. "Controlled Study of Imipramine and Morphine in Chronic Pain Due to Cancer (abstract)," *Proceedings of the American Society of Clinical Oncology* 5:237, 1986.

World Health Organization. *Cancer Pain Relief and Palliative Care*. Report of a WHO expert committee. World Health Organization Technical Report Series, 804:1-75. Geneva: World Health Organization, 1990.

RESOURCES

Suggested journals

Anesthesia and Analgesia, Williams and Wilkins Co., 351 W. Camden St., Baltimore, MD 21201-2436.

Clinical Journal of Pain, Lippincott-Raven, Philadelphia.

Journal of Pain and Symptom Management, Elsevier Science, Inc., New York.
Pain, Elsevier Science Publishers (Biomedical Division), Amsterdam.
Pain Forum, Churchill Livingstone, Inc., Avenue of the Americas, New York, 10011.

Suggested textbooks and reference books

Bonica, J.J. *The Management of Pain*, 2nd ed. Baltimore: William & Wilkins, 1990.

Cousins, M.J., and Bridenbaugh, P.O., eds. *Neural Blockade in Clinical Anesthesia and Management of Pain*, 2nd ed. Philadelphia: Lippincott-Raven, 1988.

Merskey, H., and Bogdukn, eds. *Classification of Chronic Pain*, 2nd ed. Seattle: IASP Publication, 1994.

Raj, P.P., ed. *Practical Management of Pain*, 2nd ed. St. Louis: Mosby-Year Book, 1986.

Wall, P.D., and Melzack, R., eds. *Textbook of Pain*, 3rd ed. New York: Churchill Livingstone, Inc., 1994.

Suggested resources for acute pain

Acute Pain Management Guideline Panel. *Acute Pain Management: Operative or Medical Procedures and Trauma. Clinical Practice Guideline.* AHCPR Pub. No. 92-0032. Rockville, Md.: Agency for Health Care Policy and Research, Public Health Service, U.S. Department of Health and Human Services, February 1992.

Ferrante, F.M., and VadeBoncover, T.R., eds. *Postoperative Pain Management.* New York: Churchill Livingstone, Inc., 1993.

Ready, L.B. and Edwards, W.T., eds. *Management of Acute Pain: A Practical Guide.* Seattle: IASP Publication, 1992.

Sinatra, R.S., et al., eds. *Acute Pain—Mechanisms and Management.* Seattle: Mosby-Year Book.

Suggested resources for cancer pain

Jacox, A., et al. *Management of Cancer Pain.* Clinical Practice Guideline No. 9, AHCPR Publication No. 94-0592. Rockville, Md: Agency for Health Care Policy and Research, U.S. Department of Health and Human Services, Public Health Service, March 1994.

National Cancer Institute. NCI Workshop on Cancer Pain. Bethesda, Md: September 14-15, 1990.

Patt, R.B., ed. *Cancer Pain.* Philadelphia: Lippincott-Raven, 1993.

World Health Organization. Cancer Pain Relief and Palliative Care. Report of a WHO expert committee World Health Organization Technical Report Series, 804:1-75. Geneva, Switzerland: World Health Organization; 1990.

CHAPTER 8

Complementary therapies

Suzanne L. Howell, RN, PhD

Complementary pain therapies are gaining in popularity among the general public as well as among members of the health care professions in the United States. Many people today are concerned about the overuse of drugs and surgery for conventional pain management and about the "just have to live with it" sentence when conventional therapy fails. Americans are turning toward more self-management of their health problems. Over-the-counter herbal and homeopathic remedies, once limited to health food stores, are now appearing on the shelves of ordinary pharmacies and grocery stores. Many contemporary publications give lay people and health care professionals alike clear, concise, practical information on effective alternative but medically sound techniques for relief of chronic pain (Burroughs and Kastner 1993; Ford 1994). Consumer organizations such as the People's Medical Society make previously unavailable medical information accessible to people so they can make informed decisions about their health care. (See Resources, page 283.)

Understanding complementary therapies

Why is education about complementary pain therapies essential for health care professionals? The primary reason is that people use these therapies and the majority of patients do not inform their conventional health care providers of that use (Eisenberg et. al 1993). The failure of allopathic providers to encourage discussion of complementary therapies that patients may use on their own is not in patients' best interest and could be harmful.

Paradigm, from a Greek word meaning "to compare," refers to a model, a frame of reference through which people perceive, understand, and interpret the world. People often fear and disparage therapies based on a paradigm that they do not understand or have not experienced (Heubscher 1994). When conventional clinicians understand the operative paradigms of complementary therapies, they are better able to evaluate these therapies critically and decide whether to incorporate them into their practice or to provide appropriate educational materials and referrals for patients. Many low-risk complementary pain-relief methods can help suffering patients whereas the often slow-moving scientific process seeks to confirm or refute them. Complementary therapies can often supplement conventional care, thereby greatly expanding the patient's repertoire of effective pain-relieving techniques. (See *Complementary therapies for migraine headache*, page 256.)

This chapter introduces some common complementary therapies for pain and presents current scientific evidence regarding their efficacy and safety. A wealth of sound information about these therapies is also available through networking with other health care professionals, holistic health and wellness centers, natural food stores, special-interest publications for general readership such as *Yoga Journal*, new journals for health care professionals, such as *The Journal of Alternative and Complementary Medicine* and *Alternative Therapies in Health and Medicine*, and professional associations, such as the American Holistic Medical Association and the American Holistic Nurses' Association.

Western and Eastern paradigms of medicine

Although the majority of complementary pain therapies can be explained using the Western paradigm of medicine, a more comprehensive understanding can be reached through an appreciation of Eastern medicine, which offers a more consistent rationale for their use. In the conventional Western model, illness and pain arise from distinct, causal entities that are separate from the material and nonmaterial entities that make people unique individuals. Western medicine studies the physical functioning of separate body parts, organs, and systems. The Western paradigm tends to be more effective when a disease or pain etiology is definite and clear, such as bacterial infections or fractured bones.

A holistic philosophy, which falls within the Eastern paradigm of medicine, assumes that each individual is a unique, complex balance of physical, mental, and spiritual energies. Illness and pain are viewed as only a part of a complex energy imbalance that manifests itself in all aspects of the patients' life. For diagnosis, the holistic practitioner relies

PATIENT HISTORY

Complementary therapies for migraine headache

Amy L., a 23-year-old woman, suffered from attacks of migraine headaches approximately 2 to 3 times per week. In addition to conventional medical treatment, she requested instruction in relaxation techniques. Because Amy was enthusiastic about learning complementary pain therapies, her therapist was able to help her change many of her lifestyle habits, such as deleting known migraine-trigger foods from her diet, getting adequate sleep, walking approximately 15 minutes per day, and beginning a yoga program. Neuromuscular therapy was initiated to relieve trigger points in her upper back. For her daily use, the therapist recorded a 10-minute relaxation exercise with *Rocky Mountain Suite* as background. She also practiced meditation, visualizations, and affirmations. The therapist also provided therapeutic touch.

When Amy arrived at her usual therapy session, she reported that a migraine was beginning and was already a 5 on a 10-point scale. Based on Amy's previous visualizations, the therapist knew that Amy saw her pain as a green spiked ball. Through hypnotic suggestion, the therapist taught Amy to progressively relax her muscles and then visualize a pain thermostat, which she could turn down to change the color and texture of the "pain ball." Following hypnotic suggestion, the patient turned the dial down until she reached 3, a number which she reported changed her pain to a soft, furry blue ball. Amy learned to perform this self-hypnosis routine to alleviate her migraines. She also began taking feverfew capsules daily. Although practicing these techniques is time-consuming, she is pleased with the results. She feels more in control.

primarily on clinical observation and rarely looks further than the patient himself, in contrast with the high-technology diagnostics of Western medicine. Comprehension of the overall pattern of imbalance, with the symptom as part of it, is the objective of Eastern medicine.*

In the Eastern paradigm, effective therapies alter patients' unbalanced energy flows. These therapies, which have been used in China, Japan, and India for thousands of years, are based on the view that health and disease reflect changing patterns in life energy, called *chi* or *qi* in China, *ki* in Japan, and *prana* in India, which flows by way of channels, called *meridians,* over the body surface and into the interior organs. Fundamentally, health (absence of pain) represents a balanced, unimpeded energy flow, and disease (pain) results from a blocked or imbalanced flow. According to author and practitioner Theodore J. Kaptchuk, "The Chinese (Eastern) system is not less logical than the Western, just less analytical."

---

* For a comprehensive yet readable text on Chinese medicine, see *The Web that Has No Weaver: Understanding Chinese Medicine.* (New York: Congdon & Weed, 1983) by Ted J. Kaptchuk. Dr. Kaptchuk, a Doctor of Oriental Medicine (O.M.D.) who was educated in Macau, writes from a Western perspective and practices traditional Chinese medicine in the United States.

Although viewed by many practitioners as opposites, Western and Eastern pain therapies complement each other. Eastern medicine can frequently alleviate many types of pain that fail to respond to Western techniques. When a precise etiology evades Western medicine—for example, chronic low back pain, Eastern pain therapies may indeed be more effective.

Benefits and limitations

A recent intensive research study of the lives of women with various chronic pain syndromes reported that 13 of the 14 participants used numerous complementary pain therapies with diverse perceptions of their effectiveness. The women who experienced the most pain relief actively used complementary therapies. One woman said, "I think that I get well a lot faster when I'm valued and when I'm part of my healing. One of the things I've learned is that I'm really in charge of my health." Another woman added, "It's up to you if you want to put the work and effort into making your life as good as possible."

In contrast, the women who experienced little or no benefit from the complementary pain therapies described their desires for more immediate and passive pain relief. For example, one woman described her management preference for headaches in this way: "I'm not against the idea that relaxation techniques, biofeedback, or whatever work, it's just that I don't think that I want to take the time with it. To me—and this is probably wrong thinking—[I prefer] going in and popping a pill in [my] mouth and in 20 or 30 minutes having a little relief." (Howell, *Nurse Practitioner Forum*, 1994).

Exclusive reliance on conventional medicine for chronic pain severely limits patients' options for pain relief and fosters ongoing frustrations between patients and health care providers, because most states curtail opioids for pain other than that caused by cancer. Although most complementary therapies offer the benefits of expanded pain-relief options and the promotion of self-care as a positive value, two limitations of these therapies are that they require time to learn and practice and the beneficial effects are often delayed. Also, although complementary pain therapies are typically less expensive than conventional allopathic care, most patients must pay for these therapies themselves because insurance companies seldom provide reimbursement.

Although the complementary therapies covered in this chapter can be effective for a wide range of patients, they are best administered, prescribed, or taught by licensed practitioners or experienced, credentialed lay people. Also, some of these therapies may require expert adaptation before use with infants, children, and pregnant or lactating women.

Nutrition and medicinal plants

Naturopathy, or "nature cure," stresses health promotion and disease prevention through various natural means, notably nutritional programs and herbs. Although the term *naturopathy* was not used until the late 19th century, its roots can be traced back to Hippocrates (circa 400 B.C.). It arose in the 18th and early 19th centuries in reaction to the "heroic," but often fatal, conventional medical practices of the time, such as blood letting and toxic mercury dosing. In the United States, Benedict Lust began using the term "naturopathy" in 1902 to cover a group of complementary healing therapies that he envisioned as the future of natural medicine, namely, nutritional therapy, botanical medicine, homeopathy, acupuncture, physiotherapy, counseling, and lifestyle modification. Naturopathy prospered in the United States until the mid-1930s when the development of more effective, less toxic allopathic therapies and technological advances in surgery made its practice less prevalent.

According to naturopathic philosophy, the key to successful therapy is a high level of patients' involvement in their own healing. Naturopathy, as well as many other complementary therapies, is based on the following principles:

• Discover and eliminate the primary cause of disease or pain.
• Use the most natural, nontoxic, and least invasive forms of therapy available.
• Treat the whole person.
• Teach the individual to develop a healthy diet and lifestyle.
• Support the body's own healing abilities.

Recent reference books on natural medicine provide a wealth of information and enough scientific data to dispel the common thought that natural medicine is unscientific (Murray and Pizzorno 1991). Although naturopathic remedies are generally safe, some therapists also use regular colonic irrigations that may cause significant fluid and electrolyte imbalances.

Nutrition

Although diet in general does not have much effect on pain perception, some dietary considerations may influence pain by inhibiting certain biochemical events associated with inflammation (Murray and Pizzorno 1991). Also, in specific conditions, certain foods may initiate a pain response. For example, alcohol (especially red wine) cheese, chocolate, citrus fruits, shellfish, and cured meats are often triggers for migraine headaches.

Some foods are associated with pain alleviation in certain chronic diseases. For example, berries and cherries having red-blue or black skins are rich in bioflavonoids, substances known to inhibit the formation of inflammatory compounds (Havesteen 1983; Middleton 1984). Liberal consumption of bioflavonoids, such as a half pound of cherries, preferably fresh, has been reported to ease the pain of gout and of rheumatoid arthritis (Ford 1994). Chronic pain sufferers may be deficient in vitamins A, B-complex, C, D, or E as well as in calcium, magnesium, or zinc. Eating a wide variety of fruits, vegetables, legumes, whole grains, some sunflower seeds, and a few nuts each day should provide a diet sufficient in the necessary vitamins and minerals (Ford 1994). Daily supplements of B-complex vitamins (100 mg), vitamin C (500 mg), and magnesium (200 mg) are generally considered safe (Graham and MacLean 1993). However, megavitamin therapy can cause toxicity or other side effects. For example, megadoses of vitamin C or niacin may exacerbate gout.

The metabolization of animal fats and the fatty acids found in vegetable oils other than olive and canola produces substances that may intensify the inflammation response. In contrast, the fatty acid eicosapentaenoic acid (EPA), a component of certain fish oils, inhibits formation of substances associated with inflammation (Strasser et al. 1985). Eating fatty, cold-water fish results in a significant EPA intake and possible inhibition of the inflammatory process. However, cod liver oil is not recommended because it "is neither an approved additive nor an approved drug, nor is it on the FDA list of foods 'generally regarded as safe'." (Graham and MacLean 1993). Oils from fish livers may contain toxic levels of vitamins A and D.

Scientific evidence for using the amino acids tryptophan and phenylalanine to produce mild analgesia by increasing pain tolerance thresholds is mixed. Reviews and studies published in the early 1980s, especially those by Seltzer and colleagues, confirmed the value of these two amino acids in controlling chronic pain (Seltzer et al. 1981, 1982, 1982-83, 1985; Budd 1983). However, more recent research, controlled studies with experimentally induced and chronic pain, indicates that tryptophan and phenylalanine have no significant analgesic effect when compared to placebos (Walsh et al. 1986; Mitchell et al. 1987). Because of a contaminated batch of tryptophan, the FDA currently does not allow tryptophan to be sold in the United States. Diets that include whole grains, starchy vegetables, and small amounts of meat or dairy foods provide sufficient amino acids for pain control (Graham and MacLean 1993).

Herbology

According to the World Health Organization, approximately 80% of the world's population relies on herbal remedies for health care. (Murray 1992). Before the mid-19th century, all remedies for chronic ailments, pain, and infectious disease were derived from plants that were believed to have spiritual as well as curative powers (Jackson 1986). Throughout history many herbs have been used for pain allevi- ation, and scientific analyses have shown that many of them are remarkably effective (see *Selected herbal remedies for pain*, pages 262 and 263). Although the popularity of medicinal plants in the United States declined with the growth of the pharmaceutical industry, 25% of all prescription drugs contain ingredients from plants (Murray and Pizzorno 1991).

In the West, a renewed interest in herbology has followed the development of technology for studying the pharmacologic mecha- nisms of whole medicinal plants. "In general, isolated and refined drugs are much more toxic than their botanical sources." (Weil 1988, page 99). The intensity of a drug's effect is determined more by how fast its concentration in the bloodstream and target organs increases than by the amount taken. One natural safeguard present in plants is the slower release of the drug into the bloodstream, which facilitates the onset of therapeutic actions before higher concentrations produce toxic effects. Secondary compounds found in whole plants may pro- vide balancing effects that attenuate any harmful actions of the dom- inant compound. Additionally, an herb often corrects the underlying cause of pain.

The science of herbs is central to Chinese medicine.* A Chinese medical practitioner chooses from a repertoire of some 500 common classical prescriptions that can rebalance various disharmonies in patients' energy patterns (Kaptchuk 1983). A prescription commonly contains 5 to 15 substances and is usually in the form of a drink but may also be available in pills, powders, tinctures, and poultices. The contemporary identification of chemical components of Chinese herbs has facilitated understanding of how these remedies act upon certain painful conditions, particularly arthritis. The herbs commonly used have an "adaptogenic" action, meaning they promote resistance to the ill effects of stress by supporting adrenal gland function. Patients receiving steroid drugs for arthritis can greatly benefit when Chinese

---

* The World Health Organization, in cooperation with the Institute of Chinese Materia Medica, recently produced *Medicinal Plants in China*, which lists (by Latin, Chinese, and English names) 150 species of the most commonly used Chinese medicinal plants, their indications, and dosages. It is available from WHO Distribution and Sales, 1211 Geneva 7, Switzerland.

herbal medicines are added to their conventional regimes. The herbs enhance the effects of the steroids, thus reducing the amount of steroid needed and minimizing side effects (Tsung and Hsu 1987).

Current studies of herbs

The pain-relieving effects of a number of traditional herbs have been reported in contemporary literature. Among those that have been studied are bromelain, cayenne, ginger, curcumin, and feverfew. Bromelain, first introduced as a therapeutic agent in 1957 (Murray 1992), shows anti-inflammatory effects in a variety of clinical studies. For example, one double-blind controlled study of oral surgery patients found bromelain significantly superior to a placebo in reducing both postoperative swelling and pain duration (Tassman et al. 1965).

Cayenne *(Capsicum frutescens)* contains capsaicin, a substance that causes depletion of substance P and other peptides (Murray 1992). Plants of the *Capsicum* genus have been used as food additives and probably as pharmacologic agents for thousands of years. Drawing from an ancient Aztec remedy of honey mixed with chili for mouth lacerations, oncologists at the Yale Cancer Center treat mouth pain in cancer patients with candy that contains capsaicin. Numerous recent studies have demonstrated analgesia with capsaicin taken orally, applied topically, injected under the skin, or applied to the mucous membranes of the nose and mouth (Fusco et al. 1994).

The aqueous extract of ginger potently inhibits the formation of the inflammatory compounds prostaglandin and thromboxane, an effect that may explain the historical use of ginger as an anti-inflammatory agent (Murray 1992). In one clinical study, seven rheumatoid arthritis patients who had received only temporary relief from conventional drugs received treatment with ginger. All patients reported substantial improvement in pain relief and joint mobility as well as decreased swelling and morning stiffness (Srivastava and Mustafa 1989).

Curcumin may be the most potent known botanical anti-inflammatory compound (Murray 1992). In one study, the anti-inflammatory action of curcumin in patients with postoperative inflammation was comparable to potent nonsteroidal anti-inflammatory drugs yet had substantially reduced toxicity (Satoskar et al. 1986). Curcumin may be preferable to aspirin for arthritis patients prone to vascular thrombosis (Srivastava et al. 1986). The use of bromelain in conjunction with curcumin may provide the greatest therapeutic advantage due to bromelain's anti-inflammatory action and its possible enhancement of curcumin absorption (Murray 1992).

Preparations of fresh or dried feverfew leaves are widely consumed in Great Britain as a remedy for migraines and arthritis. Extracts of feverfew have actually been shown to inhibit the synthesis

Selected herbal remedies for pain

Herbal remedy (Chinese name) (Botanical name)	Key uses	Comments
Bromelain (Ananas comosus)	An anti-inflammatory, smooth-muscle relaxant used in inflammation, sports injuries, oral surgery, episiotomy, painful menstruation	Protein-digesting enzyme (proteolytic enzyme) obtained from the pineapple plant. Effective in virtually all inflammatory conditions. Nontoxic and well tolerated in chronic use.
Cayenne pepper (Capsicum frutescens)	A selective, long-lasting analgesia used in migraine and cluster headaches, post-herpetic neuralgia, post-mastectomy syndromes, diabetic neuropathy, trigeminal neuralgia, osteoarthritis and rheumatoid arthritis, phantom - limb pain, psoriasis	Pungent ingredient of red peppers that first irritates then desensitizes peripheral nociceptive fibers. Does not impair sensitivity to other noxious stimuli. Applied topically. May cause severe burning sensation, which may become more bearable after 1st or 2nd week of treatment. Burning side effects may be managed by applying 5% lidocaine ointment to smaller skin areas before treatment, by reducing frequency of application, or by using oral analgesic regularly in first few days. Topical application is safe, but optimal concentration remains unknown. *Warning:* Avoid eye contact. Wash hands after each application and use rubber gloves or applicators. Do not open or cut capsule. Avoid contact with broken or irritated skin.
Curcumin (Curcuma longa)	An anti-inflammatory used in rheumatoid arthritis	Derived from tumeric, the major ingredient in curry powder. Action is comparable to potent nonsteroidal anti-inflammatory drugs, but toxicity is substantially less.
Feverfew (Tanacetum parthenium)	An anti-inflammatory used in migraine headaches, rheumatoid arthritis	Taken prophylactically for migraine attacks. To work effectively, must be taken daily and over an extended period. Some reported withdrawal symptoms such as joint stiffness, nervousness, or sleeplessness. Used by large numbers of people for many years without reports of toxicity. *Warning:* Do not take during pregnancy. Do not take if allergic to ragweed. In some people, feverfew may lower blood pressure, increase appetite, or cause diarrhea.
German chamomile (Matricaria chamomilla)	An anti-inflammatory, antispasmodic, analgesic used in intestinal spasms or cramps	*Warning:* Do not take if allergic to ragweed, asters, or chrysanthemums.

Selected herbal remedies for pain *(continued)*

Herbal remedy (Chinese name) (Botanical name)	Key uses	Comments
Chinese or Korean ginseng (Jen-shen; Hung-shen) (*Panax ginseng*)	An adaptogenic stress resistance, adrenal-enhancing remedy used in rheumatoid arthritis	Perhaps the most famous medicinal plant of China; broad range of nutritional and medicinal properties. Counteracts any shrinkage of adrenal glands by corticosteroid drugs often used in treatment of rheumatoid arthritis. *Warning:* Take according to directions. Ginseng abuse syndrome includes hypertension, euphoria, nervousness, insomnia, skin eruptions, and morning diarrhea.
Licorice (Kan-tsao) (*Glycyrrhiza glabra*)	An adaptogenic, anti-inflammatory that inhibits breakdown of adrenal hormones by liver. It inactivates herpes simplex and is used in rheumatoid arthritis and in oral and genital herpes lesions	One of most popular components of Chinese medicine. Enhances action of bupleuri; the two are almost always used together in Chinese herbal formulas. *Warning:* Long-term use can cause hypertension due to high sodium content.

of inflammatory compounds to a much greater degree than aspirin (Murray 1992). Several well-documented British studies indicate that prophylactic feverfew use may reduce the incidence of migraine as well as diminish the pain of attacks that do occur (Johnson et al. 1985; Murphy et al. 1988). In the Johnson study, 17 patients who normally ate fresh feverfew leaves daily as prophylaxis against migraines participated in a 6-month-long double-blind, placebo-controlled trial of the herb. Eight of these patients received capsules of freeze-dried feverfew, and the other nine received a placebo. The placebo subjects showed a significant increase in the frequency and severity of the headaches, nausea, and vomiting. Those who took feverfew capsules showed no increase in the frequency or severity of their headaches.

Many other herbs are used in treating painful conditions. Dosage and administration information has not been provided because these herbs are nonprescription products and may be taken according to individual labeling instructions. Special precautions are in order for the Chinese herbs. In the United States, ginseng extracts are quite safe due to good quality control (Murray and Pizzorno 1991). Chinese herbal remedies should be purchased only through reputable dealers who can assure quality control and therapeutic consistency.

Instances of toxicity and even fatalities have been reported because of use of unregulated herbal products. For example, *chuifong toukuwan*, also known as Chinese Black Ball, initially produces marked improvement in rheumatoid arthritis and similar joint and muscle pains, but the drug's potentially toxic levels of corticosteroids and lead negate its benefits (Goldman and Meyerson 1991). Also, this drug has been shown to test positive in drug-screenings for benzodiazepines, particularly diazepam ("Chinese Medicinal Plants," *Chronic Pain Letter* 1991). Recently, two fatalities due to aconitine poisoning followed the ingestion of a "street-obtained" Chinese herbal medicine. Analysis of the preparations confirmed the presence of aconitine-containing herbs in quantities far exceeding the maximum recommended dosage (Dickens et al. 1994).

Aromatherapy

Aromatherapy, better known in Great Britain and Europe than in the United States, is the therapeutic use of aromatic essential oils distilled from the flowers, stems, leaves, roots, or fruits of plants. These highly concentrated, volatile oils are the most potent form of herbal remedies. By 3000 B.C. the Egyptians were using aromatic oils as medicines, cosmetics, and religious artifacts as well as to embalm the dead. Today these oils are applied to the skin through massage, hot or cold compress, or as a bath additive. Therapeutic effects are also claimed for oils that are inhaled via a vaporizor or diffusion device. Various pain-relieving properties are attributed to aromatic oils; for example, both benzoin and lavender oil may be applied to the skin around arthritic joints for temporary pain relief.

Scientific interest in the therapeutic aspects of essential oils began in the 1920s and is credited to René Maurice Gattefossé, a French perfume chemist who applied oil of lavender to his own badly burned hand and noted that the fresh wound healed within a few hours (Davis, 1991). In addition to their dermatologic effects, Gattefossé claimed that inhaled or topically applied oils affected metabolism, nerves, digestive organs, and endocrine glands (Jackson 1986). Since Gattefossé coined the term aromatherapy in 1928, other French doctors and scientists have continued his research. One English hospital currently uses lavender oil applied with sterile gauze as a treatment for burns.

Although aromatherapy is growing in popularity, current scientific justification in clinical practice is lacking. A recent study conducted in England and reported in a 1994 issue of the *Journal of Advanced Nursing* is apparently the first published account of a controlled aromatherapy clinical evaluation. The study examined the role of lavender oil, known for its antiseptic and healing properties, in relieving postpartum perineal discomfort. Of the the 635 women randomly and blindly assigned to use one of three different bath additives to reduce perineal discomfort (pure lavender oil, synthetic lavender oil, or a placebo), those using lavender oil recorded lower average discomfort scores with no side effects (Dale and Cornwell 1994).

Today aromatherapy employs several hundred essential oils, frequently used in combination for specific ailments. Many are chemically unstable and should be stored properly to prevent alteration. They will react with light, heat, plastic, and metals other than stainless steel. Also, some oils have pharmacologic effects that could exacerbate other ailments; for example, rosemary oil (*Rosmarinus officinalis*) is a central nervous system stimulant and should not be used by patients with hypertension or epilepsy.

Homeopathy

Homeopathy formally dates from 1810 when Samual Christian Hahnemann, a German physician, published *Organon of Medicine* in reaction to the "heroic" medicine of the time. In his text, he set forth the experimental and theoretical basis of homeopathy. His rules for drug testing are still applicable today. For example, he believed that drug experiments should be performed on healthy bodies and tested on both men and women.

Homeopathic physicians are licensed MDs with postgraduate work in homeopathy. Homeopaths believe people get sick or respond to injuries in individual ways, showing unique symptom patterns instead of specific "disease entities." Homeopathy is derived from Greek word *homeos*, meaning similar, and *pathos*, meaning disease. Once a symptom pattern is clear, the homeopath uses the rule "like cures like," meaning that the patient's symptom pattern is matched with the one substance that most closely reproduces those symptoms in the normal person. The patient receives microdoses of the very substances that would, in large doses, elicit his symptoms in healthy patients. The majority (80%) of homeopathic medicines are derived from plants. Others are derived from minerals, such as flint and sulphur, or from animal products, such as sponge, honey, and snake venom. Before a remedy can be recognized as an official homeopathic medicine and entered in *The Homeopathic Pharmacopeia of the United States* it must be tested scientifically on healthy human beings under a double-blind procedure to determine the specific symptoms it causes. Controlled studies on the actual efficacy of homeopathic remedies for specific painful disorders are quite scarce. (See *Homeopathic medicines for pain.*)

Paradoxically, homeopathic theory contends that substances become *more* potent as remedies the more they are diluted and made less concentrated. The dosage and administration of homeopathic medicines are determined by their X- or C-potencies, with the higher number of dilutions indicating higher potency. The lower potencies (6X 12X, 6C, 12C) are most suitable for self-medication because they have general effects and are helpful for symptoms of acute conditions. Chronic conditions requiring medium (30X, 30C) to high (200X or greater) potencies should be treated by professional homeopaths.

Bodywork

Bodywork includes complementary therapies that emphasize manipulation of joints, skin, and underlying tissues, stretching and movement exercises, and energy balancing. These therapies are distinguished from conventional physical therapy and rehabilitative exercise by their intentions to engage simultaneously the body, mind, and spirit. With these types of techniques, the patient's mind (and for some therapies, the therapist's mind as well) is focused in a meditative way on body movement, skin and muscle sensations, and relaxed breathing. Bodywork should be administered only by licensed practitioners or experienced laypersons with credentials. Particular caution is in order when applying these therapies to infants, children, and pregnant women.

Osteopathic craniosacral therapy

Osteopathy, meaning "bone treatment," emphasizes the relationship of body structure to organic function. Manipulating all bone joints, even the relatively immobile cranial joints, is believed to promote healing by enhancing blood circulation and balancing nerve function. Currently osteopaths not only manipulate joints, but also prescribe the same drugs as conventional medicine. All states recognize a Doctor of Osteopathy (DO) degree as legally equivalent to an MD

Although only a small percentage of osteopaths currently practice craniosacral therapy, the technique was introduced more than 50 years ago by osteopathic physician John E. Upledger (1983). Although the fact of craniosacral motion is still in question, craniosacral theory states that the normal skull constantly expands and contracts at its sutures in order to promote circulation of cerebrospinal fluid. Craniosacral therapy involves gentle, noninvasive

Homeopathic medicines for pain

Medication	Key uses	Comments
Arnica montana (Leopard's bane)	Bruises, arthritis, rheumatism, backache, lumbago, sprains, strains	Apply as a gel externally to affected area. Use as soon after injury as possible. If skin is broken, use calendula gel instead. For maximum relief, use along with an internal remedy. Relieves pain and swelling. Reduces black-and-blue marks.
Belladonna (Deadly nightshade)	Earaches, headaches	Relieves a wide variety of headaches.
Bryonia alba (Wild hops)	Headaches, arthritis, rheumatism	Relieves headaches and muscle aches.
Calendula officinalis (Marigold)	Abrasions, burns	Apply as a gel externally to affected area. Gel protects the injury, relieves pain, and promotes healing. For best results, use along with an internal remedy.
Cantharis (Spanish fly)	Burns	Take before blisters form.
Chamomilla (Chamomille)	Infant colic, infant teething	Relieves colic accompanied by gas. Relieves irritability that accompanies teething.
Rhus toxicodendron (Poison ivy)	Arthritis, rheumatism,, lumbago, sciatica, sprains, strains	Relieves arthritic pain that is worsened by rest and relieved by continual motion. Relieves pain along tendons and muscles. Relieves sciatica that worsens after rest and cold exposure and improves with warmth and exercise. Relieves pain and stiffness that follows recovery from muscle strain or sprain.

Adapted from *The Family Guide to Self-Medication: Homeopathic.* (1988). Boericke & Tafel, Inc. Used with permission.

skull manipulation to promote cerebrospinal circulation and realignment of these bones, thereby reducing chronic pain and improving mental function. This therapy claims to be effective for temporomadibular joint pain as well as for chronic head or neck pain associated with muscle tension. Therapists generally receive training in special workshops. Although conventional medicine has yet to recognize the existence of the craniosacral system and its pathophysiologic significance, a 1988 survey of accredited entry-level physical therapy programs in the United States showed that 15 (16%) of the 95 respondents included a unit on craniosacral therapy in their curricula (Ehrett 1988).

Chiropractic

Chiropractic manipulation is essentially the same as that used in osteopathy but is restricted to the spine. Spinal manipulation can immediately relieve some types of acute musculoskeletal pain, sometimes with one session producing an instant and lasting cure, but is less successful with chronic problems. Chiropractors must complete 4 years of postgraduate training for the Doctor of Chiropractic (DC) degree and must pass state-licensure examinations.

Chiropractors deliver a substantial amount of health care in the United States. In a recent study of insurance claim forms for all fee-for-service chiropractic visits, investigators discovered that spinal manipulation accounted for 61% of services provided and that 42% of visits were for back pain (Shekelle and Brook 1991). Another current study found that annually, approximately 5% of the total population use chiropractic services, which were delivered by about 45,000 chiropractors at a cost of approximately $2.4 billion in 1988 (Shekelle et al. 1992). About 32% to 45% of visits were for low back pain, with 5 to 18 visits per painful episode. This same study reviewed research on spinal manipulation for low back pain published from 1952 to 1992 and concluded that chiropractic was effective for acute low back pain and when compared with other conservative treatments showed an increased probability of recovery at 2 to 3 weeks. However, research data were insufficient to demonstrate the efficacy of chiropractic for chronic low back pain. Physicians and other primary health care providers should be aware of possible dangers of chiropractic treatment for patients with severe spondylitic changes, osteoporosis, fractures, tumors, ankylosing spondylitis, infections, or signs of nerve root pressure (Shvartzman and Ableson 1988).

Swedish massage

Evidence of massage therapy has been found in prehistoric cave drawings. Today, more than 30 different therapies involve touching or manipulating the body to reduce stress, relieve pain, decrease muscle tension and spasm, improve blood circulation and lymphatic drainage, enhance energy, and restore a sense of well-being. Because all massage stimulates blood circulation and lymph flow, it is contraindicated for patients with cancer, heart conditions, recent serious operations, open wounds, fever, bacterial or viral infections, or nausea. Massage should also be avoided over areas of broken or bruised skin, varicose veins, deep vein thrombosis, acute trauma, as well as the abdomen during the first three to four months of pregnancy. It is also not appropriate for persons with severe emotional or mental problems.

Swedish massage, developed around 1800 as the first organized massage system, uses six basic strokes:

- effleurage: long, gliding strokes toward the heart
- petrissage: squeezing, kneading, and wringing of muscles
- friction: compressing by moving superficial tissue over deep tissue
- tapotement: brief, brisk, and alternating striking of the tissues, such as cupping and tapping
- joint range of motion
- vibration and traction: continuous shaking movements to the tissues with the hand (Russell 1994).

Swedish massage is relaxing and passive for the patient and may incorporate massage oils, including aromatherapy oils, as well as music and mental relaxation or meditative techniques.

Neuromuscular therapy

Neuromuscular therapy, also known as trigger point therapy or myotherapy, restores balance between the nervous and musculoskeletal systems by manipulating trigger points, areas of highly localized muscle pain associated with ischemia (Russell 1994; Prudden 1980). When palpated, trigger points often produce both local and referred pain thought to result from an accumulation of metabolic wastes associated with ischemia. Trigger points are especially common in muscles subjected to repetitive motion, whiplash injuries, and strain from poor body mechanics.

Neuromuscular therapy begins with application of moist hot packs and Swedish massage followed by systematic palpation for trigger points, which typically feel like firm peas. A 6- to 12-second hard compression (it's supposed to hurt!) of the trigger point with a finger, an elbow, or a T-bar (a wooden-handled dowel with a rubber tip) alters tissue hyperirritability. (See *Application of neuromuscular therapy,* page 270, for examples of these techniques.) Release of compression followed by massage of the area improves circulation and metabolic waste removal. To further promote waste removal and prevent muscle soreness, patients should follow treatment with several glasses of water and a warm bath. Neuromuscular therapy requires patient participation in finding trigger points. Patients can also massage trigger points themselves. For inaccessible areas, such as the back, rolling on a small, hard ball placed on the floor can be effective.

Acupressure and shiatsu

Acupressure predates acupuncture and was used in Chinese medicine as long ago as the fifth century B.C. The therapist relieves pain through the application of firm, deep finger pressure over acupuncture points, a technique that redirects and unblocks the flow of *chi*.

Application of neuromuscular therapy

Neuromuscular therapy techniques include the application of concentrated pressure to trigger points. Release of the compression followed by massage of the trigger point aids in removal of metabolic waste and alters the tissue irritability associated with these points.

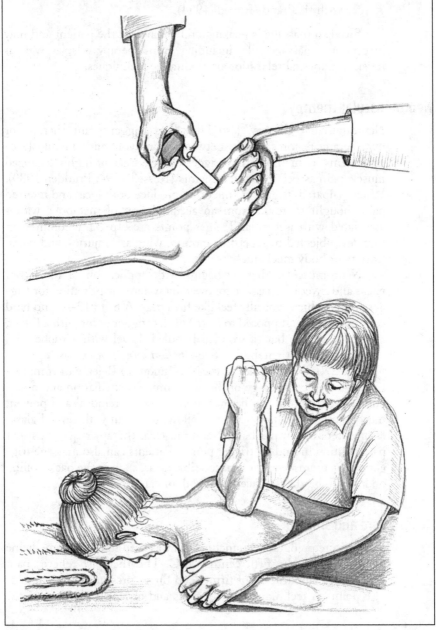

Western medicine posits that acupressure blocks pain through stimulation of large peripheral nerve fibers and promotion of endorphin release.

Acupressure points for treatment of headache, page 272, shows some of the acupressure treatment points for frontal headache. Treatment begins by applying pressure at tender points on the head, called *ah shi* for "ouch," and continues with pressure at other related acupuncture points, including points in the hands, feet, and legs (Kenyon 1988). Acutely painful conditions usually require two or three treatments administered hourly until pain abates, but chronic conditions may require up to 20 treatments two or three times week.

Shiatsu, a traditional Japanese massage based upon the same philosophy as acupressure, literally means "finger pressure." Practitioners also use palms, elbows, knees, and feet to apply stronger pressure. Clients also receive passive muscle stretching to increase flexibility.

Therapeutic touch

In therapeutic touch (TT), a modern version of the laying-on of hands, therapists use their hands to balance the energy fields of those who are ill. Although therapeutic use of the hands is an ancient and universal practice historically associated with Eastern philosophy, modern TT can be learned by anyone, regardless of religious background or personal beliefs. First introduced in 1974 by Delores Krieger, professor of nursing at New York University, and Dora Kunz, a healer, therapeutic touch can elicit a profound, generalized relaxation response and relieve pain (Kreiger 1979). Janet Quinn, an internationally recognized researcher in therapeutic touch, has provided a comprehensive review of research studies documenting the effectiveness of therapuetic touch for a variety of conditions (1988).

In TT, three basic assumptions operate:

- Human beings are energy fields.
- Illness and pain result from an imbalance in those energy fields.
- An energy transfer occurs between individuals when one person intends to help the other.

Because therapists work with energy fields, physical contact is unnecessary, although it is often used. The ability to perform TT is considered a natural human ability that can be developed by any healthy person who intends to help and heal. Many TT workshops are held throughout the United States each year, and the use of such therapy has grown rapidly among nurses for one reason: it seems to work (see *Use of therapeutic touch,* page 273).

(Text continues on page 274.)

Acupressure points for treatment of headache

Some of the acupressure points used to treat frontal headache are shown here. To apply pressure effectively, therapists use finger pressure plus a variety of other techniques, for example, a matchstick vigorously massaged over various points on the ear.

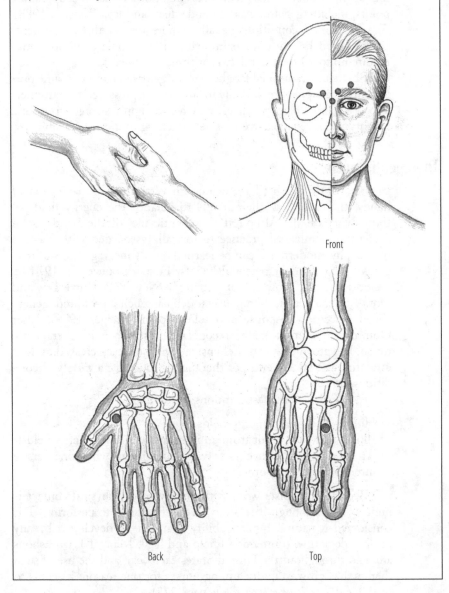

Front

Back   Top

PAIN MANAGEMENT PRACTICE

Use of therapeutic touch

1. The therapist first centers himself to be sensitive to the patient's body, mind, emotions, and spirit.
2. The therapist then assesses the patient's energy field by passing the hands over the patient's entire body, keeping them 2" to 6" above the patient. This focused assessment allows energy imbalances to be felt by the therapist as warmth, tingling, coldness, hollowness, or heaviness.

3. Following assessment, the therapist uses focused concentration and hand movements to adjust the areas of energy imbalance. For example, the therapist attempts to clear areas of blocked energy, cool off warm areas, warm up cool areas, and add energy where it is felt to be low.

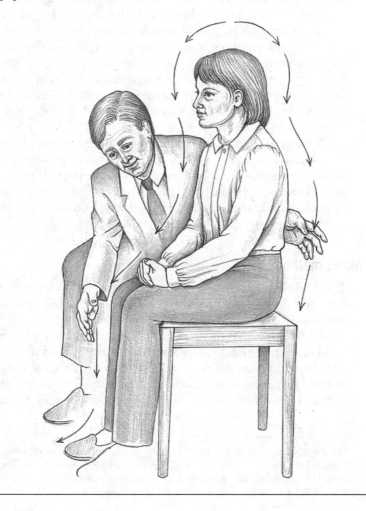

Yoga and tai chi chuan

Yoga, which means "union" or "harmony," developed in ancient India. Tai chi chuan is a system of dance-like movements developed centuries ago by Chinese Taoist monks. Both of these ancient techniques combine sophisticated postures, movements, breathing, and meditation to integrate body and mind. In the United States, instruction in these techniques usually focuses on movement and breath control to increase overall physical health and reduce stress. Both effects help to alleviate musculoskeletal pain, particularly back pain. (See *Pain relief with yoga.*)

The exercises of hatha yoga, in particular, take each joint through its full range of motion while strengthening, stretching, and balancing all body parts. Because the exercises start with gentle stretches and breathing techniques, hatha yoga is ideal as an active relaxation and exercise program for sedentary people with stiff muscles. Practiced over time, yoga promotes strength and flexibility and improves posture, body mechanics, circulation, and respiration. A 1993 survey of back pain patients reported that 51% of those practicing yoga dramatically increased their long-term relief, and another 42% obtained moderate long-term benefits ("Yoga: Full-Body Conditioning," *Chronic Pain Letter* 1993).

Because all bodies are unique, yoga exercises should be specifically tailored to patients' strength, flexibility, and habitual posture.* Yoga postures should be performed only to the point of tension, not pain. However, individualizing these movements for safe use requires a thorough understanding of therapeutic yoga, preferably taught by a skillful Iyengar-style yoga teacher (see Resources, page 283).

Feldenkrais method

The Feldenkrais method of body-mind integration through movement was developed by Moshe Feldenkrais, an Israeli electrical and mechanical engineer, as a result of his interest in body mechanics (1990). The Feldenkrais therapists guide patients through a precise set of corrective muscle movements individually designed to repattern the neuromuscular system and alter faulty habitual movement patterns that exacerbate musculoskeletal pain. The movements are performed in a slow, easy manner without strain or pain. Specialized

---

* In *Back Care Basics: A Doctor's Gentle Yoga Program for Back and Neck Pain Relief,* Mary Pullig Schatz presents a medically sound yoga program for prevention and treatment of musculoskeletal pain. Her program focuses on yoga for individuals with back and neck strain, spinal arthritis, osteoporosis, scoliosis, and premenstrual syndrome.

Pain relief with yoga

The following quotations illustrate the experiences of two patients practicing yoga for painful conditions: severe phantom-limb pain of the arm and postoperative pain following extensive knee surgery respectively (Howell 1994).

"There was a woman in the class who did what she called American yoga. When I did it with her, whatever she had put together worked. I could do it even with one arm. I went to bed that night and I slept like a baby. Whatever we did worked . . . I think it was very simple. It was not anything that are these difficult stances."

"I began the yoga exercises very aware of the aching and stiffness in my healing knee. Then I became aware of not feeling any difference between the two sides of my body. As I did the relaxation, I 'saw' myself as a warm yellow glow surrounding my body."

training is required for Feldenkrais Guild certification. Therapists call themselves teachers and refer to clients as students. By retraining students in new patterns of muscle use, practitioners alleviate pain and promote recovery from such diverse conditions as whiplash and repetitive-movement disorders.

Mental and spiritual therapies

The creative mental and spiritual responses to pain often take the form of a search for meaning, strength, and hope. The core of healing often lies in the meaning that is added to the lives of people who suffer with pain and not in the rapidity with which the pain is relieved and the body restored to strength. Wishing to be fixed and rid of the pain as rapidly and with as little bother as possible may actually delay healing, inhibit long-lasting pain relief, and prevent patients from finding personal significance in the pain. The therapeutic benefits of mental and spiritual methods arise from patients' careful attention to body, mind, and spirit as well as from their efforts to integrate the whole being with all aspects of the painful condition.

Centering

"Life is an art, and centering is a means" (Richards 1993). Centering, a mental process of personal quieting, brings into focus the sensations, thoughts, emotions, and will. To become centered is to eliminate mental distractions and achieve quietude, a sense of peace, and access to the intuitive inner self. Centering encourages an open, receptive, and perceptive state of consciousness in which people can hear inner answers or wisdom from God or from other spiritual guides. The practice of centering promotes body-mind-spirit integration. Francelyn Reeder, associate professor of nursing at the University of Colorado, emphasizes that once people have experienced the inner self, chosen a peaceful place within, and practiced, they can center themselves in about 30 seconds. To learn centering, people may listen daily to audio-taped instructions until the skill becomes automatic (see *Guide for centering*).

Meditation and prayer

Meditation is the focusing and holding of attention on one thing for a given period. It produces a relaxed physiologic state evidenced by reduced rates of metabolism, pulse, and respiration, coupled with a wakeful and highly alert mental state.

Many different types of meditation exist. Some focus on a strictly mental object of attention whereas others employ certain actions or body movements as the focus of attention. One structured, purely mental meditation involves counting the breath. The meditator breathes in, exhales, and mentally counts "one," repeats this pattern up to a count of four, and then starts over at one. The pattern is continued for an allotted time period. An example of an unstructured mental meditation is thinking about a subject and concentrating on those thoughts and feelings for 15 minutes. Meditations centered on body movement awareness include as Eastern forms, hatha yoga and tai chi, and as a Western form, Feldenkrais. Action meditations include the Western Christian traditions of singing and prayer and the Eastern traditions of archery, flower arrangement, and karate.

Lawrence LeShan, a psychotherapist and meditation teacher, emphasizes that the basis for selecting a meditation should be whether it makes the individual feel better (more "put together" and less fragmented) when it is done than when it is not done (1974). A good meditation teacher can assist people in their progress, but numerous clearly written educational materials and audiotapes are available for self-instruction.

Through prayer, patients experience the spiritual aspects of healing and the awareness of God as a source of strength and comfort. Prayer may be particularly important for patients with chronic pain. A woman with constant back pain described her daily prayers as follows: "There were many, many times that I would say, 'Life just isn't worth living like this.' At my lowest points I would close my door and have a good talk with God, cry some tears and say, 'I can't tolerate this any longer.' And it was as if He would say, 'Yes, you can, with my

PAIN MANAGEMENT PRACTICE

Guide for centering

The text below can be recorded by the therapist and replayed by people who wish to learn the skill of centering. In recording this script, allow several minutes of silence to elapse between each major step in the centering process.

Take a few deep breaths and as you let them out, let the concerns of the day go for now. Now get comfortable and close your eyes. Take in a deep breath and as you blow it out, become aware of your body and let any areas of tension flow out with your breath. Notice your thoughts—you can let them just flow by for now. Let go and flow with your own special feelings as you become calm, relaxed, peaceful. Get a sense of coming to a deeper place within yourself—your center. Pay attention to any images that come into your mind, feel the sensations, hear the sounds, smell the air.

Now take another deep breath and as you let it flow out, just sink down deep within yourself until you reach a point of calm. Continue to breathe deeply and let the air flow out. Take a few moments to just be in your calm place. Allow yourself to experience it. Follow it, trust it, flow with it, make it your own place. This is your space, your place, your center. While you flow with it, stay in contact with your place, but let your awareness just flow. Don't worry about which way it's going. Take in a few more deep breaths and just let them flow out. Now that you are in your peaceful place, go with it and listen to anything that comes to you.

Now while still feeling that peaceful sensation, move around just a little bit, slowly, and start coming back to this room. While remembering that feeling of being in your calm centered place, move around a little more, and open your eyes. Now carry with you those feelings of being calm, peaceful, and centered. They are yours.

strength,' and I would get up and go for another couple or three hours" (Howell 1994).

Affirmations and visualization

Affirmations are personal statements that are spoken aloud and written down in order to influence the subconscious mind to create a desired result (Gawain 1978). They should be phrased as positive, "now" statements such as, "I'm enjoying my exercise and I'm healthy and full of vitality," as opposed to "I'm trying to exercise more and I'm not as tired and in as much pain." Visualization is the creation of a clear mental image of the goal to be manifested followed by the regular focus of attention on that image. Picturing the desired result strongly enhances a verbal affirmation. When performing guided visualization with patients, therapists should incorporate images described by the patients so as to encourage their active participation in their own healing. Pain relief and healing may be enhanced by visualizing positive change at the cellular level. Because visualization may evoke traumatic emotional experiences, it should be facilitated only by a competent practitioner.

Music

The effects of music on the body have been studied for many years. Because of its multidimensional qualities, music touches individuals physically, emotionally, socially, and spiritually. Beginning in the 1960s, documented clinical evidence established that music therapy can provide improvement in a variety of acutely and chronically painful conditions. For example, serene and tranquil classical music produced a relaxing effect on emotional upset and excessive pain during childbirth, while music with a rhythmic beat reduced fatigue during labor. Calm, soothing music can promote the muscular relaxation to alter pain perception.

Other research has demonstrated the pain-relieving effects of music for patients with malignant and noncancerous types of chronic pain. In a recent experimental study of music therapy for cancer pain, nearly three-fourths of the patients experienced at least some pain reduction and almost one-half experienced a moderate to great decrease in pain (Beck 1991). In a similar study of women suffering from rheumatoid arthritis, pain was decreased while listening to 20 minutes of self-selected music and remained significantly decreased during the following 2 hours (Schorr 1993). Research emphasizes the therapeutic importance of assessing patients' preferences and allowing them to select their own music.

Composer Steven Halpern's music promotes balance of body, mind, and spirit. It lacks recognizable rhythm, melody, and harmony, making it an excellent adjunct to meditation, massage, and yoga (1985). John Beaulieu, musician and music therapist, works on the premises that music affects life energy and that healing music should match the energetic needs of the patient (1987). Music that is healing for one person might not be healing for another. All healing occurs when intuition and rational thinking are brought into balance with each other, so healing is aided when personal taste is set aside to experience the many different qualities of music, especially rhythm. In many hospitals, soothing music and guided relaxation tapes are available and are prescribed for patients. (See Resources, page 283.)

Use of a diary

Keeping a pain diary or journal can place present situations into the perspective of both past and future while encouraging contact with creative and spiritual sources (Progoff 1975). A reflective journal uses open-ended questions or suggestions that require a written response or an artistic expression such as poetry or a drawing. Patients who keep pain journals often gain insights into the ways in which life events and relationships precipitate or exacerbate the experience of pain. Many patients recognize for the first time that they are not taking very good care of themselves and that their lack of personal attention both increases pain and undermines feelings of general well-being. Also, sometimes patients who ordinarily describe their pain as being constant are able to identify and experience more clearly the more pleasant aspects of their lives.

Hypnosis

Hypnosis is a naturally occurring altered level of consciousness in which the patient focuses attention on one thought or object and becomes so absorbed that he enters a trancelike state (Zahourek 1990). While in this state, the patient's perceptions and sensations can be enhanced, modified, or changed either by a therapist or, with practice, by the patient himself. The components of hypnosis are induction (focusing attention), relaxation and absorption, and hypnotic suggestions.

Since acceptance by the Council on Mental Health of the American Medical Association in 1958, hypnosis and hypnotic techniques have become recognized as powerful methods for effective relief of myriad acute and chronic pain conditions. Although hypnosis is not magic, the results are often dramatic. For example, patients have experienced analgesia with little or no pain medications while undergoing surgery, debridement of burns, and childbirth. A recent study by Brian Kiernan will surely impact future research into the effects of hypnosis in pain control. This study offers concrete evidence that hypnosis affects pain, not only in the higher brain centers responsible for perception and interpretation of stimuli, but also by reducing afferent impulse transmission at the spinal cord level (1995).

Although controversy exists among the experts, hypnotic techniques are used today by clinicians in all disciplines. Unfortunately, the use of hypnosis for entertainment purposes has inhibited complete professional acceptance of it as a therapy. Only the expert clinical hypnotherapist should attempt hypnosis with individuals experiencing mental or emotional problems, such as severe depression or suicidal tendencies. The first prerequisite of ethical and professional use of hypnosis is adequate education and training. Workshops and courses are offered across the country.

REFERENCES

Beaulieu, J., and Quasha, G. *Music and Sound in the Healing Arts: An Energy Approach.* Barrytown, N.Y.: Station Hill Press, 1987.

Beck, S.L. "The Therapeutic Use of Music for Cancer-related Pain," *Oncology Nursing Forum* 18(8):1327-37, November-December 1983.

Bud, K. "Use of D-phenylalanine, an Enkephalinase Inhibitor, in the Treatment of Intractable Pain," *Advances in Pain Research and Therapy* 5:305-308, 1983.

Capacchione, L. *The Well-Being Journal: Drawing on your Inner Power to Heal Yourself.* San Bernadino, Calif.: Borgo Press, 1989.

Cassar, M.P. *Massage Made Easy.* Allentown, Pa: People's Medical Society, 1995.

Cherkin, D.C., and MacCornack, F.A. "Patient Evaluations of Low Back Pain Care from Family Physicians and Chiropractors," *Western Journal of Medicine* 150:351-55, 1989.

"Chinese Medicinal Plants," *Chronic Pain Letter* 8(1):2, 1991.

Cowmeadow, O. *The Art of Shiatsu.* Rockport, Maine: Element, 1992.

Dale, A., and Cornwell, S. "The Role of Lavender Oil in Relieving Perineal Discomfort Following Childbirth: A Blind Randomized Clinical Trial," *Journal of Advanced Nursing* 19(1):89-96, January 1994.

Davis, P. *Aromatherapy: An A-Z* (revised ed). Essex, England: C.W. Daniel, 1995.

Dickens, P., et al. "Fatal Accidental Aconitine Poisoning Following Ingestion of Chinese Herbal Medicine: A Report of Two Cases," *Forensic Science International* 67(1):55-58, June 28, 1994.

Ehrett, S.L. "Craniosacral Therapy and Myofascial Release in Entry-Level Physical Therapy Curricula," *Physical Therapy* 68(4):534-40, April 1988.

Eisenberg, D.M., et al. "Unconventional Medicine in the United States: Prevalence, Costs, and Patterns of Use," *New England Journal of Medicine* 328(4):246-52, January 28, 1993.

Feldenkrais, M. *Awareness through Movement: Health Exercises for Personal Growth.* San Francisco: Harper, 1990.

Ford, N.D. *Painstoppers: The Magic of All-Natural Pain Relief.* West Nyack, N.Y.: Parker, 1994.

Fusco, B.M., et al. "Preventative Effect of Repeated Nasal Application of Capsaicin in Cluster Headache," *Pain* 59(3):321-25, December 1994.

Gawain, S. *Creative Visualization: Use the Power of Your Imagination to Create What You Want in Your Life,* 2nd ed. Novato, Calif.: New World Library, 1995.

Goldman, J.A., and Myerson, G. "Chinese Herbal Medicine: Camouflaged Prescription Anti-inflammatory Drugs, Corticosteroids, and Lead," *Arthritis & Rheumatism* 34(9):1207, September 1991.

Graham, T.O., and MacLean, H. "Nutrition, Weight, and General Well-Being," in *Every Woman' Health: The Complete Guide to Body and Mind,* 5th ed. Edited by MacLeah, H. Garden City, N.Y.: Doubleday Book & Music Clubs, 1993.

Halpern, S. *Sound Health: The Music and Sounds that Make Us Whole.* New York: Harper & Row, 1985.

Havsteen, B. "Flavonoids, a Class of Natural Products of High Pharmacological Potency," *Biochemical Pharmacology* 32(7):1141-48, April 1983.

Howell, S.L. "Natural/Alternative Health Care Practices Used by Women with Chronic Pain: Findings from a Grounded Theory Research Study," *Nurse Practitioner Forum* 5(2):98-105, June 1994.

Howell, S.L. "A Theoretical Model for Caring for Women with Chronic Nonmalignant Pain," *Qualitative Health Research* 4(1):94-122, February 1994.

Howell, S.L. *Validating Women's Experiences of Living with Chronic Nonmalignant Pain.* Unpublished doctoral dissertation. University of Colorado, Denver, 1991.

Hsu, H-y, and Tsung, P-K. *Arthritis and Chinese Herbal Medicine.* New Canaan, Conn.: Keats Publishing, Inc., 1996.

Huebscher, R.R. "What is Natural/Alternative Health Care?" *Nurse Practitioner Forum* 5(2):66-71, June 1994.

Jackson, J. *Scentual Touch: A Personal Guide to Aromatherapy.* New York: Fawcett Book Group, 1987.

Johnson, E.S., et al. "Efficacy of Feverfew as Prophylactic Treatment of Migraine," *British Medical Journal Clinical Research Ed.* 291(6495):569-73, August 1985.

Kaptchuk, T.J. *The Web that Has No Weaver: Understanding Chinese Medicine.* New York: Congdon & Weed, 1993.

Kastner, M., and Burroughs, H. *Alternative Healing: The Complete A–Z Guide to Over 160 Different Alternative Therapies.* La Mesa, Ca: Halcyon, 1993.

Kenyon, J.N. *Acupressure Techniques: A Self-Help Guide.* Rochester, Vt.: Healing Arts Press, 1988.

Kiernan, B.D., et al. "Hypnotic Analgesia Reduces R-III Nociceptive Reflex: Further Evidence Concerning the Multifactorial Nature of Hypnotic Analgesia," *Pain* 60(1):39-47, January 1995.

Krieger, D. *The Therapeutic Touch: How to Use your Hands to Help or to Heal.* Englewood Cliffs, N.J.: Prentice-Hall, 1979.

LeShan, L. *How to Meditate: A Guide to Self-Discovery.* New York: Bantam, 1984.

Macrae, J. *Therapeutic Touch: A Practical Guide.* New York: Alfred A. Knopf, 1988.

McBride, R.L. "Legal, Religious, and Professional Issues," in *Clinical Hypnosis and Therapeutic Suggestion in Patient Care.* Edited by Zahourek, R.P. New York: Brunner/Mazel, 1990.

Middleton, E. "The Flavonoids," *Trends in Pharmaceutical Science* 5:335-38, 1984.

Mitchell, M.J., et al. "Effect of L-tryptophan and Phenylalanine on Burning Pain Threshold," *Physical Therapy* 67(2):203-205, February 1987.

Murphy, J.J. "Randomized Double-Blind Placebo-Controlled Trial of Feverfew in Migraine Prevention," *Lancet* 2(8604):189-192, 1988.

Murray, M.T. *The Healing Power of Herbs: The Enlightened Person's Guide to the Wonders of Medicinal Plants,* 2nd ed. Rocklin, Calif.: Prima Publishing, 1995.

Murray, M.T., and Pizzorno, J.E. *Encyclopedia of Natural Medicine.* Rocklin, Calif.: Prima, 1991.

Progoff, I. *At a Journal Workshop: Writing to Access the Power of the Unconscious and Evoke Creative Ability.* New York: Dialogue House, 1992.

Prudden, B. *Pain Erasure: The Bonnie Prudden Way.* New York: Ballantine, 1985.

Quinn, J.F. "Building a Body of Knowledge: Research on Therapeutic Touch 1974-1986," *Journal of Holistic Nursing* 6(1):37-45, 1988.

Richards, M.C. *Centering in Pottery, Poetry, and the Person.* Middletown, Conn.: Wesleyan University Press, 1969.

Russell, J.K. "Bodywork—the Art of Touch Massage, Neuromuscular Therapy, Trager, and Bowen Work," *Nurse Practitioner Forum* 5(2):85-90, June 1994.

Satoskar, R.R., et al. "Evaluation of Anti-Inflammatory Property of Curcumin (Diferuloyl Methane) in Patients with Postoperative Inflammation," *International Journal of Clinical Pharmacology, Therapy and Toxicology* 24(12):651-54, December 1986.

Schatz, M.P. *Back Care Basics: A Doctor's Gentle Yoga Program for Back and Neck Pain Relief.* Berkeley, Calif.: Rodmell, 1992.

Schorr, J.A. "Music and Pattern Change in Chronic Pain," *Advances in Nursing Science* 15(4):27-36, June 1993.

Seltzer, S. "Pain Relief by Dietary Manipulation and Tryptophan Supplements," *Journal of Endodontics* 11(10):449-53, October 1985.

Seltzer, S., et al. "The Effects of Dietary Tryptophan on Chronic Maxillofacial Pain and Experimental Pain Tolerance," *Journal of Psychiatric Research* 17(2):181-86, 1982-1983.

Seltzer, S., et al. "Perspectives in the Control of Chronic Pain by Nutritional Manipulation," *Pain* 11(2):141-48, October 1981.

Seltzer, S., et al. "Alteration of Human Pain Thresholds by Nutritional Manipulation and L-tryptophan Supplementation," *Pain* 13(4):385-93, August 1982.

Shekelle, P.G., et al. "Spinal Manipulation for Low Back Pain," *Annals of Internal Medicine* 117(2):590-98, October 1, 1992.

Shekelle, P.G., and Brook, R.H. "A Community-based Study of the Use of Chiropractic Services," *American Journal of Public Health* 81(4):439-42, April 1991.

Shibata, S., et al. "Chemistry and Pharmacology of Panax," *Economic and Medicinal Plant Research* 1:217-84, 1985.

Shvartzman, P., and Abelson, A. "Complications of Chiropractic Treatment for Back Pain," *Postgraduate Medicine* 83(7):57-58, 61, May 15, 1988.

Siegel, R.K. "Ginseng Abuse Syndrome," *JAMA* 241(15):1614-15, April 13, 1979.

Srivastava, K.C., and Mustafa, T. "Ginger (Zingiber officinale) and Rheumatic Disorders," *Medical Hypotheses* 29(1):25-28, May 1989.

Srivastava, R., et al. "Effect of Curcumin on Platelet Aggregation and Vascular Protacyclin Synthesis," *Arzneimittel-Forschung* 36(4):715-17, April 1986.

Strasser, T., et al. "Leukotriene B5 Is Formed in Human Neutrophils after Dietary Supplementation with Icosapentaenoic Acid," *Proceedings of the National Academy of Science of the United States* 82(5):1540-43, 1985.

Upledger, J.E., and Vredevoogd, J.D. *Craniosacral Therapy II: Beyond the Dura.* Seattle: Eastland Press, 1987.

Walsh, N.E., et al. "Analgesic Effectiveness of D-phenylalanine in Chronic Pain Patients," *Archives of Physical Medicine & Rehabilitation* 67(7):436-39, July 1986.

Weil, A. *Health and Healing.* Boston: Houghton Mifflin, 1995.

Wytias, C.A. "Therapeutic Touch in Primary Care," *Nurse Practitioner Forum* 5(2): 91-97, June 1994.

Yamasaki, H. "Pharmacology of Sinomenine, an Anti-Rheumatic Alkaloid from Sinomenium Actum," *Acta Medica Okayama* 30(1):1-20, February 1976.

"Yoga: Full-Body Conditioning Practice Increases Flexibility and May Ease Pain," *Chronic Pain Letter* 10(3):1, 6, 1993.

Zahourek, R.P. *Clinical Hypnosis and Therapeutic Suggestion in Patient Care,"* New York: Brunner/Mazel, 1990.

RESOURCES

American Association for Music Therapy
P. O. Box 80012
Valley Forge, PA 19484
(215) 265-4006

American Association of Naturopathic Physicians
P. O. Box 20386
Seattle, WA 98102
(206) 323-7610

American Holistic Medical Association
American Holistic Nurses' Association
4101 Lake Boone Trail, Suite 201
Raleigh, NC 27607
(919) 787-5181

American Massage Therapy Association
1130 W. North Shore Avenue
Chicago, IL 60626-4670
(312) 761-2682

American Society for Clinical Hypnosis
2200 E. Devon Avenue, Suite 291
Des Plains, IL 60018-4534
(708) 297-3317

B.K.S. Iyengar Yoga National Association
of the United States, Inc.
4090 Forest Hill Drive
La Canada-Flintridge, CA 91011

People's Medical Society
462 Walnut Street
Allentown, PA 18102
(610) 770-1670

International Foundation for Homeopathy
2366 Eastlake Avenue East, Suite 301
Seattle, WA 98102
(206) 324-8230

Nurse Healers Professional Association
1827 Haight Street, Suite 157
San Francisco, CA 94117

Suggested music
Daniel Kobialka: *Timeless Motion* (Li-Sem)
Larkin: *O' Cean* (Sonia Gaia)
Mike Rowland: *The Fairy Ring* (Music Design)
Solitudes: *Rocky Mountain Suite* (Dan Gibson)
Windham Hill: *Sampler '86* (Windham Hill)
Wind Machine: *Voices in the Wind* (Silver Wave)
Lind Institute: *Music for Imagining* (Lind Institute)

CHAPTER 9

Cancer pain management

Julie Hammack, MD

Cancer pain is a worldwide problem. In the United States, over 547,000 deaths from cancer occurred in 1995 alone, and it has been estimated that 70% of patients with advanced cancer report moderate to severe pain that warrants the use of opioid medications. Applying these prevalence rates to worldwide cancer statistics, 3 million of the over 4 million patients who died from cancer in 1993 and 16 million surviving cancer patients experienced moderate to severe cancer-related pain—a total of 19 million patients! (Bonica et al. 1990.) Pain is also present at the time of diagnosis in 20% to 50% of patients, and 30% experience pain while receiving cancer therapy as a result of the malignant disease or its treatment. Good to excellent relief from pain could be obtained in 95% of these patients if their physicians were skilled in the use of analgesic drug therapy and aware of the indications for anesthetic and neurosurgical analgesic procedure. Despite this, only 50% of cancer patients in the United States who are experiencing pain receive adequate pain control (Bonica et al. 1990).

A number of barriers to relief of cancer pain exist. One problem is poor communication between patients and their caregivers regarding pain intensity and its impact on quality of life. Patients may not complain of pain unless questioned. They may assume that pain is an expected consequence of malignant disease or that by "complaining" they may distract their physicians from primary treatment of the cancer. Many patients equate pain with progression of their tumors or a bad prognosis and thus fear discussions about pain with their caregivers. Lastly, as members in a "just say no" society, patients may believe that addiction, or psychological dependence, is an inevitable result of opioid use. Uninformed physicians and nurses sometimes foster this mistaken belief.

Many recent studies have demonstrated a startling prevalence of misconceptions regarding opioid use and cancer pain management among physicians, nurses, and other health care workers. The problem is not a deficiency of compassion or competence but a lack of education in cancer pain control. Opioid use in treating cancer pain is not well covered in most medical or nursing school curricula. There is a tendency to adhere to the Physicians' Desk Reference-recommended dosage for fear that higher doses of drug even in tolerant patients may produce life-threatening adverse effects. Few medical or nursing personnel are aware of the wide variations in the amount of drug required to control pain among different individuals. Furthermore, medical training in Westernized countries has focused on the treatment of disease, with less emphasis on the relief of symptoms such as pain. Ill-informed medical and nursing students will become ill-informed doctors and nurses. If these attitudes are to change, there must be intervention at all levels of training of health care providers as well as improved education of patients.

The goal of this brief chapter on cancer pain management is to encourage caregivers to do the following:

- *Recognize that pain has a major destructive impact on the quality of life in patients with cancer.* Good to excellent relief can be obtained in most patients with currently available modalities. Learn to inquire regularly about pain intensity and quality, and record the information in patients' records.
- *Learn the importance of establishing a "pain diagnosis" and carefully search for the etiology of the pain.*
- *Understand opioid and adjuvant drug use.* Learn appropriate dosing and dose escalation. Understand and differentiate between tolerance, physical dependence, and psychological dependence. Learn how and when to convert from one opioid to another or from one route of administration to another.
- *Consider the full range of therapeutic options in the treatment of cancer pain.* Know the indications for making correct choices among the following treatment options: type of analgesics, routes of administration, nerve blocks, epidural administration of opioids or local anesthetics, neurosurgical procedures such as cordotomy. Be able to "triage" patients to the appropriate subspecialist in pain management when necessary.

Establishing a pain diagnosis

There is a tendency to consider cancer pain as a single diagnostic entity. A recent study performed in Memorial Sloan-Kettering Cancer Center revealed that evaluation of cancer-related pain identified previously unsuspected conditions (predominantly metastatic or recurrent tumor) in 64% of patients. Previously unsuspected neurologic disorders were found in 36%, and an unsuspected infection was discovered in 4% (Gonzalez et al. 1991). A thorough assessment of cancer pain thus may have a significant effect on the staging of the underlying tumor and on subsequent anticancer therapy.

Pain is a frequently encountered symptom in neurology and general medicine, and the diagnostic approach to pain is much the same as it is for any other symptom. However, pursuing a pain diagnosis differs from pursuing a conventional diagnosis in that the pain physician seeks to treat not only the underlying cause of the symptom, which may or may not be amenable to therapy but also the pain itself. The pain history emphasizes the onset, quality, severity, location, ameliorating and exacerbating factors, and associated symptoms. The physical examination should include a complete neurologic assessment. Diagnostic studies such as X-rays, computed tomography (CT) scans, and magnetic resonance imaging (MRI) will depend on the findings.

Cancer pain mechanisms

Cancer patients may experience pain as a direct result of tumor invasion; as a reaction to antineoplastic therapy, such as surgery, radiation, or chemotherapy, or as a problem unrelated to cancer or its therapy, although this is the case for a minority of patients. These pain syndromes may be further subdivided into nociceptive, neuropathic, and idiopathic mechanisms. Nociception refers to pain produced by injury to soma (bone, muscle, dura, fascia, skin, blood vessels) or viscera (pleura, peritoneum, organ capsules, hollow viscus). Damage to these structures activates peripheral nerve fibers, which are sensitive to noxious stimuli. Neuropathic pain results from direct injury to the central or peripheral nervous system, which then produces aberrant discharge of nerve fibers in pain pathways. Idiopathic pain refers to syndromes in which the underlying cause or mechanism of discomfort cannot be discovered. By definition, this is a diagnosis of exclusion. Idiopathic pain syndromes, such as fibromyalgia, are fairly common in the general population without cancer. This type of pain is quite rare in patients with cancer, however, and should never be diagnosed without a thorough investigation of alternate causes of pain.

Pain syndromes related to direct tumor invasion

Three types of pain result from tumor invasion: nociceptive somatic pain, nociceptive visceral pain, and neuropathic pain. With nociceptive somatic pain, the most commonly encountered pain arises as a result of bone metastases. Nociceptive visceral pain is thought to arise from distension or pressure on nociceptive fibers in the organ capsules, the pleura, or the peritonium. Neuropathic pain arises from tumor invasion of any structure in the nervous system. Patients with neuropathic pain typically experience a variety of sensations in addition to pain, such as numbness, tingling, or burning.

Nociceptive somatic pain

Bone metastases are among the most common causes of cancer-related pain. Bone periosteum is exquisitely sensitive to infiltration or stretching by tumor, although bone marrow is relatively insensitive to pain. This pain is typically well-localized, sharp, and constant. Bone metastases in some locations may produce pain that is felt in distant sites. Metastatic bone pain is typically worse when the involved bone is stressed. It is often relieved to some degree by nonsteroidal anti-inflammatory drugs (NSAIDs), which block the production of prostaglandins that may play an important role in pain related to bone metastases.

Base of skull syndromes

Bone metastases are commonly seen in the vertebrae, pelvis, femur, and skull. Patients may have multiple areas of bone metastasis and multiple areas of pain. Five different metastases to the base of the skull are described here.

Jugular foramen syndrome. Pain from metastasis to this region is typically dull and constant and referred to the occiput (back of the head) or postauricular (behind the ear) region. There may be associated sharp, lancinating pain, so-called glossopharyngeal neuralgia in the throat or ear. Deficits of cranial nerves IX, X, and XI are common, causing dysphagia, dysarthria, and weakness of the trapezius and sternocleidomastoid muscles. Pain from a metastasis to the jugular foramen may be exacerbated by neck flexion.

Orbital syndrome. Pain secondary to a metastasis to the bony orbit is localized behind, above, or around the eye. It is dull and constant and may be worse when lying down or with eye movement. It may be associated with visual loss and palsies of cranial nerves V1, V2, III, IV, and VI and may produce diplopia, facial numbness, and proptosis.

Clivus syndrome. The clivus is the bony ridge between the pituitary sella (sella turcica) and the foramen magnum. Metastasis to this bone often refer pain to the top of the head (vertex), which is worse with neck flexion. A number of cranial nerves (VI and XII) travel in the vicinity of the clivus and thus may be compromised, depending on the site of metastasis.

Parasellar and middle cranial fossa syndrome. Symptoms may closely resemble those of an orbital syndrome (see above) secondary to involvement of structures within the cavernous sinus located just behind the bony orbit. Proptosis, however, is less frequent. Pain in the face, diminished corneal sensation, and weakened chewing muscles secondary to trigeminal ganglion involvement are common with metastasis to the bone of the middle cranial fossa

Occipital condyle syndrome. The occipital condyles join the skull to the cervical vertebrae. Metastasis produces dull, constant occipital pain that worsens with neck movement. Tongue weakness and wasting with fasciculations (visible, involuntary contractions of groups of muscle fibers) are common secondary to involvement of cranial nerve XII within its exit canal in the occipital condyle.

Appropriate imaging procedures for skull base lesions include plain X-ray and bone scan, CT scan with bone windows, or MRI including special base of skull, orbital, or cavernous sinus views, as required to locate the lesion

Vertebral syndromes

Malignant involvement of vertebrae typically produces pain located over the vertebrae affected by the metastasis. This type of pain is worse with percussion or movements that apply stress to the spine. Spine pain is often worse at night secondary to the lengthening of the spine and stretching of the periosteum after several hours of resting in a reclining posture.

Reclining also increases intraspinal pressure. Extension of tumor into the epidural space around the spinal cord may compress nerve roots, producing neuropathic pain radiating into the arms, legs, or around the chest or abdomen "like a belt or band," depending on the spinal level involved. Evidence of spinal cord injury (cord compression due to metastasis in the epidural space) with limb weakness, sensory loss, and bowel and bladder dysfunction may or may not be present. A caregiver should suspect epidural cord compression in any cancer patient with persistent spine pain, especially if evidence of nerve root or spinal cord injury is present. This constitutes a neurologic emergency requiring high-dose corticosteroids, MRI or myelogram, and emergency radiation therapy or neurosurgery.

Vertebral involvement at some levels may produce unique patterns of pain radiation, which can be deceptive. Metastasis to T12 or L1, for instance, may produce pain radiating to the iliac crest or to the sacroiliac joint. This may result in inappropriate imaging of the pelvis or sacrum and failure to diagnose the actual site of disease. C7 or T1 involvement may produce pain that is felt between the shoulder blades.

Nociceptive visceral pain

Malignant involvement of viscera is common in lung, GI, and genitourinary malignant disease, although virtually any cancer may produce visceral metastases. Most organ tissue is not supplied by pain-sensitive nerve fibers, although their surrounding capsules, pleura, and peritoneum are. Hence, pain may be experienced when these pain-sensitive structures are directly involved by tumor by means of the tumor's seeding of the pleura or peritoneum, when organ capsules are distended, as in metastases to the liver or spleen, or when hollow viscus are distended, as in bowel, biliary, or ureter obstruction.

Visceral nociceptive pain is poorly localized, constant or intermittent, and often associated with symptoms of visceral dysfunction, such as nausea, dyspepsia, vomiting, jaundice, dysuria, dyspnea, and so forth. Pain secondary to distention of a hollow viscus is often colicky or cramping and may be felt over the entire abdomen or chest wall. Visceral pain is usually worse with palpation of the involved organ or with maneuvers that stretch irritated structures, for example, deep inspiration in the case of pleural malignancy. Diagnostic studies are tailored to individual patients and obviously may include plain chest or abdominal X-rays, body CT, intravenous pyelogram (IVP), colon X-ray, upper GI series, and so forth.

Neuropathic pain secondary to tumor invasion

Tumor may invade structures at all levels of the nervous system, producing discomfort that patients might have difficulty describing. Neuropathic pain may be sharp, jabbing, and sudden or dull, gnawing, and constant. Burning, tingling, "pins and needles," numbness, and "stretching" are qualifiers that patients use to describe this pain. Allodynia, the perception of pain when a nonpainful stimulus is applied, is characteristic and may cause the light touch of garments or bedclothes to be excruciatingly uncomfortable. Weakness, sensory loss, or autonomic impairment, including bowel or bladder incontinence, loss of sexual function, inappropriate diaphoresis, and skin temperature changes may be present.

Brain tissue itself is not pain-sensitive, although stretching (as with raised intracranial pressure secondary to brain tumors) or irritation of the surrounding dura (leptomeningeal metastasis) may produce somatic nociceptive pain. Rarely, an injury to the thalamus may produce a neuropathic pain syndrome.

Epidural spinal cord compression is a neurologic emergency that begins with spine pain in more than 90% of patients. Pain originating from vertebral body involvement may be referred to a site distant from its origin (see "Vertebral syndromes" above). Thoracic vertebrae metastases are more common and often are associated with pain around the chest or abdomen due to compression of thoracic roots. This may prompt an inappropriate and fruitless evaluation of the heart or GI tract.

Patients with cervical and lumbosacral epidural metastases may develop pain in arms or legs secondary to nerve root compression. Although pain is usually the first symptom, most patients have some degree of weakness, sensory loss, or bowel and bladder dysfunction at the time of diagnosis. This is regrettable, because the risk of permanent neurologic injury is greater in patients who have developed neurologic symptoms in addition to pain, even if appropriate treatment is instituted. Prompt diagnosis is imperative. Any patient in whom the diagnosis of epidural metastasis is suspected should receive 100 mg of I.V. dexamethasone (a corticosteroid, which will reduce tumor swelling), plain X-rays of the entire spine, and an MRI or myelogram. Treatment consists of radiation therapy to the area of epidural tumor. Surgery is reserved for those who do not have a known malignancy (to make a tissue diagnosis), for those with radiation-insensitive tumors, and for those who have previously received radiation and cannot be re-radiated. A simple laminectomy (removal of a vertebral lamina to allow access to the tumor) is usually ineffective because most epidural tumor is located anteriorly and the spinal cord is not adequately decompressed by such an approach. The favored procedure is a combined anterior and lateral or posterior approach with vertebrectomy (excision of a vertebra), bone graft, and rod stabilization.

Peripheral nerve involvement is less common, although intercostal neuropathies are frequent with chest wall invasion by lung or other tumors. Tumors of the limb (osteogenic sarcoma) may produce solitary or multiple mononeuropathies.

Plexus invasion

The brachial plexus is an important neural structure located above the apex of the lung through which nerve fibers travel as they pass from the cervical spine into the arm. Tumors at the apex of the lung or in nearby lymph nodes may invade and damage the brachial plexus. Patients first develop neuropathic pain and loss of sensation in the armpit, which may spread down the inner arm to the little finger. Weakness in the muscles of the hand may also occur. A supraclavicular mass may be felt. CT scan or MRI through the upper chest both adequately visualize the brachial plexus. MRI has an added advantage in that it may be used to visualize the cervical epidural space as well. Electromyography (EMG) is helpful, in selected cases, to delineate the extent of neurologic involvement.

Lumbosacral plexus involvement by colon, urinary tract, gynecologic, or prostate tumors produces severe constant or lancinating pain in the buttock or leg. There may be associated weakness, sensory loss, and reflex changes, depending on the area of the plexus involved. Bowel, bladder, and sexual dysfunction indicate either bilateral plexus involvement or extension of tumor into the spinal epidural space with an associated cauda equina syndrome. CT or MRI are both adequate imaging techniques, one having no clear advantage over the other. Myelography or MRI of the spine should be considered in those patients whose mass extends paraspinally and in those with bowel, bladder, or sexual dysfunction.

Pain syndromes related to cancer therapy

Chronic pain can result from surgery, radiation, or chemotherapy agents used in the treatment of cancer. Four well-characterized postoperative pain syndromes are caused by injury to a peripheral nerve or plexus. These are postmastectomy pain, postthoracotomy pain, post-amputation pain, and post–radical-neck-dissection pain. Pain syndromes that arise subsequent to radiation therapy result from destruction of tissue within the field of administered radiation. Post-chemotherapy pain is commonly associated with chemotherapy agents that damage peripheral nerves or with reactions to the corticosteroids that are frequently part of multidrug chemotherapy regimens.

Postsurgical pain

Postmastectomy pain occurs in 4% to 10% of women undergoing mastectomy, although it can occur following a simple lumpectomy or following a thoracotomy (procedure to open the chest). Postmastectomy pain is neuropathic and is caused by the formation of a posttraumatic neuroma (abnormal nerve regrowth) of the inter-costobrachial nerve, a sensory branch of T1 and T2 nerve roots supplying the anterior chest wall and axilla. The discomfort is described variously as a burning, tingling, constricting constant pain, sometimes with a sudden, sharp, jabbing component in the anterior chest wall, posterior upper arm, and axilla. In addition, patients with this syndrome usually experience sensory loss in this distribution and sometimes marked allodynia. A trigger point may be found along the mastectomy scar. Arm movement typically accentuates the pain, predisposing patients to immobility and adhesive capsulitis (frozen shoulder). Postmastectomy pain usually develops within a few weeks of surgery, although on occasion it may be delayed by as long as 6 months.

Postthoracotomy pain is neuropathic pain, beginning soon after surgery, and resulting from traction or cutting of one or more of the intercostal nerves with or without formation of a neuroma. Rib resection or traction on the rib and its neurovascular bundle is the usual mechanism of nerve injury. Pain is located along the incision, which may display exquisite point tenderness, and is often burning and constricting with or without a lancinating component. Marked allodynia may be present, making even the light touch of garments unbearably painful. Three groups of patients with postthoracotomy pain have been identified. The first and largest group includes those patients in whom the normal postoperative thoracotomy pain resolves by the second month after surgery. In those patients in whom incisional pain subsequently recurs, it is due to recurrent tumor in most cases. The second group contains patients whose postthoracotomy pain steadily increases in intensity following surgery. In these patients as well, recurrent tumor or infection is the most likely cause. The third group consists of patients whose pain remains stable or decreases over a protracted time period. Unless pain later increases in intensity, this pattern is not associated with recurrent malignancy in most patients. Clearly, a high index of suspicion must be maintained in patients undergoing thoracotomy for malignant tissue whose incisional pain increases in intensity or recurs after the initial postoperative period. A thorough search for infection or recurrent tumor should be made in these patients.

Postamputation pain

Two distinct pain syndromes may result from amputation of a limb. Stump pain is usually experienced in the distal stump along the incision and is secondary to traumatic neuroma formation. Trigger points along the scar are usual. Pain is often burning or lancinating and may make the wearing of a leg or arm prosthesis unbearable. Phantom pain is a painful sensory experience which the patient localizes to the now missing limb. The "phantom limb" may assume unusual postures and may be experienced as swollen or misshapen. Pain is often severe, burning, or tingling. Phantom pain usually decreases with time and is maximal during the first few weeks postoperatively. As the pain resolves, the perceived phantom limb is felt to shrink or telescope into the stump. Interestingly, severe phantom pain is more likely if the limb is painful prior to the amputation. Preoperative epidural lumbar local anesthetic infusion significantly reduces the incidence of phantom pain.

Neck and shoulder neuropathy

Pain that occurs after radical neck dissection is neuropathic neck and shoulder pain resulting from injury to the cervical plexus and cervical nerves at the time of surgery for head and neck cancers. Pain is often described as burning or constricting with or without a lancinating component, which may radiate into the external auditory canal. Pain may also result from muscular imbalance due to removal of the sternocleidomastoid and strap muscles. Symptoms similar to thoracic outlet syndrome (arm pain and paresthesias of the fingers due to compression of the brachial plexus nerve trunks) or suprascapular nerve entrapment (dull, aching shoulder blade discomfort with weakness of external rotation and abduction of the shoulder) may occur secondary to "droopy shoulder." Escalating pain in a patient after radical neck dissection with or without episodes of syncope (from invasion of the carotid sinus) suggests recurrent tumor or soft tissue infection. The latter may be surprisingly indolent and unassociated with fever and it can respond dramatically to empiric antibiotic therapy directed against oral anaerobes. The diagnosis of soft tissue infection may be difficult in tissues already red and indurated by radiation and surgery. Appropriate imaging studies (CT or MRI) assist in making the diagnosis.

Postradiation pain

During and immediately after treatment, radiation therapy may cause a short-lived pain syndrome related to mucosal injury within the field of administered radiation. Mucositis of the mouth and esophagus is seen after radiation for head and neck or cervical spine tumors. Inflammation of the anus and rectum is a common cause of postradiation pain in the case of pelvic tumors of the prostate, uterus, or colon. Oral swishes of a local anesthetic such as viscous lidocaine for oral mucositis and a low-fiber diet with use of a rectal steroid for proctitis may be all that is required for relief, although opioid analgesics may be required if pain is severe.

Acute radiation-induced skin reactions are common. They are usually managed with moisturizing lotion and mild oral analgesics. Necrosis of bone within the radiation field may occur and be an ongoing source of pain. Rarely, radiation-induced tumors may develop many years later and manifest themselves as a painful lump within the previous radiation port. These are often malignant sarcoma tumors of the nerve sheath that may present with neuropathic pain extending along the course of the involved nerve. Radiation-induced meningiomas, sarcomas, and gliomas may be seen if the brain was included within the field of radiation.

Radiation plexopathy

Radiation fibrosis of the brachial or lumbosacral nerve plexus may develop from 6 months to 20 years after radiation therapy is administered. Unlike invasion of the plexus by tumor, radiation plexus injury is painful in less than 25% of patients.

Radiation fibrosis of the plexus may, however, produce tingling, itching, "squeezing," sensory loss, and weakness as in malignant plexopathy. Other features may be helpful in differentiating radiation from malignant brachial plexopathy. Radiation plexopathy most commonly involves the upper part of the brachial plexus (C5 or C6 root distribution) while malignant plexopathy generally involves the lower (C8 to T1 root distribution) because the lower trunk is relatively protected from the effects of radiation by the overlying clavicle bone and is closer to the top of the lung and lymph node chain where tumors may reside. Lymphedema (swelling of a limb due to obstruction of lymph channels) of the upper extremity is more common in radiation plexopathy. CT or MRI is helpful in identifying tumor, although on occasion a surgical exploration of the area may be required.

An acute reversible plexopathy may be seen during or immediately after a course of radiation therapy to the brachial plexus. This is characterized by aching shoulder pain and tingling in the hand and forearm. Temporary weakness may be present in some arm and hand muscles. CT or MRI should be normal. Presumably this lesion is caused by acute radiation-induced loss of the nerve's myelin, which can regenerate.

Pain is similarly uncommon in lumbosacral radiation plexopathy which usually presents with tingling, sensory loss, and leg weakness with diminished deep tendon reflexes occurring 1 to 30 years following treatment with radiation. Symptoms usually begin in the lower leg and foot and may be present on both sides. Patients such as those with uterine cancer who receive radiation directly into a pelvic cavity as well as external beam therapy may be at especially high risk. Radiation necrosis of the pelvic bone with or without spontaneous pelvic bone fractures (insufficiency fractures) can accompany this syndrome.

Postchemotherapy pain

A number of chemotherapy agents may produce painful injury to peripheral nerves, often associated with sensory loss, weakness, and absence of sweating in a glove-and-stocking distribution. Vincristine commonly produces peripheral nerve injury that does not usually cause symptoms, but that may produce burning and tingling of the feet and hands associated with extreme sensitivity to touch. On occasion, vincristine may produce an acute painful injury to a single peripheral nerve; acute severe jaw pain is a common example. Vincristine may also cause an acute ileus (paralysis of gut peristalsis) secondary to autonomic nerve dysfunction. Cisplatin (Platinol), etoposide (VP-16), procarbazine (Matulane), misonidazole, Surinam, and paclitaxel (Taxol) are other agents that may produce a painful neuropathy. Symptomatic relief of these toxic neuropathies may be obtained with adjuvant analgesics (see "Analgesic drug therapy for cancer pain" below), such as amitriptyline or nortriptyline, or the use of transcutaneous electrical nerve stimulation (TENS). Usually the painful symptoms of these neuropathies improve spontaneously over time.

Corticosteroid-associated pain

Corticosteroids are commonly prescribed for cancer patients as components of chemotherapy regimens; for example prednisone is a component in the four-drug combination of cyclophosphamide, doxorubicin, vincristine, and prednisone (called CHOP) and the four-drug combination of mechlorethamine, Oncovin (vincristine), procarbazine, and prednisone (called MOPP). Corticosteroids are also used in the treatment of nausea and in the treatment of brain or spinal cord tumor swelling. Several pain syndromes have been attributed to these medications. A brief burning sensation in the perineum is noted by over 50% of patients given large bolus doses (100 mg) of I.V. dexamethasone, a synthetic corticosteroid usually administered in the treatment of epidural spinal cord compression by tumor. The cause of this effect is unknown. It usually lasts only minutes and treatment is neither available nor required. It is helpful to warn patients of this effect prior to administration of the drug.

Steroid pseudorheumatism is characterized by severe muscle and joint aches during withdrawal from steroids. This adverse effect does not appear to depend on the dosage, length of therapy, or speed of withdrawal. Although the exact pathogenesis is unknown, it is thought to be caused by sensitization of joint and muscle sensory nerve endings. Treatment is simple and effective and consists of reinstating the corticosteroid at a higher dose and slowly tapering off.

Aseptic necrosis of the head of the femur or humerus may follow the intermittent or chronic daily use of corticosteroids. Pain is typically located over the joint or its zone of referred pain (hip disease refers to the knee; shoulder pain refers to the elbow) and is made worse by movement of the involved joint. The pain may occur before changes are seen on X-rays. A bone scan or an MRI of the involved joint is useful for early diagnosis. If discovered early, the treatment of aseptic necrosis is conservative, using analgesics and tapering of the corticosteroids. Surgery may be required in those patients with actual destruction of the joint or poorly controlled pain.

Phenobarbital, a drug often used to prevent seizures in patients with primary or metastatic tumors of the central nervous system, may also cause a similar pain problem, phenobarbital pseudorheumatism, characterized by shoulder discomfort and immobility (frozen shoulder). If diagnosed promptly, this problem resolves with discontinuance of the phenobarbital. The exact cause is unknown but signs and symptoms are typical of adhesive capsulitis of the joint. If the problem becomes severe, signs of a superimposed sympathetically maintained pain syndrome (reflex sympathetic dystrophy) may develop and lead to a painful, useless limb. Some cancer patients are chronically maintained on steroids and phenobarbital for a variety of indications. The differential diagnosis of localized shoulder pain in these patients includes metastatic spread of tumor, aseptic necrosis of the humeral head, and phenobarbital pseudorheumatism.

Analgesic drug therapy for cancer pain

Analgesic drug therapy is the most common method of cancer pain management, with opioids as the mainstay treatment for moderate to severe cancer pain of all types. The World Health Organization has developed a three-step ladder for the treatment of cancer pain (see the *World Health Organization analgesic ladder*). Step 1, for mild pain, utilizes a nonopioid analgesic such as an NSAID with or without an adjuvant drug. Step 2, for mild to moderate pain, utilizes a low-potency opioid with or without an adjuvant drug. Step 3, for moderate to severe pain, utilizes a strong opioid with or without an adjuvant drug.

Selected patients may be candidates for neurosurgical or neuroanesthetic procedures designed to relieve some types of cancer pain. These approaches are generally reserved for those patients in whom drug therapy has failed or who are experiencing unmanageable side effects of drug therapy. Moreover, it is rare that complete pain relief can be obtained with these procedures alone, and most patients will continue to require supplementary opioid medication.

Nonopioid analgesics

Acetaminophen, aspirin, and other NSAIDs are the prototypes of this drug class. These drugs are usually administered orally, although acetaminophen and indomethacin are available in a rectally administered preparation and ketorolac (Toradol) is available for I.M. administration. These medications all have the advantage of safety and relative low cost, with the exception of some of the newer NSAIDs. Tolerance and physical dependence do not develop. There is a ceiling effect, however, which means that a particular dosage produces a given level of analgesia and higher doses of the drug do not produce greater pain relief.

Aspirin and other NSAIDs produce anti-inflammatory, antipyretic, and analgesic effects. Acetaminophen is equipotent with aspirin as an analgesic and antipyretic, but much less effective as an anti-inflammatory medication. Acetaminophen does not interfere

World Health Organization analgesic ladder

The World Health Organization (WHO) analgesic ladder graphically demonstrates the principle of responding appropriately to a patient's actual level of pain.

During the course of cancer, a patient's pain may increase or decrease, depending on the treatment and the patient's individual response to treatment.

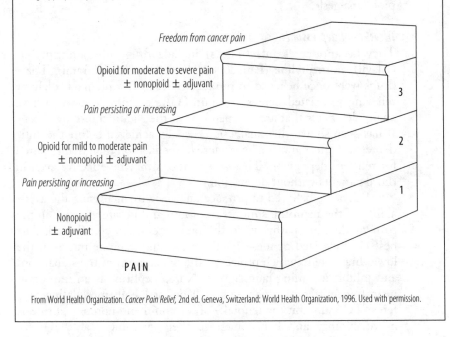

Freedom from cancer pain

Opioid for moderate to severe pain
± nonopioid ± adjuvant

3

Pain persisting or increasing

Opioid for mild to moderate pain
± nonopioid ± adjuvant

2

Pain persisting or increasing

1

Nonopioid
± adjuvant

PAIN

From World Health Organization. *Cancer Pain Relief*, 2nd ed. Geneva, Switzerland: World Health Organization, 1996. Used with permission.

with platelet function or produce stomach irritation and bleeding and hence is usually preferred. Acetaminophen is relatively contraindicated in patients with liver disease, and an overdose may produce life-threatening liver injury. Other NSAIDs share with aspirin the risk of interfering with platelet function and producing stomach irritation. In addition, NSAIDs may produce or worsen kidney failure, and they have been reported to cause confusion in elderly patients.

NSAIDs and aspirin produce analgesia by inhibiting the production of prostaglandin E_2 (PGE_2), a fatty acid derivative that sensitizes pain nerves to the effects of tissue inflammation products. NSAIDs thus play an important role in the treatment of pain due to bony metastases, in which PGE_2 production is believed to be involved. Corticosteroid medications have a similar action but should not be given together with NSAIDs due to the added risk of GI bleeding.

Adjuvant medications

Adjuvant analgesics are a diverse group of medications that have primary uses but that also, in selected cases, have pain-relieving effects. This group includes tricyclic antidepressants, anticonvulsants, neuroleptics, antihistamines, and psychostimulants, among others. Adjuvants are typically used in conjunction with an opioid or a nonopioid analgesic.

Tricyclic antidepressants

Tricyclic antidepressants (TCAs) include drugs like amitriptyline (Elavil), nortriptyline (Pamelor) and imipramine (Tofranil). These drugs were once believed to produce relief in chronic pain solely by relieving associated depression, but TCAs are now known to have analgesic effects that are independent of their antidepressant effects. It has been shown that analgesia is usually achieved before the antidepressant effect and at a lower dose of medication than that required for relief of depression. These medications may be effective even in those patients without depression.

TCAs are believed to produce analgesia by increasing the availability of the neurotransmitters serotonin and norepinephrine in the pain-modulating pathways in the brain stem and spinal cord. The best-characterized of these are the serotonergic raphe nuclei in the lower brain stem, which project to the dorsal horn of the spinal cord and inhibit incoming pain signals. Norepinephrine is an important neurotransmitter in other, less well-defined pain-modulating systems. TCAs inhibit the reuptake of serotonin and norepinephrine at nerve endings and hence increase their availability at the nerve synapses. They bind to a variety of other receptors as well and their interactions are probably more complex than has been thought.

Both nociceptive and neuropathic chronic pain may respond to the addition of a TCA. In general, visceral and somatic nociceptive pain is most responsive to opioids (see "Opioid analgesics" later in this chapter). Neuropathic pain with a component of continuous burning or tingling is the usual indication for a TCA in cancer pain. Moreover, any pain syndrome in a cancer patient accompanied by depression is likely to be benefited. Studies have confirmed the effectiveness of amitriptyline in postherpetic neuralgia (pain after shingles) and diabetic nerve disease. Other controlled studies have documented its effectiveness in muscle and ligament pain syndromes, tension headache, and idiopathic pain syndromes with or without a superimposed depression. The use of other TCAs, including nortriptyline, imipramine, and doxepin, has been supported in a number of controlled and uncontrolled studies.

TCAs are not appropriate in certain circumstances. These drugs should not be used in patients with significant heart disease, acute-angle-closure glaucoma, or an enlarged prostate because TCAs may worsen the symptoms associated with these disorders. All TCAs may produce some degree of sedation, dry mouth, and hypotension, especially when the drug is first started. The starting dose should be low and should then be increased slowly in weekly stages. Most of these medications can be given once daily, preferably at night to take advantage of the sedative effect. If a maximal dose has been reached (150 mg at bedtime for amitriptyline, nortriptyline, and imipramine) without benefit or with uncontrollable side effects, consideration should be given to a trial of another TCA. A given patient may respond to one TCA and not to another. The response cannot be predicted without a trial of medication, so sequential trials of different TCAs may be required.

Another class of antidepressants, the serotonin reuptake inhibitors (SSRIs), such as fluoxetine, paroxetine, or sertraline), has not been tested for analgesic effects. Until data on these drugs become available, the role of SSRIs in pain alleviation remains uncertain.

Anticonvulsants

Medications in this category that are occasionally used in the treatment of neuropathic pain include phenytoin, carbamazepine, valproic acid, clonazepam, and baclofen. Their precise mechanism of action is unknown, although presumably it relates to these drugs' ability to block abnormal nerve discharge. It follows that these drugs would be most effective in the treatment of sharp, shooting (lancinating) neuropathic pain. Controlled studies in neuropathic cancer pain are lacking, although these agents have been shown effective in nonmalignant, lancinating neuropathic pain syndromes, such as trigeminal neuralgia, diabetic neuropathy, and postherpetic neuralgia.

There is no support for the use of these drugs in the treatment of nonneuropathic (somatic or visceral nociceptive) pain. Similarly, there is little if any proof to suggest that these medications are useful in treating the continuous burning or tingling often noted in neuropathic pain syndromes. The use of adjuvant anticonvulsants should probably be limited to the treatment of sharp, shooting pain.

Neuroleptics

Neuroleptics have been used as adjuvants in cancer pain treatment for many years with few controlled studies to support their use. Most have effective antinausea and sedative properties and thus have a clear role in the symptom management of cancer patients.

Methotrimeprazine (Levoprome), however, has been shown to have potent pain-relieving effects similar to morphine on a milligram-for-milligram basis. Unfortunately, the powerful sedative and blood pressure lowering effects of methotrimeprazine preclude its use in patients who are not bedbound. It is an extremely useful agent in the treatment of terminal delirium and as an analgesic in bedridden patients with advanced malignant disease who cannot tolerate opioids.

No other drug in this class can be recommended as an analgesic, although the antianxiety effects of these medications may have a valuable impact on patients' perception of pain and their resulting suffering. Nausea, delirium, and anxiety are clear indications for using these drugs.

Local anesthetics
Systematically administered local anesthetics, including intravenous lidocaine or orally ingested mexiletine may be useful in some patients with neuropathic pain. Their effect probably results from inhibition of aberrant neural discharge by the blocking of sodium channels in the nerve membrane.

Corticosteroids
Corticosteroids are used in the emergency treatment of spinal cord compression related to tumor invasion of the epidural space. These drugs are also used on a short-term basis as analgesics for bone pain. Their effectiveness in these cases is due to their inhibition of arachidonic acid synthesis which in turn reduces the formation of prostaglandin metabolites. They are useful in neural compression and invasion by tumors because they reduce tumor-associated swelling. Dexamethasone is the usual drug of choice.

Chronic use of low doses of corticosteroids may improve appetite and mood in patients with advanced cancer. The chronic use of high doses of corticosteroids is often complicated by life-threatening immunosuppression, osteoporosis, aseptic necrosis of joints, gastrointestinal bleeding, and muscle weakness.

Psychostimulants
Methylphenidate (Ritalin), caffeine, and dextroamphetamine (Dexedrine) have minimal if any analgesic effects when used alone. Their most useful application in cancer pain is in the treatment of the sedation associated with opioid use because they allow better drug tolerance and escalation of opioid dose to obtain analgesia. Methylphenidate and dextroamphetamine are begun at a dose of 2.5 to 5 mg administered in the early morning and early afternoon. The dose may be gradually increased as necessary to a maximum of about 60 mg per day. These drugs may produce restlessness, anxiety, insomnia, paranoia, and confusion. Psychostimulants should be avoided in those patients with cardiac disease, delirium, or uncontrolled hypertension. Pemoline (Cylert), another stimulant, is structurally unrelated to methylphenidate but produces similar alertness with minimal cardio-

vascular effects. It is available in a chewable tablet that allows drug absorption across the oral mucosa. This is an advantage for patients unable to take oral medicines

Opioid analgesics

Opioid analgesics are indicated in the treatment of moderate to severe cancer pain of all etiologies. Expertise in using these medications is the most important skill in successful management of cancer pain. Prior to a discussion of opioid analgesia it is important to define the concepts of tolerance, physical dependence, and psychological dependence.

Tolerance refers to a state in which increasing doses of a medication are required to maintain its effect. Sometimes tolerance is desirable, as when it develops to the adverse effects of opioids, that is, sedation, depression of respiration, nausea, and constipation. Tolerance to these adverse effects develops at different rates. It usually develops quickly to respiratory depression but slowly, if ever, to constipation. Tolerance may also develop to the analgesic effect of opioids. The first signs of tolerance are usually patients' reports that the duration of analgesia from a dose of opioid has shortened. They may request more medicine before the scheduled dose and thus be mislabelled a "clock-watcher."

Clinical experience suggests that the need for increasing doses of opioids is rarely due to tolerance alone but to progression of the underlying painful disease. This is supported by the common observation of a decrease in opioid requirements when the cancer pain stimulus is lessened by surgery, radiation, or chemotherapy or when an effective alternative method of pain control is utilized. Furthermore, experience suggests that there is no limit, or ceiling, to tolerance. Patients with progressive painful disease are able to achieve and maintain pain control with escalating doses of opioids while also increasing their tolerance to the sedative and respiratory depressant effects. Skill in safely and effectively titrating opioids as needed is critically important in cancer pain management.

Physical dependence refers to the potential for development of a withdrawal syndrome if the opioid is abruptly discontinued or if an opioid antagonist such as naloxone is administered. Withdrawal symptoms are easily avoided if the opioid is gradually tapered when it is no longer needed.

Neither tolerance nor physical dependence is equivalent to addiction, which is psychological dependence. Addiction is defined as a behavioral pattern of drug abuse characterized by drug craving, using a drug for other than analgesic purposes, and overwhelming behavioral involvement in obtaining and using a drug. Confusion about the difference between physical and psychological dependence by physicians, nurses, and patients has been a tremendous obstacle to cancer pain management. Experience has shown that true addiction to opioids is extremely uncommon in cancer pain patients, even when opioids are used over a long period of time.

Principles of potent opioid use

Four rules apply to the correct usage of opioids for pain (see *Principles of opioid use*). Adherence to these basic principles ensures that patients receive correct and timely amounts of the appropriate drug for their pain. Attention to the details of managing side effects improves patient comfort and helps minimize many of the undesirable consequences of these drugs.

Appropriate drug choice

In choosing the appropriate drug for patients' pain, it is important to consider a number of important factors: the severity of pain, available routes of administration (oral, I.V., S.C., transdermal, rectal, epidural, or intrathecal), cost, previous side effects experienced by a particular patient to a given opioid, patient age, and preexisting kidney and liver function.

Patients with mild pain that has not responded to acetaminophen or an NSAID may be given a weak, or low-potency, opioid, such as codeine, oxycodone, or hydrocodone. These drugs are generally combined with acetaminophen or aspirin in commonly used preparations. Unlike strong opioids, they have a ceiling effect, in that increasing the dose past a certain point will not increase analgesic effect but will increase the likelihood of side effects. Furthermore, many of these low-potency opioids are combined with aspirin or acetaminophen, which also limits the number of tablets that can be taken in a day. Moderate to severe cancer pain of any etiology requires the use of a potent, or strong, opioid.

The oral route is preferred due to ease of administration, cost, and the good to excellent oral absorption of most opioids. In patients who cannot tolerate or cannot absorb an oral drug, an alternate route must be selected. Similarly, patients with severe uncontrolled pain may require a brief course of intravenous drug to obtain rapid pain control. They may then be switched over to the oral route. Opioids that have previously produced side effects in a given patient should be avoided.

Most opioids are metabolized by the liver into active and inactive metabolites, which are then eliminated by the kidney. Opioids and their breakdown products accumulate in patients with kidney failure and in normal elderly patients. Adverse opioid effects, such as slowing of respiration and sedation, are thus more likely to occur in these patients. Avoidance of morphine, methadone, and levorphanol is

PAIN MANAGEMENT PRINCIPLES

Principles of opioid use

Four basic principles govern the use of opioids for pain management. Adherence to these rules ensures optimal patient comfort and safety.

1. Choose the appropriate drug.
2. Begin with a low dose.
3. Titrate the dose until analgesia is achieved or until unmanageable side effects result.
4. Learn the concept of equianalgesic doses, including conversion from one route of administration to another and from one opioid to another.

warranted in elderly patients or those with renal dysfunction. An excellent alternative is hydromorphone, which has the advantage of a short half-life and no known active metabolites.

Low initial dosage

In patients who have never taken opioids or who have been exposed only to weak opioids, a starting dose should be in the range of 5 to 10 mg of the I.V. drug or 15 to 30 mg of oral immediate-release morphine given every four hours around the clock. Optional, or as-needed, doses should be made available to patients every 2 hours as a rescue for breakthrough pain. The dose of rescue medication to be made available should be 5% to 10% of the total daily opioid dose. In this way, the patient has the opportunity to obtain relief if the scheduled dose of opioid is insufficient. Rescue medication should be a short half-life, immediate-release opioid, such as morphine or hydromorphone. The number and amount of rescues used should be recorded by the patient or caregiver because it will assist the physician in dose adjustments. Analgesia given solely PRN is usually inappropriate in cancer patients because a constant blood level of opioid is required to obtain good analgesia.

Potent opioids must be dosed according to their duration of analgesic effect, which does not always correspond to a drug's half-life (see *Equianalgesic dosage of opioids*, page 304). Thus, methadone and levorphanol, although they both have long half-lives, must be given every 4 to 6 hours in order to maintain a constant level of analgesia. Unfortunately, side effects like sedation and nausea correspond more closely to drug half-life, making drugs with long half-lives problematic in elderly patients and in those with renal failure. Moreover, the time required to reach a steady state with a given opioid depends on the drug half-life, so that full assessment of analgesic efficacy and drug toxicity takes approximately $4^{1}/_{2}$ half-lives (24 hours for morphine and 5 to 10 days for methadone).

Equianalgesic dosages of opioids

Opioid	Equianalgesic dose	Half-life	Duration of action
Morphine *	10 mg I.M. or I.V. 20 to 60 mg P.O.	2 to 3.5 hr "	4 to 6 hr 4 to 7 hr
Hydromorphone	1.5 mg I.M. or I.V. 7.5 mg P.O.	2 to 3 hr "	4 to 5 hr 4 to 6 hr
Levorphanol	2.0 mg I.M. or I.V. 4.0 mg P.O.	12 to 16 hr "	4 to 6 hr 4 to 7 hr
Methadone	10 mg I.M. or I.V. 20 mg P.O.	15 to 30+ hr "	4 to 6 hr (variable)
Codeine	130 mg I.M. or I.V. 200 mg P.O.	3 hr "	4 to 6 hr "
Oxycodone	30 mg P.O.	2 to 3 hr	3 to 5 hr
Meperidine	75 mg I.M. or I.V. 300 mg P.O.	3 to 4 hr "	4 to 5 hr 4 to 6 hr
Fentanyl *Transdermal patch*	0.1 mg I.V. See page 309.	3 to 4 hr See page 309.	0.5 to 2 hr 72 hr

When converting from one route of administration to another or from one opioid to another, the equianalgesic dosages in this chart allow calculation of the correct amount of opioid. For example, in converting from 3 mg of I.M. hydromorphone to I.V. morphine, the correct dosage would be (10/1.5) X 3 mg = 20 mg of morphine.

*Relative potency of I.M.:P.O. for morphine changes from 1:6 to 1:2 or 1:3 with prolonged use.

Adapted from Foley, K.M., "The Treatment of Cancer Pain," *New England Journal of Medicine* 313:84-95 (1985). Used with permission. © 1985, Massachusetts Medical Society. All rights reserved.

Titration for optimal analgesia

Doses should be titrated until analgesia is achieved or until unmanageable side effects result. A tremendous difference in opioid requirements exists among cancer patients, even among those with similar cancers and pain diagnoses. There is no "standard opioid dose," and therapy must be individualized. Furthermore, titration is required at multiple points in patients' illnesses, depending on disease progression, which usually indicates an increased dose, and on treatment, which often allows for a decreased dose. If pain is poorly controlled with a given scheduled dose of opioid, it is helpful to determine the total opioid rescue requirement for a 24-hour period and add it to the scheduled dose. Thus, a patient with inadequate analgesia on immediate-release morphine 30 mg every 4 hours who required six rescues of 15 mg immediate-release morphine in a 24-hour period could be safely escalated to a dose of 45 mg every 4 hours with rescues of 15 to 30 mg every 2 hours as needed. For patients receiving I.V. opioid infusions, escalation of dose may also be accomplished by calculating the rescues used in a 24-hour period and increasing the infusion accordingly. If more rapid escalation is required due to poorly controlled pain, an increase in the infusion rate by 50% every 6 to 12 hours is generally safe if the patient is awake and alert and shows no sign of respiratory depression. Close monitoring of vital signs is required in any patient on an opioid infusion, especially after an increase in the dose of opioid.

Equianalgesic dosage

Equianalgesic dosage and conversion from one route of administration to another and from one opioid to another are vitally important concepts. The knowledge of equipotency is crucial when switching from one opioid to another or from one route of administration to another. Relative analgesic potency is the ratio of two analgesics required to produce the same level of analgesia and can be obtained by consulting a conversion table. For the commonly used strong opioids, 10 mg of I.M. or I.V. morphine are used as the standard for comparison. The equianalgesic table provides guidelines for switching from one drug to another and from one route of administration to another.

The equianalgesic table should serve as a reference point but should not be interpreted as a table of standard doses. As stated earlier, dosage is likely to vary among patients and optimal dosage of any opioid should be individualized. When converting an opioid-tolerant patient from one strong opioid to another, the equianalgesic dosage obtained using the conversion table is reduced by 50% for initial administration because tolerance for side effects between opioids (cross-tolerance) may not be complete. In addition, when converting to methadone, the equianalgesic dosage should be reduced by 60% to 80%, because cross-tolerance appears to be especially incomplete between other strong opioids and methadone.

Management of opioid side effects

Adverse effects of opioids include sedation, nausea, constipation, respiratory depression, and myoclonus. No opioid is better or worse with respect to another in this regard, with the exception of meperidine. Meperidine has a metabolite, normeperidine, that is toxic to the central nervous system (CNS). In a given patient, however, one opioid may produce an side effect that another does not. The occurrence of particular side effects cannot be predicted ahead of time unless the patient has experienced previous side effects from the drug.

Most opioid side effects are manageable. Constipation, a common effect to which tolerance either never develops or is incomplete, is best avoided by starting stool softeners at the same time the opioid is started. Sometimes, stronger agents like bowel stimulants, enemas, and osmotic agents are needed.

Respiratory depression

Fortunately, rapid tolerance develops to the slowed respirations caused by opioids. These drugs act directly on the brain stem's respiratory centers and suppress respiratory rate and volume. With long-term opioid use, this is rarely a problem unless the dose is increased too rapidly. Respiratory depression, if it develops, often parallels the degree of drug-induced sedation. Thus, stimulating patients by speaking to them, turning on the radio or TV, or turning on the room lights may be sufficient to alert him and speed up breathing until tolerance develops.

More severe respiratory depression may require artificial ventilation and the I.V. administration of a drug (naloxone) to counteract the effects of the opioid. Naloxone should be given very carefully, by diluting one ampule (0.4 mg) in 10 to 50 ml of saline and administering by slow injection just until the sedation and respiratory depression improves. Especially in overdose with a long half-life opioid, a continuous slow infusion of naloxone may be required. An acute withdrawal syndrome should be avoided because it may be extremely uncomfortable and sometimes excruciatingly painful to the cancer patient using opioids for pain. Aspiration of stomach contents may occur, especially in the unconscious patient. Naloxone administration in patients on meperidine may pose a particular risk. Removing the sedating effect of meperidine may unmask the effects on the CNS of its metabolite, normeperidine, producing convulsions. Unconscious patients should be intubated prior to the administration of naloxone to protect the airway.

Tolerance to sedation from opioids usually develops over a period of days. If tolerance is incomplete or patients are unwilling to wait, a trial of a psychostimulant is useful. Simple measures such as a strong cup of coffee or espresso or a caffeinated soda twice a day at 8 a.m. and 1 p.m. are usually tolerated and inexpensive, and they eliminate the need for a prescription stimulant. If these measures are ineffective, then methylphenidate, dextroamphetamine, or pimoline may be tried. The usual starting dose of methylphenidate or dextroamphetamine is 2.5 to 5 mg twice a day and may be gradually increased to a daily maximum of about 40 to 60 mg per day. Pimoline is available in a chewable tablet that is absorbed across the oral mucosa. Contraindications for these medications include uncontrolled hypertension, unstable angina, and a history of irregular heartbeat.

Nausea and myoclonus

Opioids produce nausea via three different mechanisms, each of which may be discovered by taking a nausea history. First, opioids directly stimulate an area in the brain stem called the vomiting center. The stimulation usually produces nausea that is continuous and not particularly worsened by eating or changing position. It is best relieved by a phenothiazine such as prochlorperazine. Second, opioids also reduce stomach-emptying. This type of nausea is typically much worse after eating and is best treated with metoclopramide. Third, opioids sensitize the vestibular apparatus in the inner ear, producing nausea similar to motion sickness, which is much worse with changes in position. This variety of nausea is treated most effectively with scopolamine or meclizine, common remedies for motion sickness.

Myoclonus is an abnormal, rapid, involuntary jerking of muscles that is a common side effect of all opioids. In its lesser form, myoclonus is characterized by accentuated "sleep jerks," most prominent during drowsiness and light sleep. They may be quite disturbing to patients and can require treatment. Clonazepam, a relative of diazepam, at a starting dose of 0.25 mg taken orally twice a day is usually helpful but may be very sedating.

Clearly, most opioid side effects are manageable, either by reassuring the patient while waiting for tolerance to develop or through the use of symptom-controlling medications. If side effects persist despite treatment, then switching to another opioid is warranted. Usually with perseverance and trials of different opioids, a drug can be found that provides good analgesia without unmanageable side effects.

Potent opioids used in cancer pain

Potent opioids are the mainstay of analgesic therapy for moderate to severe cancer pain of all etiologies.

Morphine

Morphine serves as the standard strong opioid against which other drugs are compared. It is recommended as the drug of choice by the World Health Organization Cancer Pain Relief Program.

Morphine is metabolized in the liver into active (morphine-6-glucuronide, or M6G) and inactive (morphine-3-glucuronide) products. Little morphine is excreted unchanged. Morphine and its metabolites are eliminated by the kidney predominantly as morphine-3-glucuronide. Morphine's half-life in young adults is 3 to 4 hours. The half-life of M6G is considerably longer, perhaps as long as 12 to 24 hours. The metabolite M6G is approximately four times more potent than morphine and is an important contributor to the analgesia derived from one dose of morphine. It also probably plays a significant role in the production of side effects to morphine, such as sedation, nausea, and respiratory depression, especially in patients with renal failure and in elderly patients, who cannot excrete the drug promptly.

In opioid-naive patients, the relative potency of I.V. to oral morphine is 1:6, with 1 mg taken I.V. equaling 6 mg taken orally. With long-term administration over 1 to 2 weeks, the potency ratio becomes 1:3 because continued oral intake of morphine results in increased conversion to the potent M6G form by the liver.

This is only a rough guideline. Individual patients might well require more or less morphine when moving from one route of administration to another. This truth emphasizes the importance of individualizing treatment.

Hydromorphone

Hydromorphone (Dilaudid) is a relative of morphine and is approximately six times more potent per milligram than morphine. Its oral to parenteral ratio is 5:1. Hydromorphone has no known active metabolites. Its analgesic duration of action is 4 to 6 hours, and its half-life is 2 to 3 hours. The more rapid clearance of this drug from the body makes it an extremely useful alternative to morphine in patients with kidney disease and in elderly patients. It is an excellent second-line drug for patients with poor pain control and uncontrollable side effects from morphine.

Levorphanol

Levorphanol (Levo-Dromoran) is another relative of morphine, but it is approximately five times more potent than hydromorphone. It has a half-life of 15 hours and a duration of analgesia of 4 to 6 hours, with excellent oral absorption and an oral to parenteral ratio of 2:1. It should be administered every 4 to 6 hours. Because of its long half-life and high potency, it should be used with caution and titrated with equal care in patients with kidney failure and in elderly patients, in whom drug and metabolites will accumulate, often producing difficult-to-control side effects.

Methadone

Although best known for its ability to suppress withdrawal symptoms in the physically dependent population, methadone is a potent and useful analgesic in patients with cancer pain. At 15 to 48 hours, it has the longest half-life of any of the currently available opioids. Unfortunately, despite the long duration of many of its opioid side effects, the duration of analgesia is nearly the same as that of morphine, often necessitating dosing every 4 to 6 hours for pain control. When used exclusively to prevent withdrawal and not for analgesia, it may be given as infrequently as every 72 hours. As with morphine and levorphanol, methadone use can be a problem in elderly patients and patients with kidney failure because the inevitable gradual accumulation of drug causes side effects.

I.V. methadone is equianalgesic, milligram per milligram, with morphine. Methadone's oral absorption is much better than morphine, however, with an I.V. to oral ratio of 1:2. When converting from another strong opioid to methadone, cross-tolerance for side effects is often incomplete, and the calculated initial methadone dose should be reduced by a factor of 3 or 5 and then adjusted over time to achieve the best analgesia. When methadone is used as the principal around-the-clock analgesic, shorter-acting opioids, such as morphine or hydromorphone, should be used as rescue medication. Unfortunately, because of its association with addicts, oral methadone may be difficult to obtain in neighborhood pharmacies, and patients may be reluctant to use it.

Fentanyl

Fentanyl (Sublimaze and Duragesic) is a synthetic relative of meperidine. When administered I.V., it is 100 times as potent as morphine. The half-life of fentanyl is 3 to 4 hours, with a duration of analgesic effect of 1 to 2 hours. In the past, it has been commonly used as an anesthetic agent and postoperative analgesic. Fentanyl is not available in oral form but is available in solution for I.V., epidural, and intraspinal administration. Recently, fentanyl has been marketed in a transdermal formulation as a patch, which produces continuous drug release through the skin over a period of about 72 hours. This novel route of delivery has been especially useful in patients unable to take oral medications.

When administered by the transdermal patch, fentanyl takes 6 to 12 hours to reach analgesic serum levels and 24 hours to reach steady state. Thus, transdermal fentanyl should not be used in the management of acute pain because it takes too long to reach analgesic serum levels and its dose adjustment is slow. Furthermore, despite its short half-life when administered I.V., a drug reservoir develops in the fat beneath the skin, resulting in a prolonged drug effect even after the patch is removed. This may become a problem if side effects such as respiratory depression or sedation develop because it may take several days after patch removal before these undesirable effects recede.

Fentanyl comes in 25, 50, 75, and 100 mcg/hour patches. A usual starting dose in an opioid-naive patient is 25 to 50 mcg/hr. Initial predictions were that I.V. and transdermal fentanyl would be equal in potency. In fact, transdermal fentanyl is probably 20 times more potent than I.V. morphine, so that 10 mg of parenteral morphine is equivalent to 500 mcg of transdermal fentanyl, or a 100 mcg/hour patch is equianalgesic with 36 to 60 mg of oral morphine every 4 hours. No oral preparation of fentanyl is currently available, and morphine or hydromorphone should be used as rescue medication in patients maintained on fentanyl patches.

Meperidine

Meperidine (Demerol) is not appropriate for chronic administration in cancer pain. It is included in this discussion only to discourage its use. Meperidine's half-life is 3 to 4 hours. Its metabolite, normeperidine, has a longer half-life of 12 to 16 hours. Normeperidine is a potent CNS excitotoxin. Long-term administration of meperidine, especially in elderly patients or those with kidney dysfunction, results in normeperidine accumulation in the blood. Normeperidine can produce seizures, tremor, myoclonus, and confusion, effects that are not eliminated by the administration of naloxone. In fact, naloxone may counteract the sedating effects of meperidine, unmask the activity of normeperidine, and lead to hard-to-manage seizures. Even in patients with normal kidney function, repeated administration of doses as low as 250 mg/day may produce side effects from normeperidine.

Rare reports of fever, muscle rigidity, seizures, and death have been reported with single doses of meperidine in patients receiving monoamine oxidase inhibitors, which are occasionally used as antidepressants. This interaction has not been reported with other opioids. There is no therapeutic advantage of meperidine over other opioid analgesics, and there appear to be a number of reasons not to use this drug.

Low-potency opioids used in cancer pain

Low-potency opioids are appropriate analgesics for patients with mild to moderate cancer pain that has not responded to NSAIDs. The most commonly used low-potency opioids are discussed below.

Codeine

Codeine is the prototype low-potency opioid recommended by the World Health Organization for the management of mild to moderate cancer pain. It is related structurally to morphine and has a high oral to parenteral ratio of 2:1. Codeine's half-life is 2 to 4 hours and its duration of effect is 4 to 6 hours. Most of its analgesic activity is due to its conversion by the liver into morphine. Doses greater than 200 mg are usually associated with significant nausea and vomiting, producing a ceiling effect in its use. It is often combined with aspirin or acetaminophen, which in themselves have dose-limiting side effects on the stomach and liver, respectively. Although 200 mg of oral codeine sulfate is equal to 10 mg of I.V. morphine, conversion is not generally made between low- and high-potency opioids. If transition to a potent opioid is made, the patient who has developed tolerance to a low-potency opioid is assumed to be potent-opioid-naive.

Oxycodone

Oxycodone (Percocet and Percodan) is also a relative of morphine with good oral absorption. It is more potent than codeine; 30 mg of oral oxycodone is equivalent to 10 mg of I.V. morphine. Side effects do not usually produce the same analgesic ceiling as that of codeine, and oxycodone at higher doses is sometimes given along with the strong opioids for management of moderate to severe cancer pain.

Propoxyphene

Propoxyphene (Darvon) is a methadone relative that is one-half to two-thirds as strong as codeine. Its half-life is 3 to 6 hours, but its breakdown product, norpropoxyphene, has a half-life of 24 hours or more. Norpropoxyphene has side effects like normeperidine and may be toxic to the heart at very high levels. This drug should be avoided in elderly patients and in those with kidney dysfunction.

Neuroanesthetic and neurosurgical procedures

About 10% to 15% of patients with cancer pain cannot obtain adequate pain relief with use of the previously described analgesics. Some of these patients experience unmanageable side effects that prevent upward titration of an opioid, which is often required to maintain analgesia in progressive disease. In these patients, surgical or anesthetic methods of pain control should be considered. Such procedures should be reserved for patients who have failed medical therapy. Rarely do they produce enough relief to allow for complete independence from the use of analgesic medications.

Neuroanesthetic procedures include blocking a nerve by injecting it with local anesthetic or destroying a nerve by injecting it with phenol. Blocking an intercostal nerve may be very helpful in patients with chest wall pain, and a celiac plexus block can provide excellent relief of abdominal pain in patients with pancreatic cancer. Continuous epidural administration of opioids is sometimes indicated, and in these cases the epidural catheter necessary for delivery of the drug is placed by an anesthesiologist.

Neurosurgical procedures include cutting nerves (neurolysis) at the level of the nerve root or within the spinal cord in the dorsal root entry zone. This may be especially helpful in patients with brachial plexopathy or chronic neuropathic pain from shingles. On rare occasions, a cut in the pain pathways of the spinal cord (or cordotomy) may relieve pain that is confined to the lower extremities.

These neuroanesthetic and neurosurgical procedures are not useful in patients with pain unrelated to cancer because of their often temporary effect. Furthermore, these procedures are not without risk and are often expensive. They should be reserved for patients with specific pain problems and for those who have failed an adequate trial of medical treatment. A full discussion of these techniques is beyond the scope of this chapter. A general description of some common neuroanesthetic and neurosurgical techniques for pain alleviation appears in Chapter 7.

Other adjunctive therapies

Depression and anxiety are common in patients with cancer and may have a significant impact on quality of life, adding to the suffering associated with cancer pain. Psychological interventions aimed at treating depression and anxiety often have a beneficial effect on pain tolerance. Cognitive-behavioral therapy that employs such techniques as visualization and relaxation training may be very useful in the treatment of multiple symptoms related to cancer, including pain and the anticipatory anxiety associated with chemotherapy or radiation treatments.

The techniques employed by physical therapy may be a useful adjunct in the treatment of cancer pain. Transcutaneous electrical nerve stimulation (or TENS) is often helpful in treating a variety of pain syndromes, especially neuropathic pain. Heat, massage, and orthotic devices also may enhance analgesia. Lymphedema, swelling of an arm or leg due to lymphatic obstruction by radiation-induced fibrosis or tumor, may be relieved by pressure stockings, pneumatic devices, and wraps.

Conclusion

Pain is a common symptom associated with all stages of cancer. The underlying cause must be sought in each patient in order to best treat the pain and to manage malignant disease. Most patients can achieve good pain relief if their medical caregivers are skilled and knowledgeable in the diagnosis of cancer pain and the use of opioid and nonopioid analgesics.

Treatment of cancer pain must be tailored not only to the pain syndrome but also to the individual patient. A "cookbook" approach is inappropriate and usually ineffective. Regular, around-the-clock dosing of medication, escalation of drug to achieve analgesia or to the point of unmanageable side effects, and trials of alternate agents until an effective drug is found are the principles of effective cancer pain management. Unfortunately, many health care professionals are unfamiliar with the appropriate use of opioids and have unfounded fears of tolerance and addiction.

Each cancer patient with pain deserves a comprehensive evaluation, treatment of the underlying cause of pain if possible, and rational selection of an appropriate analgesic. Frequent reassessment, titration of drug, management of drug side effects and occasionally a switch to another analgesic may be required. A multidisciplinary approach with psychiatry, physiatry, neurosurgery, and anesthesia may be required in patients who fail to respond to pharmacologic therapy alone.

REFERENCES

American Pain Society. *Principles of Analgesic Use in the Treatment of Acute Pain and Chronic Cancer Pain. A Concise Guide to Medical Practice*, 3rd ed. Skokie, Illinois: American Pain Society, 1992.

Bonica, J.J., et al. *The Management of Pain*, 2nd ed. Baltimore: Williams & Wilkins, 1990.

Cherny, N.I., and Portenoy, R.K. "Cancer Pain Management: Current Strategy," *Cancer 72*(11 supp.):3393–3415, December 1993.

Foley, K.M. "The Treatment of Cancer Pain," *New England Journal of Medicine* 3132:84–95, July 11, 1985.

Gonzalez, G.R., et al. "The Impact of a Comprehensive Evaluation in the Management of Cancer Pain," *Pain* 47:141–44, 1991.

Lang, S.S., and Patt, R.B. *You Don't Have to Suffer: A Complete Guide to Relieving Cancer Pain for Patients and Their Families*. New York: Oxford University Press, 1995.

Portenoy, R.K. "Adjuvant Analgesics in Pain Management," in *Oxford Textbook of Palliative Medicine*. Edited by Doyle, D., et al. Oxford: Oxford University Press, 1993.

Ventafridda, V., et al. "A Validation Study of the WHO Method for Cancer Pain Relief," *Cancer* 59(4):850–56, February 15, 1987.

CHAPTER 10

Management of acute pain

Asteghik Hacobian, MD
Carol A. Warfield, MD

Acute pain can be defined as pain of recent onset. Among the causes of acute pain are trauma, burns, inflammation, infection, cancer, exacerbation of a chronic medical disorder, and surgery. Because acute pain may be a useful sign of an underlying problem, careful initial evaluation of any patient in acute pain is crucial. After the cause has been diagnosed, proper treatment of the pain as well as of the underlying cause is mandatory. Medical literature contains ample reports indicating past and present inadequacies in the treatment of patients in acute pain, but proper treatment is essential for the prevention of further complications of the underlying problem.

This chapter addresses postoperative pain, acute pain caused by trauma or burns, and common syndromes, such as acute low back pain, acute chest pain, and acute abdominal pain. The end of the chapter covers acute episodic pain that is associated with a disease or disorder.

Postoperative pain

Any type of injury to tissues causes pain. Acute pain usually disappears after the body heals from the injury, but initially it may be accompanied by the classic signs of autonomic nervous system hyperactivity, such as tachycardia, hypertension, sweating, abnormal dilation of pupils, and so forth. Postoperative pain is related to substances released from tissues as a result of trauma. Surgery, no matter how skillfully performed, causes local tissue damage and thus release of the biochemical mediators of inflammation, such as bradykinin, substance P, and prostaglandins. In the absence of treatment, sensory input from injured tissues is transferred by the pain-carrying A-δ and C fibers to spinal cord neurons in the dorsal horn of the spinal gray matter and then to the brain. The painful stimuli sensitize the pain receptors, an effect that persists after surgery and causes postoperative pain. Recent studies have shown that after a brief painful stimulus, long-standing changes occur in the cells associated with spinal pain pathways (Dubner and Basbum 1994). These findings support the clinical observation that pain, once established, is hard to control. Preemptive analgesia is employed to prevent unmanageable pain. (See "Preemptive analgesia for postoperative pain" later in this chapter.)

Few studies have been made of the incidence, duration, and intensity of pain experienced by postoperative patients. The most important factors that affect the intensity of postoperative pain are the type of surgery performed, the psychological makeup of the patient, the patient's preparation for anesthesia and surgery, the amount of intraopertive trauma, the skill and expertise of the surgeon, the presence of serious complications related to surgery, and, most important, the quality of postoperative care (Bonica 1990).

Postoperative pain is more severe after surgery on the abdomen, thorax, kidneys, spine, major joints, especially the knee, and large bones. After these surgeries, movements that place tension on the incision, such as deep breathing, coughing, or extensive body movements, increase the amount of postoperative pain. The type of incision also makes a difference. For example, for a cholecystectomy, a subcostal incision results in less pain than a midline incision. A transverse abdominal incision causes less nerve damage than a midline abdominal incision. After joint surgery, reflex spasms of the muscles also increase the amount of pain. Superficial operations on the neck, hand, limbs, chest, and abdomen cause less severe pain in most patients. Exceptions include burn patients who have had split thickness skin grafting and patients who have had radical mastectomies. These patients might be dealing with psychological issues that complicate the experience of pain.

The psychological makeup of the patient has a significant influence. Anxiety, fear, uncertainty, and feelings of helplessness about the operation make the pain experience worse (Chapman 1978). Surgical and anesthetic management also make a big difference. Preoperative preparation of the patient by the anesthesiologist and the surgeon will help to alleviate the patient's fear and anxiety. The intraoperative skill of the surgeon, extent of the surgery, degree of surgical trauma, and anesthetic technique are all factors influencing the degree of postoperative pain (Bonica 1990).

Inadequate treatment of postoperative pain

Postoperative pain has been treated inadequately in the past. Bonica points to a 1973 study by Marks and Sacher showing that in 75% of the patients with acute and chronic pain, the pain was not relieved by opioid treatment. When histories of these patients were carefully examined, the common finding was that only about 50% to 60% of the effective dosage of opioids was prescribed by the house physicians, and that nurses then administered only about 40% to 50% of that dose. In addition, most of the analgesics were given on an as-needed basis (Marks and Sacher 1973).

Clinical surveys continue to document situations in which routine orders for postoperative I.M. injections ordered as needed (PRN) leave more than half the patients with an increased amount of pain. Bonica talks about his own experience with pain: "I have had similar experiences following three of eleven hip operations and four ear plastic procedures, which produced severe, sometimes excruciating pain that was inadequately treated because an insufficient amount of opioids were given. This was in contrast to my experience with the other eight hip operations, a cholecystectomy, and several other surgical procedures, managed with regional analgesia that was continued postoperatively, provided effective relief, and permitted early ambulation." (Bonica 1990).

The major reason for inadequate pain management was thought to be insufficient education of health care providers about pain in general. This, in combination with the realization that adequate and timely postoperative pain management leads to better outcome and less morbidity, prompted the development of formal pain programs in major medical centers in the United States. The first program was established by Brian Ready and colleagues at the University of Washington Department of Anesthesia. Pain-management services have now become an essential part of almost every acute care facility in the United States. They provide patients with effective relief on a 24-hour basis. Teaching hospital fellowships now provide physicians with advanced training in control and treatment of both acute and chronic pain. The acute pain-management team usually consists of an anesthesiologist in a teaching hospital, a resident or pain fellow, and a clinical nurse specialist. The team sees all patients on daily rounds, evaluates their levels of pain, determines patients' satisfaction with treatment, and makes required adjustments.

In the past, postoperative pain was viewed as an inevitable event that patients should stoically endure. It is now clear that postoperative pain should be treated effectively and that patients should not suffer because of inadequate pain treatment. The physiologic risks associated with inadequate treatment of postoperative pain are greatest in frail patients, patients with other illnesses, those undergoing major surgical procedures, and the very young and very old.

Pain assessment

Pain is subjective and quite difficult to quantitate. In order to assess severity of pain, a number of standard scales and scoring systems have been developed. The most commonly used is the visual analog scale, a 10-cm line that offers a visual representation of the range of pain intensity. One end of the line represents no pain and the other end, the worst pain the patient can imagine. Patients are asked to mark the line at the point representing the level of pain they are experiencing. On the visual or verbal numerical scale, patients report the level of pain from zero to ten, zero indicating no pain and ten indicating the worst pain. The verbal rating scale is the simplest. Here, patients rate their pain intensity as "no pain," "mild," "moderate," or "severe," but this scale may have limitations because it offers a restricted choice of words (Deschamps et al. 1988).

Drawings are another way of describing pain. Here patients are asked to shade in the areas of a human figure that correspond to pain areas. Children older than age 8 can complete this successfully. The Faces Scale is especially good for use with preverbal children (see *Faces scale for pain assessment in young children*, page 356).

Options for controlling postoperative pain

Current technology and understanding of pain management offer a number of strategies for the management of postoperative pain, including the following:

- preemptive analgesia
- systemic administration of nonopioid and opioid analgesics
- patient-controlled analgesia
- epidural opioids or local anesthetic injected either intermittently or via continuous infusions
- neuronal blockade with local anesthetics injected via a catheter
- transcutaneous electrical nerve stimulation
- behavioral therapy.

Preemptive analgesia for postoperative pain

Animal studies have recently shown that injury to nociceptive nerve fibers causes changes in the central nervous system that persist long after the painful stimulus has been removed. These CNS changes may be prevented by administering an analgesic or a regional blockade prior to the injury. These findings are the basis for preemptive analgesia. Numerous studies document the efficacy of preincisional analgesia in reducing postoperative pain (Woolf and Chong 1993; Ejelersen et al. 1992). For example, one study shows that preincisional infiltration with a local anesthetic decreased postoperative analgesic requirements after herniorraphy (Tverskoy et al. 1990). Another study, which focused on administering epidural fentanyl prior to thoracotomy incision, shows much lower postoperative pain scores than when the epidural fentanyl was given after the incision (Katz et al. 1992).

Systemic medications for postoperative pain

Management of postoperative pain makes use of opioid and nonopioid analgesics administered orally or via a number of different parenteral routes.

Nonopioid analgesics for postoperative pain

Nonopioid analgesics include a variety of medications, such as aspirin and salicylate salts, acetaminophen (Tylenol), and other NSAIDs. After minor surgical procedures, NSAIDs alone can relieve pain. When insufficient to control pain, they can be used with opioids to decrease opioid requirements significantly. NSAIDs work, it is assumed, by decreasing the levels of inflammatory mediators at the site of injury. Recently, it has been shown that NSAIDs act centrally as well as peripherally to decrease inflammation. Their mechanism of action is through the inhibition of the enzyme cyclooxygenase, which is necessary for production of prostaglandins, one of the mediators of inflammation.

NSAIDs differ from opioid analgesics in several ways. They do not produce tolerance or physical or psychological dependence. Despite the fact that they act centrally, they do not cause sedation or ventilatory depression, both of which are common with opioids. In addition, they do not interfere with the bowel or bladder function as opioids do.

Aspirin, the oldest nonopioid analgesic available, can irritate the GI mucosa and interfere with platelet function. Bleeding is one of the most common side effects. Aspirin hypersensitivity can manifest itself in two ways: as a respiratory manifestation, such as asthma or rhinitis, or in a more generalized reaction that may include pruritis, wheals, angioneurotic edema (edematous skin changes such as hives), hypotension, and shock. Patients who are sensitive to aspirin may also have cross-sensitivity to other NSAIDs. Some salicylate salts, such as choline magnesium trisalicylate, do not affect platelets and have few other side effects.

Acetaminophen is a nonsalicylate with the same analgesic potency as aspirin but very little anti-inflammatory effect. Its mechanism of action is not clearly understood. It does not affect platelet function or disturb gastric mucosa. It should be avoided in patients with history of alcohol abuse or liver disease, since it can cause hepatotoxicity in this population, even when given in usual doses.

NSAIDs are especially useful for bone pain. Some NSAIDs have the same analgesic potency as aspirin, and others are more potent (see *Nonopioid analgesics: Dosage and efficacy as compared with aspirin*, pages 320 and 321). If a patient does not respond to a particular NSAID at a maximum dose, then trial of another NSAID is a good therapeutic option.

The side effects of NSAIDs include inhibition of normal blood clotting and irritation of the gastric mucosa. All NSAIDs except acetaminophen and salicylate salts inhibit platelet function by reversibly inhibiting cyclooxygenase, the enzyme that initiates the multistep conversion of arachidonic acid to various prostaglandins. Aspirin inhibits the enzyme irreversibly; the inhibition lasts for the life of the platelet, about 7 to 10 days. Platelet-inhibiting effects of other NSAIDs automatically reverse themselves once the drug is discontinued. Since NSAIDs also produce gastric mucosal irritation, patients with a history of ulcer disease are more vulnerable to gastric side effects. Dyspepsia or minor GI complaints can be an early sign of those side effects and should be noted because serious GI bleeding can occur without any warning signs or symptoms. Some propionic acid derivatives, such as ibuprofen, naproxen, and ketoprofen, have fewer GI side effects than other NSAIDs. Misoprostol (Cytotec), a prostaglandin analogue, that inhibits gastric acid secretion, may be used with NSAIDs to afford some protection against development of ulcer disease.

NSAIDs can also cause severe renal side effects. Patients especially at risk for development of renal problems are those with a history of congestive heart failure, kidney disease, liver disease, intravascular volume depletion, those taking diuretics, and elderly patients.

Most NSAIDs are available only in oral form. The only one approved by the FDA for I.M. use is ketorolac (Acular).

Opioids for postoperative pain

Opioids are the mainstay of treatment for acute postoperative pain, especially after extensive surgical procedures that normally cause moderate to severe pain. Opioids produce analgesia both centrally and peripherally by binding to specific opioid receptors. Of the different types of opioid receptors, the mu receptor is the most important for clinical analgesia. Delta and kappa receptors are also involved in analgesia that is achieved at the spinal cord.

Opioids are classified as full agonists, partial agonists, and mixed agonist-antagonists. Full agonists produce maximal analgesia when

(Text continues on page 322.)

Nonopioid analgesics: Dosage and efficacy as compared with aspirin

Drug	Average analgesic dose (mg)	Dose interval (hr)	Maximum daily dose (mg)
Acetaminophen	500 to 1,000 P.O.	4 to 6	4,000
Salicylates			
Aspirin	500 to 1,000 P.O.	4 to 6	4,000
Diflunisal	1,000 P.O. initially, 500 P.O. subsequently	8 to 12	1,500
Choline magnesium trisalicylate	1,000 to 1,500 P.O.	12	2,000 to 3,000
Propionic acids			
Ibuprofen	200 to 400 P.O.	4 to 6	2,400
Naproxen	500 P.O. initially, 250 P.O. subsequently	6 to 8	1,250
Naproxen sodium	550 P.O. initially, 275 P.O. subsequently	6 to 8	1,375
Fenoprofen	200 P.O.	4 to 6	800
Ketoprofen	25 to 50 P.O.	6 to 8	300
Indoleacetic Acid			
Indomethacin	25 P.O.	8 to 12	100
Pyrroleacetic acid			
Ketorolac	30 to 60 I.M. initially, 15 to 30 I.M. subsequently	6	150 first day, 120 thereafter
Anthranilic acid			
Mefenamic acid	500 P.O. initially, 250 P.O. subsequently	6	1,500

** Compared with 650 mg aspirin

From *Principles of Analgesic Use in the Treatment of Acute Pain and Cancer Pain*, 3rd ed. American Pain Society, 1992. Adapted with permission.

Analgesic efficacy **	Plasma half-life (hr)	Comments
Comparable to 650 mg aspirin	2 to 3	Available as suppository
	0.25	Due to risk of Reye's syndrome, do not use in children under 12 with possible viral infection; rectal suppository available
500 mg superior to 650 mg aspirin, with slower onset and longer duration	8 to 12	Initial dose of 1,000 mg significantly shortens time of onset
Longer duration of action than 650 mg aspirin	9 to 17	
Superior at 200 mg to 650 mg aspirin	2 to 2.5	
	12 to 15	
275 mg comparable to 650 mg aspirin, with slower onset and longer duration; 550 mg superior to 650 mg aspirin		
Comparable to 650 mg aspirin	2 to 3	
Superior at 25 mg to 650 mg aspirin	1.5	
Comparable to 650 mg aspirin	2	Not routinely used due to high incidence of side effects; rectal and I.V. forms available
In the range of 6 to 12 mg morphine	6	
Comparable to 650 mg aspirin		In the United States, use restricted to intervals of 1 week

they bind to a specific type of receptor. Partial agonists produce a submaximal analgesic response regardless of dosage level. Mixed agonist-antagonists activate one type of receptor and also inhibit another type of receptor. The most commonly used agonist-antagonist drugs are pentazocine (Talwin), butorphanol (Stadol), nalbuphine, and buprenorphine. They have a characteristic ceiling effect (analgesic properties), after which increased doses do not produce increased analgesia. The antagonist properties of these drugs have been used to advantage to provide postoperative analgesia with fewer side effects, such as respiratory depression. A mixed agonist-antagonist should not be given to patients who are receiving mu opioid agonists because the agonist-antagonist may cause a withdrawal response and increase the pain.

In order to use opioids properly, consciously choose the particular drug, the route of administration, the initial bolus dose, and the frequency of administration. The dosage should be individualized according to the needs of patients. Although the oral route is the most convenient, it is not useful for patients who are not allowed oral intake, and, because peak drug concentration occurs about 30 minutes to 2 hours after ingestion, the oral route is inappropriate when rapid pain control is necessary. I.M. injection can be used as a temporary measure when other routes of administration are not possible, such as when there is no I.V. access, but the variable absorption rate from the muscle and the pain and muscle damage of repeated injections make this a poor choice. I.V. bolus administration provides the most rapid onset of relief, with the peak effects of morphine occurring after 15 to 30 minutes. I.V. infusion provides a steadier plasma level of the drug as well as the option of rapidly titrating the dosage to achieve quick pain control during episodes of pain exacerbation.

To increase analgesia using the I.V. route, an initial bolus dose can be given, followed by an increase in the I.V. infusion rate. Without the initial bolus dose, an increase in analgesia may take 12 hours or more. It is important to remember that the optimal analgesic dose varies among patients. The best guide to adequate dosage is patients' comfort.

Patients with constant acute postoperative pain must receive analgesics around the clock, not PRN. A PRN order results in prolonged delays while a nurse answers the call, checks the order book, prepares the drug, and administers it. The unavoidable delay increases the amount of medication required for pain control. In addition to around-the-clock administration, a separate PRN order should be available for breakthrough pain.

Awareness of the side effects of opioids is important in order to treat them appropriately. Sedation, nausea, vomiting, pruritis, constipation, and respiratory depression are the most common side effects of opioids. For patients who are too sedated, the best strategy is to decrease the dose and increase the frequency. Nausea and vomiting can be treated with appropriate antiemetics, such as prochlorperazine, metoclopramide, and droperidol. Pruritis can be treated with antihistamines and constipation with laxatives. Respiratory depression is a true risk of opioid therapy, and patients should always be monitored for respiratory rate, depth and pattern of respiration, and state of arousal. Monitors such as pulse oxymetry are extremely useful in the immediate postoperative period and in patients especially at risk for respiratory depression, such as premature infants, neonates, or patients with baseline ventilatory compromise. Respiratory depression or coma from opioid overdose should be treated with an opioid antagonist such as naloxone. In adults, this would require I.V. boluses of 0.1 mg until the desired effect is reached.

Caregivers should note that *opioid tolerance and addiction among patients first given opioids for controlling postoperative pain is very rare.* Recent research has shown that addiction is *not* a concern *when opioids are used for control of acute pain* (Porter and Jick 1980; Perry and Heidrich 1982). Addiction is overwhelming involvement with obtaining and using a drug for its psychic effects, not for approved medical reasons. Fear of addiction is very common among physicians, nurses, and patients and often results in undertreatment of patients' pain. Caregivers should reassure patients and health care workers alike that the risk of addiction is almost nonexistent in the acute postoperative pain treatment setting. A difference exists between addiction and tolerance. Tolerance is the need for a larger dosage of an opioid to achieve the same analgesic effect caused by physiologic changes in the body. Physical dependence, which is different from addiction, is the occurrence of withdrawal symptoms at the sudden cessation of opioid administration. It is an involuntary reaction and can be avoided by tapering the dosage of the opioid over time.

Morphine, the standard opioid to which other opioids are compared, is a naturally occurring compound and an agonist at mu, kappa, and delta receptors. An unsettled issue is whether or not morphine causes smooth muscle spasm of the biliary tree and thus is contraindicated for analgesia in procedures involving the biliary system. Meperidine, another mu agonist, is commonly used for postoperative pain. Meperidine is metabolized to normeperidine, which is toxic and is excreted via the kidneys. In healthy patients, normeperidine has a half-life of 15 to 20 hours although it is prolonged in elderly patients and in those with compromised renal function. The toxic effects of normeperidine include cerebral irritation and range from dysphoria to convulsions. The effects can be observed in young healthy patients if prolonged high doses of meperidine are given postoperatively. The use of meperidine is contraindicated in elderly patients and in those with renal failure. Its use is limited to a short postoperative course for young healthy individuals, especially those who cannot tolerate other opioids, such as morphine or hydromorphone.

PCA for postoperative pain

Patient controlled analgesia (PCA) is safe and has received strong support from patients. It has been widely used in recent years. PCA permits patients to control their own medication by means of repeated self-administration of doses of opioids within prescribed limits. The PCA device consists of a microprocessor-controlled pump that can be programmed for dose, time between doses, maximum allowable dosage per unit time, and baseline infusion rate. The device is attached to the patient's I.V. line, and whenever he wishes, he can self-administer opioids by pressing a button. Although the basal rate of infusion is set by caregivers, the demand dose is under the control of the patient who can press the demand button whenever he feels or anticipates pain. Because PCA allows an opioid to be given at short time intervals, pain control is better than it is when large doses are given every 3 to 4 hours. Patients have varying requirements for opioids even after the same type of surgery, and PCA corrects for individual differences in tolerance and pharmacodynamics as well as for inaccurate pain assessment by caregivers.

Usually the side effects of opioids occur at higher concentrations than those used to treat pain. Thus, patients are able to find an analgesic range that can keep them comfortable without causing side effects. Postoperative pain increases with any kind of movement, deep breathing, or coughing so patients can use the PCA device to infuse an adequate opioid dose before engaging in any type of movement. Patients using PCA have superior analgesia and receive less medication than patients who are being treated with injections on an as-needed basis. Patients usually titrate the analgesic so that they have fewer side effects, and they usually accept a mild degree of pain because they are aware that they can press the button and receive more pain medication at any time. The interval between the perception of need for increased pain relief and the actual pain relief is decreased when the patient self-administers the opioid. An overall decrease in pulmonary complications has been reported in patients using self-controlled morphine following intra-abdominal and intrathoracic procedures (Bonica 1990).

Not all patients are suitable candidates for PCA therapy. It is inappropriate for elderly patients who get confused easily, patients who are forgetful, patients who cannot follow instructions, and for very young patients . People other than the patients themselves should not be allowed to press the dosage-delivery button. A major safety feature of PCA is that once sedated, patients cannot press the button for opioid delivery; this minimizes the risk of overdose. Such protection is voided if nurses or family members press the delivery button for already drowsy patients (see *Solutions to problems with PCA,* page 326).

Epidural analgesia for postoperative pain

Epidural analgesia has revolutionized the postoperative care of surgical patients, especially those undergoing major thoracic or intra-abdominal procedures and those with poor ventilatory reserve. The epidural space is filled with connective and adipose tissue and is located between the dura mater (the outermost covering of the spinal cord) and the connective tissues covering the vertebrae and ligamenta flava. Local anesthetics and opioids injected into the epidural space produce an epidural block. By means of an indwelling catheter placed preoperatively by an anesthesiologist, analgesics can be delivered into the epidural space. This technique can create profound analgesia by delivering drugs directly to the spinal nerves involved in transmitting pain signals.

Postoperative epidural analgesia has dramatically changed the care of intrathoracic and intraabdominal surgical patients. It is not uncommon to walk into these patients' rooms on the first postoperative day and find them comfortable because they have minimal pain upon movement. This high level of postoperative analgesia has strong implications for postoperative recovery and pulmonary function. The lack of pain enables these patients to take deep breaths, cooperate with respiratory care staff during physical therapy, and improve their pulmonary function. Thus postoperative epidural analgesia has greatly decreased the morbidity associated with these surgeries.

Opioids and local anesthetics, when used simultaneously in the epidural space, have a synergistic effect. Continuous administration of a dilute solution of a local anesthetic combined with a low dose of opioid provides more efficient analgesia with fewer side effects, such as motor blockade or respiratory depression, than equianalgesic doses of either agent alone.

Technical problems with epidural analgesia

The principal problem associated with epidurals is loss of analgesia due to technical difficulties such as catheter migration, kinking, or slippage. With migration, the tip of the catheter comes out of the epidural space. There are several ways to prevent this:

- Ensure that the catheter is inserted at least 3 cm into the epidural space.
- Secure the catheter at the site of insertion with transparent adhesive film such as Tegaderm and adhesive tape.
- At the time of insertion, tunnel the catheter (insert it into the skin several inches away from the actual epidural entry site).

PAIN MANAGEMENT PRACTICE

Solutions to problems with PCA

Although patient-controlled analgesia (PCA) has the advantage of allowing the patient to self-manage the analgesics prescribed for pain, it is not a perfect pain-management solution for all patients. For example, it is not suitable for patients with confused mental states or for very young children. To solve common problems that arise with PCA, the following actions are suggested:

Problem	Suggested actions
Patient complains of increased pain	• Administer boluses until patient is comfortable. • Increase the demand dose. • Increase basal rate of infusion, if necessary.
Patient too drowsy, sedated, or confused	• Stop any basal rate. • Decrease or stop the demand dose. • Look for other causes of drowsiness, such as decreased oxygenation or fluid or electrolyte imbalance. • Notify the physician in charge.
PCA pump nonfunctional or unavailable	• Change to another pump. • Administer I.M., I.V., or P.O. opioids.

The acute pain team should closely follow patients with postoperative epidural analgesia. Catheter sites should be checked at least once a day for kinking, slippage, and tenderness with erythema. At the end of treatment, the catheter should be removed by an anesthesiologist or a pain specialist to ensure that the tip is intact. The role of the nursing staff is important in the daily care of patients with epidural catheters. Nurses should be adequately trained and should know which medications are appropriate for epidural administration, what complications are associated with epidural analgesia, and what needs to be done in case of a problem.

The most widely used epidural solution at Harvard University teaching hospitals is a mixture of 0.1% bupivacaine and fentanyl (3, 4 or 10 mcg/ml). Fentanyl is the opioid of choice because of its shorter duration of action and its lipophilia (solubility in lipids). The lipid solubility is important because it tends to bind the drug locally to the spinal cord receptors and prevent drug migration cephalad to the brain. A high incidence of delayed respiratory depression has been observed with epidural morphine. Because of its hydrophilic nature, morphine tends to spread cephalad and reach the respiratory centers in the brain with resulting respiratory depression. In infants less than 1 year old, fentanyl is omitted because infants have a higher sensitivity to the respiratory depressant effects of fentanyl. In children ages 1 to 7, 3 mcg of fentanyl is used. The opioids are entirely eliminated from the epidural solution used in elderly frail patients (Ballantyne and Borsook 1996).

The most common side effects of epidural analgesia using a combination of opioid and local anesthetic are pruritis and urine retention. Pruritis can be treated with antihistamines; urine retention may require an indwelling urinary catheter. Nausea is a rare side effect associated with epidural fentanyl, but if present, it usually responds to antiemetics. Sedation may be a problem in elderly patients, but it usually responds to the lowering of the infusion rate or the elimination of the opioid from the solution. Epidural analgesia can also affect gut motility and prolong postoperative ileus (loss of bowel motility). Some surgeons will not allow its use in their patients for this reason. Another side effect, seen usually in hypovolemic patients, is hypotension which can be treated by volume replacement or administration of ephedrine.

A very rare complication of epidural analgesia is the development of epidural abcess or hematoma. Cardinal signs and symptoms of an epidural abcess are severe back pain, fever, leukocytosis, and neurologic deficits. This is a medical emergency. Evacuation of an epidural hematoma or abscess can prevent the development of permanent neurologic deficits, so any patient with the above signs and symptoms should be referred to a neurosurgeon for immediate evaluation and intervention.

Neuronal blockade for postoperative pain

Nerve blocks (injection of a local anesthetic around nerves) performed before or during surgery can provide adequate analgesia during the early postoperative period. Infiltration of surgical wounds with local anesthetics also greatly reduces postoperative pain. These intraoperative techniques of neuronal blockade can decrease later analgesic requirements and can sometimes eliminate the need for postoperative pain medicine. This technique is particularly useful in children who do not tolerate opioid medications as well as adults.

Occasionally prolongation of a postoperative neuronal blockade is indicated. It can be accomplished by use of continuous infusions of local anesthetics via special catheters, for example, continuous infusion of anesthetics through interpleural catheters for thoracic and upper abdominal surgery or the continuous delivery of anesthetics to the brachial plexus for hand surgery in which postoperative physical therapy is indicated (Ballantyne and Borsook 1996).

TENS for postoperative pain

Transcutaneous electrical nerve stimulation (TENS) is helpful in reducing pain in certain patients. It consists of passing a low-voltage electrical stimulus through a series of electrodes placed at the site of pain. TENS is not an alternative to postoperative drug analgesia, but its use may decrease the opioid requirement for some patients. Its developement grew out of the gate-control theory of pain, which states that stimulation of large-diameter afferent nerve fibers inhibits the transmission of pain by closing the spinal gating mechanism for nociception.

Behavioral therapy for postoperative pain

The goal of behavior therapy is to provide patients with strategies for dealing with postoperative pain. Careful preoperative psychological preparation of patients greatly lessens their subsequent pain. The learning of simple relaxation techniques can help some patients manage postoperative pain. Other strategies, such as music-assisted relaxation, breathing techniques, and thinking about peaceful images have been helpful in some instances.

Trauma pain

Trauma, especially trauma resulting from high-speed motor vehicle accidents, is one of the most common medical emergencies. Patients involved in trauma often have multiple fractures and need pain control. The issue of pain control becomes more complex when there is evidence of head trauma or respiratory complications. Intracerebral hemorrhage, epidural hematoma, meningitis, and bleeding into the subarachnoid space produce severe headache. Balancing an appropriate level of patient conciousness with pain relief may be a challenge.

Orthopedic trauma

Trauma to bones and soft tissues causes significant pain, but that pain can be useful because it prevents movement of the injured site and thus decreases the likelihood of further damage. Sometimes immediately after trauma, patients feel little or no pain, and their injuries become apparent only some time later.

Two kinds of pain follow trauma. The first is immediate pain, which is sharp and nociceptive. That is followed by deep, persistent pain which is due to a local inflammatory reaction in a joint, the associated capsule, a muscle, or the associated fascial compartment. The increased pressure associated with local edema can cause ischemia of the nerves and resulting pain. The pain can also be due to release of inflammatory mediators, such as bradykinin or prostaglandins. This is probably why the anti-inflammatory medications are effective in relieving orthopedic trauma pain. In taking a history and performing the physical examination, the origin of the pain—whether it is muscle, soft tissue, tendon, or bone must be identified.

Management of orthopedic trauma pain

One of the initial steps in management of musculoskeletal trauma is splinting, which immobilizes the injured area and provides the opportunity to rest it so that swelling may decrease. This in itself can cause dramatic pain relief. In the case of a displaced fracture, the initial management is to reduce it. If the fracture is unstable, then external (cast or traction) or internal (plating) fixation may be used. Despite these stabilizing procedures, additional pain medications are usually needed. Once a diagnosis is made, the pain should be brought under control, particularly because inadequate relief of acute pain may increase the likelihood of subsequent development of chronic pain.

For management of acute orthopedic pain, both NSAIDs and opioids are good choices. Given together they have increased efficacy. The systemic route is the preferred one initially because it allows faster onset of relief. Peripheral nerve blocks and regional analgesia also are useful, especially in lower-limb injuries. Local anesthetic blockade can be used in rib fractures where splinting may interfere with ventilation.

Some people argue against the use of epidural analgesia for situations in which there are any risks for the development of compartment syndrome (neuromuscular damage caused by trauma-related swelling of a group of muscles within a single fascia). The argument is that increased pain, which is one of the first signs of compartment syndrome, can be masked by regional analgesia, thus delaying diagnosis of this orthopedic emergency.

Certain fractures are more amenable to local nerve blocks. For example, fractures around the ankle can be managed by local blockade. In the arm, Colle's fracture (fracture of the lower end of the radius) is amenable to local blockade, whereas pain from injuries to fingers or toes can be controlled by ring blocks.

Burn pain

Burn pain is one of the most severe and prolonged types of pain. More than 2 million burn injuries occur every year in the United States. Of these, most are caused by thermal burns from flames, hot liquids, and so forth. Chemical and electrical burns are less common. Around 3%

of all burn injuries are so severe that they require hospitalization (Choiniere 1994).

The degree and severity of a burn is determined by the depth and extent of tissue damage. First-degree burns involve the superficial layer of the skin (the epidermis) and heal within 1 to 2 weeks without scarring. They usually generate a mild to moderate amount of pain. Second-degree burns involve the epidermis and some layers of dermis. This is the most painful type of burn. Here, the nerve endings are exposed and cause significant pain. Third-degree burns involve destruction of the entire epidermis and dermis. Because no nerve endings are exposed, this kind of burn is thought not to be very painful. However, since most third-degree burns are intermixed with or surrounded by second-degree burns, they, too, can be very painful. Because there are no layers of epidermis to provide cells for regeneration, a third-degree burn will not heal by itself. It requires skin grafting and involves wound contraction.

Burn management is divided into three phases. The first phase, or acute phase, is the period immediately after the traumatic event and is basically the resuscitative phase. During this period, efforts are directed toward fluid volume resuscitation, airway control, and infection prevention. Once the patient is medically more stable, the second phase, or subacute phase, begins. It involves wound debridement, skin grafting, physical therapy, occupational therapy, and so forth. During this phase, patients experience severe pain, and the input of a pain specialist may be needed. This phase is terminated by wound closure. The third phase, or chronic or rehabilitative phase, may last a long time because it involves functional rehabilitation and prevention of contractures.

Burn pain can have several etiologies. It can be related to local tissue injury, which is characterized by constant sharp pain. It can also arise as a consequence of multiple procedures, such as dressing changes and debridement. The tissue donor site for skin grafting can also be painful, and tissue regeneration and healing can be a painful process.

Characteristics of burn pain
Pain may not start immediately after injury. One study reports that about 30% of burn patients experienced an interval of no pain right after the injury (Choiniere et al. 1989). Delayed onset of pain after other types of acute injury is also reported by Melzack (1982). Wall has proposed that for a time period following an injury, pain should be inhibited to let the individual adapt through the behavioral and physiologic responses necessary for survival (1979).

Burn pain, unlike other acute pain, does not decrease in intensity over time; rather, burn pain intensity may stay the same or even increase. Among the many causes for increase in pain intensity are the return of normal nerve sensation as a result of the healing process, gradual chronic fatigue, sleep deprivation, anxiety over the outcome of healing, development of tolerance to opioids, and emergence of opioid-resistant neuropathic pain. Unfortunately, many burn patients are subject to inadequate pain management by health care professionals.

It is very important to emphasize that anxiety and apprehension play an important role in patients' responses to pain. Choiniere's study reports that anxiety and pain are interrelated in burn patients. The more anxious they are, the more pain they experience. Interestingly, increased levels of anxiety were not associated with increased pain levels during treatment procedures (1989).

Burn patients also have severe emotional and psychological problems. In contrast to many other pain states, the possibility of disfigurement or physical disability places a severe psychological burden on patients. Preexisting psychological problems are magnified after the injury and can involve psychiatric disorders, such as delirium, anxiety, depression, and the like, all of which can increase the amount of pain experienced by the patient.

Management of burn pain
Prompt cooling of the wound after a burn can decrease pain (Davies 1982). Covering the wound with a dressing may also relieve pain, but frequent dressing changes can add to pain. At some burn centers, the wound is exposed to warm, dry air, but this can cause more pain. Early debridement (removal of necrotic tissue) and skin grafting are also used to decrease the pain because they eliminate the need for later debridement of extensive amounts of tissue and the subsequent development of hypertrophied scar tissue.

Pharmacologic intervention is the primary treatment for burn pain. Opioids are the drugs of choice, but multiple factors, including fear of addiction and inadequate knowledge by health care providers about the use of opioids for this kind of pain, can make the treatment of burns inadequate. A nationwide study of 93 burn centers, which treated about 10,000 patients, reported not one case of opioid addiction (Perry and Heidrich 1982). In addition to undermedicating these patients, often no effort is made to adjust the opioid dose for development of tolerance. Most patients on opioids for serious burn pain will develop tolerance over time and will require higher doses to manage the pain. It is important to emphasize that long-term opioid treatment can cause the development of tolerance and physical dependence, which differ from psychological dependence (Jaffee 1985). As patients heal, physical dependence can easily be managed by gradual tapering of opioids to prevent appearance of withdrawal symptoms.

Many burn patients require high levels of opioids for adequate pain control. Burn patients are known to be hypermetabolic, especially in the initial stages, and thus have increased requirements for opioids. Whether this is due to altered pharmacokinetics or pharmacodynamics is not clear. *Burn patients with high opioid requirements should be given the appropriate amount of drug to control their pain.* The fear of respiratory depression frequently deters care providers from administering high doses of opioids, even though they are required to manage patients' pain. Personnel who work with burn patients should understand that if patients are experiencing severe pain, careful titration of an opioid to control the pain carries a minimal risk of respiratory depression.

Two kinds of pain are associated with burn injury: the constant pain at rest and the intermittent or incident pain associated with procedures. For mild to moderate pain, weaker opioids such as oxycodone or codeine can be used. Morphine is the prototype used for moderate to severe pain. Methadone is also used for prolonged analgesia in burn patients. Meperidine is used for moderate pain, but its use for chronic pain is not recommended because the accumulation of its metabolite, normeperidine, can cause central nervous system stimulation. Mixed agonist-antagonists are also helpful, but they should not be used for patients treated with pure agonists because they can precipitate withdrawal symptoms and the onset of previously suppressed pain.

The I.V. route is preferred for initial administration of opioids. The I.M. route is inappropriate because it produces unreliable drug absorption and is impractical for providing continuous analgesia. Later, when patients are more stable, the oral route can be used.

The management of acute burn pain immediately following the initial trauma differs from the management of burn pain during recovery. During the acute period, burn pain is best managed by intermittent I.V. medications with careful monitoring of patients' vital functions. Once patients are more stable, continuous I.V. infusion of opioids can provide excellent relief. For patients with the cognitive capacity to operate the device, PCA can provide constant relief by supplying a basal rate of infusion and then allowing a demand dose to cover pain that arises with movement or dressing changes. Epidural analgesia is often not recommended for burn patients because of the possibility of infection, especially when large areas of skin over the back are involved. For burns of the lower extremities, however, epidural administration can be an excellent analgesic option.

For pain associated with dressing changes or other procedures, shorter-acting opioids such as fentanyl are useful. I.V. ketamine, an anesthetic that also produces analgesia, has been used for years for this purpose with good effects, although a possible negative side-effect of this drug is the subsequent occurrence of unpleasant hallu-cinations or nightmares. Recently, the introduction of propofol, a lipid-soluble anesthetic, as a sedating agent during dressing changes has made a big difference. Propofol causes acute sedation but allows immediate postprocedure recovery without causing residual hangover effects. However, unlike ketamine, it does not have analgesic proper-ties and its use is more associated with episodes of apnea. Propofol is also associated with more psychomotor problems than is ketamine. For extensive painful dressing changes, general anesthesia may be an option.

Burn patients should receive treatment for the anxiety associated with this type of trauma. Anxiolytics such as the benzodiazepines can be helpful and, for some patients, behavioral approaches, such as biofeedback, relaxation training, and individual or group therapy, can also be helpful for increasing the ability to cope with pain.

Acute low back pain

Acute low back pain, a common problem, arises from many different causes. The diagnosis is usually made on the basis of the history and physical examination. Laboratory studies and radiographic imaging may help to verify the differential diagnosis.

Diagnosis and treatment of acute low back pain

A history of trauma raises the possibility of fracture in the spinal col-umn or injuries to intervertebral disks. Sudden stress in the extend-ed back may cause injury to facet joints or a pars fracture. Back pain radiating to a lower extremity is a sign of radiculopathy secondary to herniated disk. Accompanying systemic complaints, such as malaise, fever, weight loss, or change in bowel or bladder function, raise the possibility of a malignant neoplasm, infection, or spondyloarthropa-thy. Acute low back pain associated with bowel or bladder dysfunc-tion could be a sign of cauda equina syndrome (compression of the nerve roots of the lumbar spine) and such a patient should be referred to a neurosurgeon immediately.

Back pain associated with spinal fracture needs surgical inter-vention. Back pain with radiculopathy (pain or numbness in a der-matome, often indicative of pressure or disease of the associated spinal nerve root) could be a sign of herniated disk that will respond to conservative management, such as bed rest, trial NSAIDs, physi-cal therapy, or epidural steroid injections. However, the presence of any progressive neurologic loss and intractable pain calls for a surgi-cal referral.

Back pain without radiculopathy or neurologic signs could be the result of several possible etiologies, including myofacial origin (pain associated with muscle trigger points), piriformis syndrome (pain arising from a trigger point in the piriformis muscle, often mimicking sciatic pain), an annular tear (tear in the cartilaginous covering of an intervertebral disk), facet syndrome (disease of the facet joints of the spinal column), sacroiliac joint disease, and nonspecific low-back strain. In these conditions, depending on the underlying etiology, bed rest, NSAIDs, analgesics, trigger point injections, epidural steroids, or stretching exercise programs may be helpful. In the case of facet syndrome, flexion exercises, facet injections of steroids or local anesthetics, and mobilization are options for treatment. In the case of sacroiliac joint problems, NSAIDs, sacroiliac mobilization via physical therapy, or injection of a local anesthetic with steroids into the joint can be helpful.

Systemic complaints associated with low back pain need complete workups to rule out a malignant neoplasm or infection. Various laboratory studies, such as erythrocyte sedimentation rate, SMA 20 (liver and kidney function), acid phosphatase levels; radiographic studies; and bone scans help in diagnosis. Acute low-back pain could also be due to spondylosis (degenerative change in the spine) or spondylolisthesis (forward displacement of one vertebra over another). A bone scan helps in the differential diagnosis of traumatic spondylosis-spondylolisthesis. A positive bone scan would warrant orthopedic referral. If the bone scan is negative, but the slippage (vertebral displacement) is more than 50%, orthopedic referral should be considered. A negative bone scan with slippage of less than 50% indicates conservative treatment, including medications, facet joint blocks, medial branch blocks (blocks of the nerves innervating the facet joint), and bracing.

Acute chest pain

Acute chest pain can have various causes. Because the nerves supplying vital structures in the thorax (heart, esophagus, aorta, lungs, pleura, and chest wall) share the same pathways, differentiating the origin of the pain may be very difficult.

As with many painful conditions, a careful, detailed history and a physical examination are the keys to differential diagnosis. The severity, site, radiation, character, and quality of pain should be identified as well as the factors that worsen the pain or that relieve it. For example, pain aggravated by deep breathing suggests pericardial, pleural, or chest wall pathology. Associated symptoms of dyspnea and palpitations are more suggestive of cardiac problems. Tests such as ECG chest X-ray, and routine blood work also will help in differential diagnosis.

Management of acute chest pain

Acute chest pain should be treated only after the cause has been identified. The pain should be clearly identified as visceral, peripheral somatic, joint, or axial skeleton in origin. The chest pain of myocardial infarction is one of the most life-threatening and it requires emergency transfer to a hospital for medical intervention. Visceral thoracic pain is usually dull and poorly localized and often referred. The most common visceral sites associated with chest pain are the esophagus, myocardium, trachea, bronchi, pleura, pericardium, pulmonary arteries, and aorta. Treatment includes systemic opioids. Sympathetic blockade also has proven helpful.

Acute chest wall pain could be due to muscle sprain, rib fracture, or other inflammatory conditions such as costochondritis (inflammation of rib cartilage). The possibility of pneumothorax or pulmonary embolism always exists. Treatment for myofascial pain arising in the chest wall includes medications such as NSAIDs. In the case of rib fractures, thoracic epidural blockade with local anesthetics provides excellent analgesia and also improvement in breathing and prevention of splinting (muscle rigidity that develops as a guarding response to pain) during the healing process. Pain associated with vesicles in a thoracic dermatomal distribution is a typical sign of acute herpes zoster. This kind of pain must be treated aggressively to prevent development of postherpetic neuralgia. Treatment options include oral antiviral agents (acyclovir), intralesional injection with local anesthetics and steroids, and thoracic epidural injections with local anesthetics.

Emotional factors such as acute anxiety may also be manifested as acute chest pain. In these cases, systemic, organic disease should be ruled out first. Reassurance, psychological interventions, and anxiolytics may help.

Acute abdominal pain

Acute abdominal pain is frequently observed in emergency departments. It can arise from the abdominal viscera or the peritoneum or can be referred pain from, for example, a ureteral stone. Acute abdominal pain is characterized by reflex guarding and tenderness accompanied by nausea and vomiting. Sympathetic hyperactivity signs such as sweating and vagal responses such as bradycardia may also be seen.

Visceral pain is usually dull and poorly localized. It is usually due to spasm of the smooth muscle of the hollow organs. Expansion with distension of the organ and its capsule, stretch of the mesentery or vessels, and inflammation or ischemia of the bowel may all cause visceral pain. The pain due to acute pancreatitis is extremely severe. Acute pancreatitis is a common problem in the United Sates and is usually due to alcohol abuse or biliary problems (disease of the bile duct or gallbladder). Viral, idiopathic, or drug-induced pancreatitis have also been seen. Somatic pain and pain arising from the parietal peritoneum is usually sharp and can be localized or referred. Referred pain from intrathoracic organs is also common.

Diagnosis and management of acute abdominal pain

The history should focus on the location, severity, and character of the pain. Any history of coexisting diseases, such as diabetes, uremia, porphyria, sickle cell anemia, pulmonary embolism, pneumothorax, acute myocardial infarction, spinal cord compression, or psychological problems should be elicited. Acute abdominal pain is characteristically described as pain lasting longer than six hours. Pain of sudden onset is usually a sign of rupture, perforation, or embolism. Rapid onset of pain is a sign of acute inflammation, obstruction, toxic disease such as lead poisoning, or metabolic disease such as diabetes. Gradual onset of pain could be a sign of chronic inflammation, ectopic (extrauterine) pregnancy, tumor, or infarction (tissue necrosis due to disruption of circulation). Cutaneous or somatic pain is usually described as sharp, while burning pain is a sign of nerve involvement (neuralgia). In women, a careful menstrual history is essential. Tachycardia with decreased blood pressure is a sign of sepsis or hypovolemia. Guarding, rebound pain, organ enlargement, ascites (fluid accumulation in the abdominal cavity), or masses should be noted. Auscultation of the abdomen for presence of hyperactive bowel sounds or silence should be done. Rectal or pelvic examination is also very important. Laboratory tests for urinary ketones or serum electrolytes will help assess the degree of dehydration. Increased white blood cell count and fever are suggestive of infection. A decreased hematocrit level suggests chronic blood loss.

All cases of acute abdominal pain need surgical evaluation. If the pain is not useful for evaluation, then analgesics should be started. Opioids may be helpful because their constipating effects relieve pain secondary to hyperperistalsis. Hydration should also be initiated. If the patient undergoes surgery, regional analgesia with epidural local anesthetics and/or opioids can be a good choice for postoperative pain relief. Epidural opioids are especially helpful for visceral pain. PCA is also an option.

In acute pancreatitis, spasms of the pancreatic duct or sphincters can be the cause of the pain. Initial management of these patients includes IV hydration, nasogastric tube, bowel rest, opioid analgesics, and correction of electrolyte disturbances. If pain continues, a celiac plexus block (injection of a local anesthetic combined with a corticos-terioid into the celiac plexus) can decrease the pain and alter the course of the disease. The patient's overall condition should be carefully evaluated prior to a block because most of these patients are dehydrated. Inadequate hydration prior to a block can cause a decrease in blood pressure and consequent complications. Systemic opioid treatment or epidural analgesia are other options. Because substance abuse is often the cause of pancreatitis, psychological evaluation and management of substance abuse should be part of the treatment regimen.

Acute episodic pain associated with disease or disorder

Many chronic diseases and disorders are characterized by periods of symptom abatement that alternate with periods of acute pain and exacerbation of symptoms. Patients with these diseases must learn to avoid environmental factors and personal actions that increase the likelihood of a pain attack. For example, patients with gout must avoid consumption of alcohol because alcohol may temporarily reduce renal clearance of uric acid and precipitate an attack of pain and swelling in a gout-affected joint. The pain-management practitioner assists patients with chronic, painful diseases by educating them about the best strategies for reducing the frequency of pain attacks and by providing pain relief whenever an acutely painful stage of the disease arises.

Among the chronic diseases associated with bouts of acute pain are gouty arthritis; herpes zoster, which can develop into postherpetic neuralgia; sickle cell disease; and trigeminal neuralgia. The management of the acutely painful stages of these diseases is discussed here.

Acute gout

Acute gout is a painful disease of the joints caused by the deposition of crystals of sodium urate in the joint. Gouty attacks are seen in the patients with chronically elevated serum levels of uric acid, but increased uric acid levels alone will not cause gout, and most patients with elevated uric acid are asymptomatic. Gout is more commonly seen in men. These patients are also at increased risk of developing urate kidney stones. Most of them have a history of kidney stones before developing gout.

Diagnosis and management of gout

An attack of gouty arthritis usually occurs in one joint and is extremely painful. The attacks commonly involve a distal lower extremity, especially the great toe; however, the heel, ankle, knee, or an upper extremity can also be the site of crystal deposits and subsequent inflammation and pain. Attacks can be brought on by stress, surgery, excessive alcohol intake, or diet. Patients with an acute attack of gout also often have fever, an increased white blood cell count, and an elevated erythrocyte sedimentation rate. Typically, patients are pain-free between the attacks. Diagnosis is confirmed when urate crystals are found in the synovial fluid under polarized light microscopy.

Treatment of acute gout attacks should include NSAIDs to decrease the inflammation. Phenylbutazone and indomethacin are the most effective and widely used NSAIDs for acute gout. Another treatment choice is colchicine, a drug isolated from a species of the crocus plant. This drug inhibits white blood cell phagocytosis of urate crystals and ultimately the inflammatory reaction that causes the pain. The choice between colchicine and NSAIDs is made according to the practitioner's preference. Colchicine can be given orally or I.V. and is especially helpful in patients with a history of ulcer disease because it does not exacerbate ulcers. It should not be used in patients with a history of kidney disease, bone marrow dysfunction, or diarrhea. Avoidance of future attacks is accomplished by maintaining the patient on NSAIDs or on drugs that either increase the elimination of uric acid or reduce its synthesis in the body.

Acute herpes zoster

Acute herpes zoster, or shingles, is a common problem usually seen in elderly and immunocompromised patients. In the United States over 300,000 new cases occur each year (Rogozzino et al. 1982). Older patients are more likely to experience severe pain. The incidence of acute herpes zoster rises steeply with age, from 0.5 per 1000 in children to 5 to 10 per 1000 in people over age 80. The increased incidence with age has been attributed to age-related declines in immunity. With the advent of human immunodeficiency virus and the widespread use of chemotherapy, acute herpes zoster is now being seen among young people with compromised immunologic status.

Development of acute herpes zoster is caused by reactivation of varicella, the chicken pox virus. Following a patient's recovery from chicken pox, the virus remains dormant in the dorsal root ganglion of spinal and cranial nerves. A defect in normal cell-mediated immunity allows reactivation of the virus, spread of the virus along a sensory nerve, and subsequent pain and symptoms along the dermatome served by the affected nerve.

Diagnosis and management of acute herpes zoster
The diagnosis of acute herpes zoster may be very difficult in its initial stages. The pain usually appears several days, sometimes weeks, before the classical rash. After the lesions erupt, the diagnosis is very easy.

The pain of the acute herpes zoster infection is characterized by deep, usually unilateral pain confined to a dermatomal distribution and sometimes aggravated by movement or, less commonly, by breathing. The pain can be shooting, throbbing, burning, or dull. Patients may also have fever, generalized malaise, and fatigue. Hypersensitivity to pain (hyperpathia) occurs often in the involved areas.

Herpes zoster involves dermatomes of the chest in 50% of cases. Before eruption of the lesions, the acute pain in the chest may be mistaken for a variety of conditions, such as coronary artery disease (angina), pericarditis, pleurisy, appendicitis, or cholecystitis. The other common site for reactivation of this virus is the trigeminal ganglion, which supplies the sensory input to most of the face and the eye. The ophthalmic branch of the trigeminal ganglion is the most commonly affected. With increasing age the incidence of ophthalmic zoster increases. Recurrence of acute herpes occurs in approximately 5% of patients, and 50% of these infections are at the site of previous infection. The symptoms and signs of trigeminal involvement include headaches, eye-muscle weakness, double vision, and sometimes scarring and ulcerations of the cornea. In addition to the sensory component, motor paralysis may be seen in rare cases. These deficits are usually reversible over years.

The rash of herpes zoster appears in a dermatomal distribution, most commonly on the chest as grouped vesicles on an erythematous base. Around day 4 or 5 the vesicles become pustular and then collapse to form a crust by day 7 to 10. The vesicles are thought to be infectious prior to crusting. Herpes zoster can involve up to three adjacent dermatomes. In addition to clinical signs and symptoms, laboratory tests such as the Tzanck test (microscopic examination of material scraped from vesicles) may help in diagnosis. Identification of giant cells in the vesicle exudate is a nonspecific indicator of herpes zoster.

The lesions and pain usually disappear in 4 to 5 weeks. Pain persisting longer than 1 month indicates postherpetic neuralgia, a chronic painful condition characterized by hyperesthesia, anesthesia, and dysesthesia in the affected areas. Postherpetic neuralgia develops in 10% to 50% of herpes zoster patients and is sometimes very difficult to treat. The pain and associated dysesthesias are thought to be neurogenic, possibly arising from fibrosis and scarring of the nerve sheath and loss of function in myelinated fibers.

Early identification and treatment of acute herpes zoster is essential. Evidence strongly suggests that early treatment of acute herpes zoster will result in faster recovery and possible prevention of postherpetic neuralgia. A pioneering, prospective, randomized study of 1,011 patients by Pernack and Biemans divided subjects into four groups based on the location of the lesions. Patients with trigeminal herpes received injections of methyl prednisone around the trigeminal ganglion; patients with thoracic herpes received methylprednisone and lidocaine (0.5%) injected epidurally. Of 1,011 patients, 997 had excellent relief and only 14 developed postherpetic neuralgia. Of these 14, all had suffered with acute herpes zoster for more than 3 weeks. This study and other similar studies confirm the belief that early aggressive therapy is beneficial in preventing development of postherpetic neuralgia (1985). It is therefore important that primary care providers refer acute herpes zoster patients to appropriate pain facilities for early proper treatment. Unfortunately, acute herpes zoster is viewed by many health care providers as a benign condition and appropriate early therapy is frequently not initiated.

Various drug therapies and nerve blocks provide current treatment of acute herpes zoster. Among the drug therapies, antiviral agents, such as acyclovir, vidarabine, and idoxuridine have been used with some success. Most clinical trials have shown that early initial treatment is necessary. Treatment with zoster immune globulin does not change the course of the disease and is of no value in treatment of acute herpes zoster. It is used only to offer passive immunity to susceptible individuals, such as immunocompromised patients and leukemia patients who have been exposed to chicken pox. A vaccine against the varicella zoster virus has been released recently.

Other medications for treatment of acute herpes zoster include analgesics and antidepressants. Among the analgesics, NSAIDs, corticosteroids, and opioids have been used. Much success has been reported after administering systemic corticosteroids. In a meta analysis of four clinical trials, oral prednisone decreased the incidence of postherpetic neuralgia, which was defined as pain occurring 6 to 12 weeks after the acute event (Lycka 1990). Corticosteroids such as triamcinolone have been injected S.C. at the affected area (Epstein 1981), and anecdotal reports claim it to be an effective herpes zoster treatment that also decreases the incidence of postherpetic neuralgia. Various opioids are used, depending on the severity of pain. For mild pain, codeine, oxycodone, or propoxyphene are effective, but most cases of acute herpes cause severe pain and may require strong agonists, such as meperidine, morphine, or hydromorphone.

Antidepressants have also been used to decrease the pain of postherpetic neuralgia. These medications act on the CNS by preventing the reuptake of serotonin and norepinephrine. The pain-relieving effects of antidepressants typically occur at much lower doses than those needed to treat depression. Among the antidepressants, the tricyclic antidepressants are especially useful if the patient complains of inability to fall asleep because of pain. Amitriptyline (Elavil) is the most commonly used drug for this problem even though its use is sometimes limited by the side effects of drowsiness, disorientation, hypotension or hypertension, palpitations, arrhythmia, and dry mouth.

Nerve blocks include various options, such as infiltration of the lesions with local anesthetic, sympathetic nerve blocks, and epidural blockade. Local infiltration of the lesion with a corticosteroid and local anesthetic is advocated in the early stages of the disease. Sympathetic blockade appears to be effective for decreasing herpes zoster pain associated with vasospasm. Evidence to date suggest that sympathetic blockade with a local anesthetic can decrease the pain and prevent postherpetic neuralgia. Epidural blocks may also offer good relief and help to prevent postherpetic neuralgia. Nerve blocks, as with other treatment modalities, should be performed early in the course of disease for best results.

Sickle cell anemia

Sickle cell anemia, a chronic disease common especially among African-Americans, is estimated to affect over 50,000 people in the United States. About 1,500 babies are born with the disease annually (Shapiro 1989). It is characterized by unpredictable episodes of mild or severe pain followed by the return to normal status. The frequency, severity, and duration of attacks vary among patients. About 20% of patients have frequent severe attacks, some people requiring up to 30 or 40 hospital admissions per year. About half of patients have only one or two crises per year, and 30% will rarely or never experience any crises (Shapiro 1989).

Various factors determine the severity and frequency of attacks, although the exact etiology of a vaso-occlusive crisis is not clearly understood. The pathophysiology of the disease is based on the presence of abnormal hemoglobin in red blood cells (RBCs). When deprived of oxygen, it polymerizes and forces the RBC to assume a sickle shape. The abnormal cell shape causes obstruction of blood flow through the capillaries. If significant collateral circulation is involved in the obstruction, then tissue hypoxia, ischemia, and infarction follow. The painful tissue ischemia and infarction constitute a vasoocclusive crisis or sickle cell crisis.

The acute crisis usually starts suddenly, lasts 5 to 7 days, and then resolves into a pain-free period. Some patients, however, may have pain every day, with periodic acute exacerbations. The pain can arise anywhere in the body. In young children, it usually involves the lower extremities. In adults, abdominal pain is more common. Triggering events associated with vaso-occlusive crisis include fever, infection, exposure to cold temperatures, dehydration, acidosis, fatigue, stress, and menses but, in some patients, no underlying triggering event can be found.

Assessment of vaso-occlusive crises

Most patients are able to differentiate their sickle cell pain from other types of pain, which is fortunate, because there are no reliable laboratory or radiographic tests to identify vaso-occlusive crisis. The pain can occur in the absence of any signs or in the presence of normal laboratory values.

Assessing patients for anxiety and depression is essential, but the pain experience itself can lead to anxiety and depression. These patients should receive consistent care from the same health care provider so that the caregiver knows the patient and the family prior to any acute crisis. Consistent care by the same provider helps to ensure that correct decisions regarding pain management are made when a crisis arises.

It is interesting to note that psychological studies of adults and of children with sickle cell disease have shown different results. Adults with sickle cell appear to have more psychological problems than control groups adjusted for race and socioeconomic levels. In contrast, children with sickle cell are similar to control groups matched for age, race, and socioeconomic level. It seems logical that prevention of pain in children and appropriate counseling and guidance may help to minimize psychological problems in adults with this disease.

Management of sickle cell crisis pain

There is no definite treatment for sickle cell disease. Managment consists mainly of supportive therapy during acute crisis, with a major focus on pain control. Supportive treatment includes close monitoring, hydration, infection control, and so forth. The treatment of vaso-occlusive pain is a challenge, and optimal management is sometimes difficult. Obtaining a careful and thorough history in the emergency department is the initial step. The kind and dose of analgesics used in previous crises should be noted. Specific attention should be paid to any signs of infection.

Sickle cell crisis pain calls for a differential treatment approach, depending on the severity of the pain. For mild to moderate pain, acetaminophen, aspirin, other NSAIDs, and weak opioids such as codeine are used. Stronger opioids such as morphine (MS-Contin), hydromorphone, and methadone may be used for patients with severe attacks. Combinations of NSAIDs and opioids are also used. The route of administration varies with the patient's situation. If the patient has no nausea and vomiting, then the oral route is preferred. The I.V., I.M., or S.C. routes are used if the patient cannot take oral medication, but the S.C. route is not for prolonged use because of unreliable drug absorption, especially if the patient is dehydrated. Repeated I.M. injections can cause muscle damage and fibrosis in addition to the obvious discomfort of the patient.

Among I.V. agents, morphine is the first drug of choice. Meperidine is not recommended for prolonged use because of the toxicity of its metabolite, normeperidine. Normeperidine is even more slowly excreted in patients with alkaline urine, and most patients with sickle cell disease have renal tubular acidosis. However, in clinical practice it is very common to encounter patients who insist on the use of meperidine for their pain. Because it is very difficult to convince these patients to use a different opioid during crisis, these patients need education on the effects of meperidine prior to crisis.

Initially, during the acute crisis, the patient should receive a bolus of enough of an opioid analgesic adequate to decrease the pain level below 5 in a visual analog scale of 0 to 10. The patient then should be started on an I.V. infusion or on PCA. Adding an NSAID to this regimen will improve pain control, especially if there is bone pain. Most important, medications must be given around the clock, not on a PRN basis. Patients with this disease vary signficantly in their response to analgesics. Dosage must be carefully titrated to the response and may be very different from one patient to the next. If a patient's opioid requirement seems to be high, factors such as anxiety, development of opioid tolerance, especially in patients who have received multiple previous therapy with opioids, and development of neuropathic pain should be considered.

Adjuvant analgesics have been considered for managing acute sickle cell crisis. Tricyclic antidepressants require slow titrating and may require a long time before an effect is seen. They probably have no significant role in treatment of acute vaso-occlusive crisis. Benzodiazepines, however, may be helpful, especially if the patient is anxious.

All patients with sickle cell disease need a multidisciplinary approach to pain treatment. In a study conducted by Vichinsky et al., a multidisciplinary approach included support groups, psychological assessment, psychotherapy, and home visits by nurses. This strategy decreased emergency room visits by 58% and hospital admissions by 48% (1982). Education of patients and their families is an important part of the management of this disease because it decreases fear and gives patients a sense of control over their own care. Appropriate psychological management and patient education may decrease the frequency of hospital admissions for acute crises.

Trigeminal neuralgia

Trigeminal neuralgia (TN), or tic douloureux, is characterized by acute paroxysms of facial pain interposed with pain-free intervals during which the patient is completely asymptomatic. Although it occurs in younger people, the majority of patients are 50 to 70 years old. The etiology of TN is not clearly understood. Examination of the involved nerves in these patients has revealed evidence of demyelination. In some cases, the pain results from the impingement of blood vessels on the trigeminal nerve root.

A recent and exciting hypothesis offered by Rapport and Devor that TN may disappear for weeks or months and then return with ever-increasing frequency. They propose that in TN neurons of the trigeminal ganglion have been rendered hyperactive as a result of damage. A trigger stimulus sets off abnormal bursts of neural activity in these damaged neurons. After a period of excessive firing, the nerves become refractory to further spontaneous activity, and a period of pain remission begins (Rappaport and Devor 1994).

It is believed that TN affects genetically predisposed individuals.

Diagnosis and management of TN

It is important to realize that TN is a central pain state (pain is thought to arise from aberrant nerve activity in the trigeminal ganglion) without any pathology in the painful area. There are different pain patterns in TN. Some patients experience dull, aching pain in the upper or lower jaw at the onset of their disease and then later experience the paroxysmal attacks.

The characteristic pain pattern of TN is a sharp stabbing pain, usually unilateral, of abrupt onset, and restricted to the trigeminal nerve distribution. There is usually a trigger zone around the nose or upper or lower lip that is always on the same side as the pain. Any kind of stimulus to the trigger zone, even slight movement or a brush of hair, can trigger the pain. Pain may be initiated by talking, chewing, sweating, smiling, exposure to cold, hair brushing, shaving, or brushing teeth. Usually no sensory loss is associated with this condition. Sometimes, a branch of facial nerve (nervus intermedius) or glossopharyngeal nerve can be involved along with the trigeminal nerve. Nervus intermedius involvement is characterized by pain in the ear or posterior pharynx. Glossopharyngeal nerve involvement is characterized by pain in the posterior tongue, tonsillar fossa, or larynx.

It was thought that TN in patients younger than age 40 is associated with an underlying disorder, especially multiple sclerosis (MS). However, in patients of any age, if the pain is in both sides of face or there are other neurologic signs indicative of MS, then a complete workup is mandatory to rule out MS. TN is most commonly observed in the third division of the trigeminal nerve, the mandibular nerve, and least commonly seen in the first division, the ophthalmic nerve. Involvement of both the first and third divisions of the trigeminal nerve is also common. Over time, pain-free intervals of TN characteristically become shorter and shorter. Emotional and physical stress usually increase the frequency of pain attacks.

The two most effective agents for trigeminal neuralgia are the anticonvulsants carbamazepine (Tegretol) and phenytoin (Dilantin). Since TN is a central pain state, pharmacologic intervention meant to affect peripheral tissue damage is not appropriate treatment. Opioids are good options for severe attacks, but they have a limited role in the treatment of this disorder.

About 70% of patients have a good response to carbamazepine, which is the first line of treatment. Patients receiving this medication should be followed for signs of bone marrow depression, which usually occurs in the first three months after treatment begins. Other side effects include irritation of the gastric mucosa (nausea and vomiting), dizziness, ataxia, and drowsiness. The standard dosing regimen is a low starting dose that is titrated to pain relief or a maximum daily dose of 1,800 mg, whichever happens first. Phenytoin, the second choice, has side effects similar to those of carbamazepine. Complete blood counts and liver enzyme studies should be monitored carefully during therapy with both of these drugs. The dose-response curve for carbamazepine is curvilinear; for phenytoin, it is more linear. Thus, with increased doses, blood levels of phenytoin may rise much higher than blood levels of carbamazepine. Other anticonvulsants used for treatment of this condition include mephenesin and chlormephenesin. Baclofen has also been used with success. Both opioids and nonopioids can be used during acute crises.

Nerve blocks offer another option for treatment. Local anesthetics will block the pain temporarily. Phenol or alcohol blocks of the trigeminal ganglion or peripheral branches have been used extensively for prolonged relief. Surgery is another option. Peripheral neurectomies of the branches of the trigeminal nerve have been tried. The neurosurgical technique of dissecting vascular structures from the trigeminal ganglion has been successful in selected patients. Creation of lesions in the pain fibers supplying the trigger zone by means of the targeted application of radio frequency electrical current has had excellent long-term results without affecting the associated sensory fibers. Thermocoagulation of the trigeminal ganglion has been reported to relieve pain in 50% of cases with half of the patients returning for a second procedure within 1 to 5 years. The mortality rate for this procedure can be about 0.5%, usually from intracranial hemorrhage (Dubuisson 1993). Glycerol injection into the trigeminal ganglion has also been reported to provide complete relief in 90% of patients (Hakanson 1983). The time course of relief with this procedure is variable. Dubuisson reports that 20% of patients returned for a second injection after 18 months (1993).

REFERENCES

Ballantyne, J., and Borsook, D. "Postoperative Pain," in *Massachusetts General Hospital Handbook of Pain Management,* 1st ed. Edited by Boorsook, et al., 1996.

Bonica, J.J. "Post-op Pain," in *The Management of Pain,* 2nd ed. Edited by Bonica, J.J. Baltimore: Williams & Wilkins, 1990.

Chapman, C.R. "Psychological Aspects of Pain," in *Hospital Practice* (special report), IC 14, 1978.

Choiniere, M. "Pain of Burns" in *Textbook of Pain,* 3rd. ed. Edited by Melzack, R., and Wall, P.D. New York: Churchill Livingstone, 1994.

Choiniere, M., et al. "The Pain of Burns: Characteristics and Correlates," *Journal of Trauma* 29(11):1531-39, November 1989.

Davies, J.W.L. "Prompt Cooling of Burned Areas: A Review of Benefits and the Effector Mechanisms," *Burns* 9(1):16, September 1982.

Deschamps, M., et al. "Assessment of Adult Cancer Pain: Shortcomings of Current Methods," *Pain* 32(2):133-39, February 1988.

Dubner, R., and Basbum, A. "Spinal Dorsal Horn Plasticity Following Tissue or Nerve Injury," in *Textbook of Pain,* 3rd ed. Edited by Melzack, R., and Wall, P.D. New York: Churchill Livingston, 1994.

Dubuisson, D. "Neurosurgical Treatment of Pain," in *Principles and Practice of Pain Management.* Edited by Warfield, C. New York: McGraw Hill, 1993.

Ejelersen, E., et al., "A Comparison between Pre-incisional and Post-incisional Lidocaine Infiltration and Post-operative Pain," *Anesthesia & Analgesia,* 74(4):495-98, 1992.

Epstein, E. "Treatment of Herpes Zoster and Post-Zoster Neuralgia by Subcutaneous Injection of Triamcinolone," *International Journal of Dermatology* 20(1): 65-68, January-February 1981.

Hakanson, S. "Retrogasserian Glycerol Injection as a Treatment of Tic Douloureaux," in *Advances in Pain Research and Therapy,* vol. 5. Edited by Bonnica, J.J., et al. New York: Raven Press, 1983.

Jaffee, J.H. "Drug Addiction and Drug Abuse," in *The Pharmacological Basis of Therapeutics,* 9th ed. Edited by Gilman, A.G., et al. New York: McGraw Hill, 1996.

Katz, J., et al. "Preemptive Analgesia: Clinical Evidence of Neuroplasticity Contributing to Postoperative Pain," *Anesthesiology* 77(3):439-46, 1992.

Lycka, B.A. "Postherpetic Neuralgia and Systemic Corticosteroid Therapy: Efficacy and Safety," *International Journal of Dermatology* 29(7):523-27, September 1990.

Marks, R.M., and Sacher, E.F. "Undertreatment of Medical Inpatients with Narcotic Analgesics," *Annals of Internal Medicine* 78(2):173-81, February 1973.

Melzack, R., et al. "Acute Pain in an Emergency Clinic: Latency of Onset and Descriptor Patterns Related to Different Injuries," *Pain* 14(1):33-43, September 1982.

Payne, R., et al. *Principles of Analgesic Use in Treatment of Acute Pain and Chronic Cancer Pain,* 2nd ed. American Pain Society Guidelines, 1989.

Pernack, J.M., and Biemans, J. "The Treatment of Acute Herpes Zoster in the Trigeminal Nerve for the Prevention of Postherpetic Neuralgia," in *The Pain Clinic,* vol. 1. Edited by Edmann, et al. Utrecht:VNU, Science Press, 1985.

Perry, S., and Heidrich, G. "Management of Pain during Debridement: A Survey," *Pain* 13(3):267-80, July 1982.

Porter, J., and Jick, H. "Addiction Rare in Patients Treated with Narcotics" (letter), *New England Journal of Medicine* 302(2):123, January 10, 1980.

Ragozzino, M.W., et al. "Risk of Cancer after Herpes Zoster," *New England Journal of Medicine* 307(7):393-97, August 12, 1982.

Rappaport, Z.T., and Devor, M. "Trigeminal Neuralgia: The Role of Self-Sustaining Discharge in Trigeminal Ganglion," *Pain* 56(2):127-38, February 1994.

Shapiro, B. "The Management of Pain in Sickle Cell Disease," *Pediatric Clinics of North America* 36(4):1029-45, August 1989.

Tverskoy, M., et al. "Postoperative Pain after Inguinal Herniorraphy with Different Types of Anesthesia," *Anesthesia & Analgesia* 70(1):29-35, January 1990.

Vichinsky, E.P., et al. "Multidisciplinary Approach to Pain Management in Sickle Cell Disease," *American Journal of Pediatric Hematology–Oncology* 4(3):328-33, Fall 1982.

Wall, P.D. "On the Relationship of Injury to Pain," *Pain* 6(3):253-64, June 1979.

Woolf, C., and Chong, M.S. "Preemptiive Analgesia: Treating Post-operative Pain by Preventing the Establishment of Central Sensitization," *Anesthesia & Analgesia* 77(2): 362-79, 1993.

CHAPTER 11

Care of children with pain

Raeford E. Brown, Jr., MD

Pain is an important pediatric health problem. The treatment of pain in children is often considered to be of secondary importance. Failure to respond to and treat painful conditions, however, may affect the function of the patient. Postoperative pain may prolong hospitalization, reduce oral intake, and decrease mobility. Chronic limb or back pain, reflex sympathetic dystrophy, or painful neuropathies affect school performance, mood, and family interactions. Lack of treatment may occur because of questions of safety or lack of knowledge regarding the impact of the painful conditions. Pain management is an important aspect of pediatric care that is only now receiving the attention of the medical community. The purpose of this chapter is to explore common misconceptions surrounding pain in children, establish the physiology of pediatric pain, and describe some of the currently available methods to treat children with acute and chronic pain.

Common misperceptions about pediatric pain

The study of pain in children did not begin in earnest until the early 1970s. At that time it was not uncommon for medical or nursing textbooks to include statements discounting the importance of pain and pain management in children. Conventional clinical wisdom dictated that it was unsafe to treat infants and children with narcotics and, besides, "children don't feel pain anyway." Important research conducted during the past decade as well as a large body of clinical experience discounts much of the conventional wisdom (see *Pediatric pain myths*).

Pediatric pain myths

These and other clinical myths prevent timely and appropriate treatment of children, even as adults receive consistent state-of-the art therapy. Only the implementation of accurate, currently available scientific information will ensure the adequate treatment of pain in children.

Myth: Infants do not feel pain.

It had largely been taken for granted until recently that infants were incapable of feeling pain. Male circumcisions have been done during the perinatal period for at least 2,000 years. More recently, surgical procedures were commonly performed on infants without the benefit of anesthesia.

In fact, infants and children do feel pain. Infants demonstrate behavioral and physiologic, including hormonal, indicators of pain even before birth. The nervous system of the infant is sufficiently sophisticated to appreciate adverse stimuli and conduct these signals to the brain. The central nervous system reaches adult levels of maturity by 36 weeks after conception. Thus, the nociceptive response is realized in the infant.

Myth: Children tolerate pain better than adults.

Children do not tolerate pain better than adults. Despite a lack of verbal behavior, children demonstrate pain behavior in much the same way that adults do. Children beyond infancy can accurately point to the body area that hurts and can mark a painful site on a drawing. Children as young as age 3 can use pain scales to demonstrate the level of their pain. In addition, analysis of hormone levels associated with stress reveals consistently high levels in infants and children undergoing painful procedures just as are found in adults.

Myth: Children become accustomed to pain or painful procedures.

Children often demonstrate increased signs of discomfort with repeated painful procedures. Anxiety associated with painful procedures often is worse than the procedure itself. There is no reason to believe that children can become more easily accustomed to pain than adults.

Myth: Narcotics are more dangerous for children than for adults.

Opioid compounds are no more dangerous for children than for adults when they are used appropriately. Side effects such as respiratory depression are dose-dependent and can be monitored and controlled. Tolerance, the need for a larger dose of opioid to maintain an original effect, will occur in children as it does in adults. Addiction resulting from the use of narcotics for pain management in children is very rare. Narcotic compounds should be used in pediatric patients in the same way and with the same care that other potent drugs are used.

Physiologic basis for pediatric pain

Recent scientific data support the conclusion that the nervous system reaches a relatively mature state much earlier than had been previously appreciated. This maturation provides the essential physiologic basis for pain in the infant and child.

Development of the nervous system

The brain and central nervous system begin to form soon after implantation of the fertilized egg into the uterine wall, perhaps as early as 28 days after conception. This early development produces the brain stem and other control centers for the heart and vascular system. Fetal appreciation of and response to external stimuli such as pain require a relatively sophisticated cortex with completed wiring to the periphery. Based on anatomical analysis cortical structure is virtually complete by 30 weeks of gestation. Mature cortical electrical activity as measured by EEG is present by 32 to 36 weeks. Although the fetus may respond to external stimuli prior to the maturation of cortical function, these responses are probably spinal reflexes.

The peripheral circuitry necessary to conduct electrical impulses to the midbrain and cortex is mature perhaps as early as 20 to 24 weeks. Peripheral receptors are present in anatomic specimens during this same time frame. The most conservative time estimate for nervous system maturity capable of nociceptive response is 36 weeks of gestation. Many practitioners believe that this time estimate is too conservative, that physiologic maturation occurs much earlier. *Maturation of pain pathways in the human fetus and neonate* illustrates one version of fetal pain pathway development. Further investigation is required in order to clearly define this issue.

Neonatal stress response

The ability of the fetus and newborn to mount a significant response to the stress of pain undoubtedly plays an important role in outcome. The metabolic endocrine axis is active soon after birth and produces an outpouring of hormonal mediators, such as epinephrine, norepinephrine, and growth hormone. Secondary breakdown of glycogen as a result of this hormonal action produces hyperglycemia (high blood glucose levels), a common finding in stressed newborns, which may place infants at risk for such complications as intracranial hemorrhage.

The impact of the neonatal stress response on the outcome of these patients remains to be elucidated. One study of critically ill newborns revealed a significant reduction in the rate of pulmonary complications when appropriate narcotic-based anesthesia was used prior to chest wall incision. Subsequent studies support the use of potent analgesic agents to suppress the stress response for a protracted recovery period.

These data, while suggestive of the importance of adequate pain control in the critically ill newborn, do not provide more than an early picture. Further analysis with large groups of patients are needed. Because some of these studies have been done in adult patients, with indications that appropriate analgesia makes a significant impact on treatment outcome, it makes sense to replicate these and other trials in pediatric patients.

Maturation of pain pathways in the human fetus and neonate

As shown in the developmental timeline here, a fetus of 36 weeks' gestation has all the neurologic mechanisms necessary to experience nociception. Many practitioners believe that this time estimate is too conservative and that the physiologic maturation necessary for nociception occurs much earlier.

Cutaneous sensory perception

Myelination

Nerve tracts in the spinal cord and brain stem

Internal capsule

Corona radiata

Cortical maturation

Neuronal migration

Dendritic arborization

Synaptogenesis with thalamocortical fibers

EEG patterns

Intermittent

Pattern 1 EEG synchronous

Pattern 2 EEG

Pattern 3 EEG

Pattern 4 EEG

Cortical evoked potentials

20   22   24   26   28   30   32   34   36   38   40

Weeks of gestation

From Berde, C.B., et al. "Pediatric Pain Management," in *Pediatric Anesthesia*, vol. 2, 2nd ed. Edited by Gregory, G.A. Churchill Livingstone, 1989. Adapted with permission.

Uncertainties surrounding pain in children

Caregivers who work with children may find themselves asking, "Is pain adequately treated in children?" Interest in the adequate treatment of pain in children arose in the early 1970s with studies by

Eland and others (Eland and Anderson 1977). Appreciation of the lack of treatment of pain in children followed similar investigations of pain treatment in adults, and it continues to the present. Original investigations dealt only with issues of acute pain, especially postoperative pain. Numerous studies have demonstrated that children receive fewer analgesics for acute pain than do adults, if they get any at all. For similar types of acute pain children may receive less potent analgesics than the analgesics given to adults. In addition, children are often not believed when they tell health care providers that they are suffering. In an especially poignant study published by Schecter, patients in a community hospital were assigned groups depending on the type of procedure that had been done. This study demonstrated that children undergoing surgical procedures similar to those performed on adults received half of the analgesic dose by weight that adults received (Schechter et al. 1986). In the study of acute pain, these data have been borne out time and again.

Subsequently, many authors have begun to assess the adequacy of treatment of children with cancer pain as well as of those with the pain associated with other chronic diseases. Unfortunately, the analysis of pain treatment in these cases has not reached the level of sophistication that has been attained with acute pain.

Chronic pain

Children probably suffer chronic pain to much the same extent as adults. The comprehensive evaluation and treatment of such entities as reflex sympathetic dystrophy, neuropathy, and headache in children is only now reaching a mature level. Information on the use of analgesics in children suffering these and other chronic disorders is largely unavailable. The well-recognized lack of training of pediatric practitioners in the management of chronic pain disorders limits the treatment options just as it does in the situation of acute pediatric pain.

Nonpharmacologic methods for pain relief may replace or supplement analgesics in the pediatric patient with chronic pain. Treatment approaches such as stress management, hypnosis, thought-stopping, and visual imagery may reduce pain scores and improve function in otherwise helpless patients. Adolescents with chronic headache, for example, often improve when they use a diary to document the timing of headaches and when they practice stress-reduction exercises to alleviate tension in their lives. Patients with congenital hemolytic anemias may reduce the hospitalization time needed for pain control through the use of visual imagery techniques that are much like self-hypnosis. Combinations of psychological techniques can often be used as adjuncts to pharmacologic and physical approaches for managment of chronic pain in pediatric patients.

Cancer pain

Pain is common in children with cancer. Recent National Cancer Institute surveys of the prevalence of pain in childhood cancer reveal that as many as 26% of outpatients and 54% of inpatients suffer from significant pain (Miser and Miser 1989). Other surveys of children and young adults suggest that nearly 80% of respondents suffer pain prior to or after the diagnosis of cancer.

Pain in children with cancer arises from tumor invasion of soft tissue structures, nerves, and bone. In addition, and perhaps more important, the pain associated with diagnostic and therapeutic procedures affects most children who have cancer. In the National Cancer Institute surveys, 78% of children receiving bone marrow aspirations and 61% of those receiving lumbar punctures reported moderate to severe pain. Recent statements by the American Academy of Pediatrics encourage the use of conscious sedation for painful procedures and provide standards for monitoring such care.

Because of fear of the complications of treating pain in critically ill children, lack of knowledge of the prevalence of pain secondary to cancer, and community attitudes that denigrate treatment for pain alleviation, pain in the child with cancer is often considered to be of secondary importance. Epidemiologic data are required to determine the significance of pain in childhood cancer as well as the impact of treatment for pain on outcome.

Pain assessment in children

Assessment of pain in children provides the basis for treatment and offers the practitioner a picture of reality that can be compared with the experience of others. That comparison leads to changes in expectations when the practitioner treats other patients. Thus, accurate assessment may lead to the appropriate treatment of all patients.

Physiologic assessment

The earliest available pain assessment instruments for children were based on evaluation of changes in physiologic parameters. Changes in blood pressure, heart rate, respiratory rate, and oxygen saturation of hemoglobin were associated with painful and otherwise stressful procedures performed in children. However, changes in physiologic parameters, while relatively sensitive, are not specific for pain. These early studies were often done in newborns, so verbal corroboration of pain was not possible. Subsequent studies have incorporated other nonverbal behaviors in attempts to improve the validity of the assessment.

Unfortunately, an accurate and sensitive biochemical indicator of pain is not available. Though some hormones are produced in quantity during pain, the coexistence of stress or other disease states cannot be ruled out as contributing factors in these changes. Stress hormones are not reliable markers of pain in children.

Pain assessment in the preverbal child

The preverbal child in pain demonstrates behavior consistent with pain and stress. The child may grimace, cry, or hold his breath, or his skin might become mottled. These behaviors and others can be counted and cataloged in much the same way that verbal pain scores can be tabulated in adults. Several investigators have produced pain evaluation scales appropriate for preverbal children and some of them have been successfully validated (see *Modified Hanallah Pain Scale* for an example).

Pain assessment in the older child

Pain assessment in the older child is predicated on the presence or absence of language and on the developmental level. Numerous visual analog pain scales are available, some appropriate for toddlers and others appropriate for children through adolescence to adulthood. The use of age-appropriate scales is extremely important, as is familiarizing the child with the assessment instrument prior to a painful procedure. Many of these scales have been validated in older children and appear to be accurate. The *Faces scale for pain assessment in young children* and *Numerical scale for pain assessment in older children*, both on page 356, are typical examples.

Pain assessment in the developmentally delayed child

Although progress has been made in the treatment of pain in children, certain populations continue to be underserved. Children with developmental delays are often considered less likely to suffer pain primarily because of their inability to communicate it. Despite the availability of pain scales for preverbal children, assessment is seen as difficult and is often avoided.

Issues related to childhood pain

Examination of the question "Should childhood pain be treated?" involves an evaluation of legal, moral, and ethical issues as well as a determination of the importance of treatment in patient outcome.

Modified Hannallah Pain Scale

The Modified Hannallah Pain Scale is useful in pain assessment of preverbal children.

Observation	Criteria	Points
Blood pressure	+/- 10% Preoperative	0
	>20% Preoperative	1
	>30% Preoperative	2
Crying?	Not crying	0
	Crying but responds to tender loving care (TLC)	1
	Crying and does not respond to TLC	2
Movement	None	0
	Restless	1
	Thrashing	2
Agitation	Patient asleep or calm	0
	Mild	1
	Hysterical	2
Posture	No special posture	0
	Flexing legs and thighs	1
	Holding scrotum or groin	2
Verbalizes pain?	Asleep or states no pain	0
	Cannot localize	1
	Can localize	2

From Hannallah, et al. "Comparison of Caudal and Ilioinguinal/Iliohyogastric Nerve Blocks for Control of Postorchiopexy Pain in Pediatric Ambulatory Surgery," *Anesthesiology* 66:832-34, 1987. Adapted with permission.

Each of these concerns is important and plays a role in children's well-being and in family integrity. It is useful to view these considerations as the legs of an equilateral triangle (see *Three primary treatment issues in pediatric pain management,* page 357), with each aspect as important as the others in the role of ensuring adequate treatment of childhood pain.

As has been previously stated, improvement in patient outcome is only now being recognized as an important consequence of pain control. Studies in adult patients as well as limited trials in newborns,

Faces scale for pain assessment in young children

Young children vary in the capacity to understand numerical pain scales as well as in the ability to understand the meaning of various words for pain. Simple visual scales, such as the face sequence shown here, allow assessment of pain without relying on children's verbal skills or comprehension of numbers.

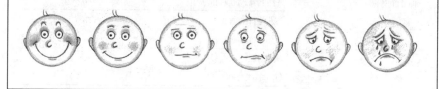

Numerical scale for pain assessment in older children

Older children can use a numerical pain scale to assist in the assessment of pain. Before using this numerical scale for pain assessment, caregivers must be certain that the child can count to 10 and can also comprehend that a higher number means more pain.

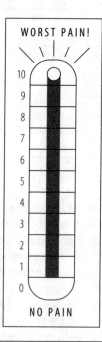

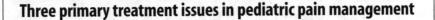

Three primary treatment issues in pediatric pain management

In deciding whether or not to treat pediatric pain, practioners must give equal consideration to legal and ethical issues, as well as to the relevance of pain treatment to patient outcome.

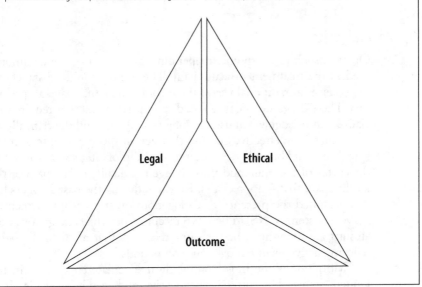

children, and adolescents strongly suggest that complications may be reduced, hospital stays may be shortened, and costs may be reduced if pain is treated appropriately.

Failure to treat pain in children is an ethical issue in that children can't protect themselves and many times are not allowed to speak for themselves. It falls then to the supervising adult to suggest or require adequate treatment of the child. The moral impetus for the treatment of pediatric pain is that since adults are entitled to treatment for pain, the treatment of children in pain is the right thing to do.

The legal right of children to have adequate treatment for pain is defined by the courts. Case law thus far has not examined this issue specifically. The position of advocate falls to the parent or guardian of the child and to the government only in the absence of a parent. The court will not dismiss the desires of the parent even if they are not in the best interests of the child. For example, a parent cannot be forced to allow the use of narcotics in a child's treatment.

Thus, the treatment of pain in a child often depends on the prevailing community standard of what is the right thing to do rather than on legal pressures or outcome analysis. As the effects of pain treatment on patient outcome become clearer, this scenario is likely to change.

Pharmacologic approaches

Pain may be safely treated in children using a wide array of pharmacologic agents. Opioids, NSAIDs, acetaminophen, and psychotropic drugs, such as the tricyclics and other classes of antidepressants, all have been used effectively to control pediatric pain.

Opioid analgesics

Opioids, such as morphine, meperidine, and fentanyl, are commonly used in the treatment of acute pain. The use of opioid substances to treat pain is a traditional use of these compounds that dates to prehistory. These drugs are safe when used appropriately, but they require specialized knowledge when used in infants, children, and the critically ill.

Opiates are effective because they act on specific receptors in the spinal cord and brain. These receptors inhibit or alter sensory input to the cortex of the brain and thus change the quality of the pain or the level of pain that is appreciated. Research during the past 20 years has demonstrated the presence of endogenous opiates within the central nervous system (CNS). The CNS receptors on which exogenous opiates act are thought to be the same receptors that mediate the pain-relieving activities of endogenous compounds.

Morphine is the most commonly used opiate compound in the United States. This drug is inexpensive and readily available. It is potent and, like other opiates, there is no ceiling (maximum dosage level) above which it does not function. Morphine may be administered parenterally or via any body orifice, given the appropriate dose adjustment. The dose of the drug is proportional to the size of the patient and the intensity of the pain. Morphine and the other opiates are most effective in the treatment of visceral pain such as that which accompanies a surgical incision. They are not as effective in the treatment of neuropathic pain syndromes, such as diabetic or peripheral neuropathy.

Common side effects of the use of morphine include respiratory depression, drowsiness, itching, nausea, and constipation. Tolerance (the need for a larger dose of drug to produce the same pharmacologic effect) occurs if the drug is used for a prolonged period, as in patients with cancer.

Addiction to narcotics is uncommon in patients with acute pain, especially in children, but addiction presents a potent source of fear among practitioners, a concern that clearly reduces the prescribing of potent narcotics for pain and, likewise, reduces patients' consumption of appropriate medications.

The efficacy of narcotics in reducing pain is dependent on the serum concentration of the drug. The serum concentration that provides maximum analgesia varies widely, and there may be a 30-fold difference in effective serum concentrations within comparable patient populations. For this reason it is difficult to predict an appropriate analgesic dose for each patient.

Patient controlled analgesia (PCA) provides the patient with the opportunity to find an effective serum level of a narcotic drug and maintain it. PCA devices incorporate microprocessors into intravenous pumps, an innovation that allows clinicians to set safe narcotic dose ranges and patients to actually administer the drug themselves. These devices have been used in adults since the 1970s and in children since the late 1980s.

PCA is effective in children, as in adults, because it provides patients with effective serum concentrations of analgesic as well as a sense of personal control over a portion of their clinical care. Children as young as age five can use PCA, and some clinicians have tried parent-controlled analgesia for children as young as 1 year. Parent-controlled or, alternatively, nurse-controlled analgesia has been a subject of substantial debate. Obviously, to ensure the safety of such children, significant alterations in routine clinical protocols are necessary.

Narcotic compounds such as morphine can also be administered directly into the CNS via epidural or intrathecal catheter placement. This technology provides potent pain relief to patients after significant surgical procedures and trauma.

Controlling pediatric cancer pain provides an example of this technique.

Nonopioid analgesics

In addition to opioid compounds, a number of other classes of drugs are available to the clinician to facilitate the treatment of pain in children. These compounds may be used alone or in combination with opiates in

---

Nonopioid drugs used in pediatric analgesia

- NSAIDs
- Acetaminophen
- Antidepressants
- Anticonvulsants
- Local anesthetics
- Neuroleptics
- Alpha agonists

---

order to achieve maximum therapeutic effect with a minimum number of side effects. Certain agents such as acetaminophen are well-known and have a long history of use in conjunction with opiates in the treatment of acute pain in children. Some drugs such as the tricyclic antidepressants are less well-known to pediatric health care providers but are extremely useful in the treatment of acute and chronic pain. The goal of this brief review is to provide information on the safe and effective use of these agents and to suggest a new approach to the pharmacologic management of pain in children. This approach advocates "coanalgesia" or the use of smaller doses of multiple analgesics in order to provide pain control. *Nonopioid drugs used in pediatric analgesia* lists the nonopioid analgesics most commonly used in pediatric pain management.

Nonsteroidal anti-inflammatory drugs

NSAIDs and acetaminophen are the most common agents used alone or in conjunction with opioids in the treatment of pain in children. Fifteen NSAIDs are currently available in the United States. In addition to salicylates, only three of these drugs are FDA-approved for use in children: ibuprofen, naproxen, and tolmetin sodium. Dosage regimens for these drugs are given in *Pediatric dosages of NSAIDs.*

NSAIDs produce analgesia at multiple sites, both in the periphery and in the central nervous system. Until recently, all pain relief ascribed to these compounds was assumed to relate to the inhibition of prostaglandin synthesis and the impact on the inflammatory process. Prostaglandins are almost certainly released during acute injury and NSAIDs are effective in blunting excess production and release. This action, however, does not fully explain the antinociceptive properties of this group of drugs. NSAIDs also produce pain relief in the absence of inflammation and there appears to be little correlation between the analgesic efficacy of a particular drug and its ability to inhibit prostaglandin synthesis. Preliminary evidence suggests that NSAIDs may modulate the central sensitization of pain pathways independent of any impact on the inflammatory process. These mechanisms are the subject of much debate and research.

Pediatric dosages of NSAIDs

NSAID	Daily dosage (mg/kg) P.O.	Frequency per day	Side effects
Ibuprofen	10 to 40	3 to 5	GI upset
Naproxen	15 to 20	2 to 3	GI upset
Tolmetin	15 to 20	3 to 4	GI upset
Choline-magnesium salicylate	40 to 60	3 to 4	Few reported
Acetaminophen*	40 to 60	6	Few reported

*Acetaminophen is commonly classed with NSAIDs; however, it differs from NSAIDs in that it lacks significant anti-inflammatory activity.

NSAIDs are divided into clinical groups according to their structural formulas. Each of the four groups (salicylates, acetic acids, fenamates, and propionic acids) contain numerous compounds. Because of the very different chemical structures, patients may respond to an acetic acid such as ketorolac and yet be unresponsive to a propionic acid such as piroxicam. Certain patients will develop nausea or other GI side effects with a particular drug or group and will be asymptomatic with an alternative agent. For these reasons, clinicians should be adept at the use of drugs in all four groups.

Side effects may seriously limit the primary use of NSAIDs as analgesics. Common side effects include GI distress, inhibition of normal platelet aggregation necessary for blood coagulation, and renal impairment. These side effects can be ameliorated or eliminated by drug or dose alterations or, in the case of minor GI upset, by the use of antacids. Certain patients, such as those with a bleeding diathesis or preexisting renal impairment, should be carefully monitored if NSAIDs are deemed necessary.

Acetaminophen, perhaps the most commonly prescribed drug for the treatment of pain in children, is often classified with NSAIDs. Although hepatic toxicity is significant when taken in large doses, acetaminophen has very few side effects when used in the therapeutic range. Acetaminophen has no effect on prostaglandins and thus no impact on the inflammatory response. The mechanism of action undoubtedly lies in the central nervous system, although scientific evidence for the exact location is scarce.

Certain guidelines should be used when choosing a NSAIDs:

• After careful assessment of the patient's renal status and consideration of the possibility of bleeding, the clinician should deter-

mine the best route of administration and identify drugs that are appropriate for that route.
- The drug chosen should be familiar to the clinician, cause no unusual effects risks for the patient, and offer duration of analgesia appropriate to the patient's pain syndrome.
- Since NSAIDs exhibit a ceiling analgesic effect, doses above those approved are usually inappropriate. A patient with a pain syndrome likely to respond to NSAIDs may benefit from switching drug classes.

TCAs and other antidepressants

Antidepressants have been used for the relief of pain since the 1950s when Seymour Diamond, a pioneer in the treatment of headache, suggested that amitriptyline (Elavil) might be useful in the treatment of headache. Subsequently, virtually all of the so-called tricyclics and numerous other classes of antidepressants have been evaluated for efficacy in the treatment of chronic pain. *Antidepressants used in pediatric pain management* gives basic information on antidepressant usage for pediatric pain.

During the past 3 years, new antidepressants such as fluoxetine (Prozac) have all but replaced TCAs in the treatment of depression. For the past 30 years, however, amitriptyline has been a mainstay in the therapy of chronic pain.

Many patients with chronic pain are depressed, but the mechanism of action of amitriptyline seems to be unrelated to its action as an antidepressant. It has been thought for some time that this class of antidepressant drugs acts by modulating the action of serotonin, a neurotransmitter in the CNS. Serotonin is present in high concentrations in the spinal cord and may act to inhibit ascending pain signals in the dorsal root ganglion or in the cord itself. This action may represent a feedback loop that acts to protect the CNS from massive overload at the time of serious trauma in the periphery.

In addition to analgesia, a second desirable effect of the antidepressants is their ability to produce sleep. Many, if not most, patients with significant pain suffer sleep disturbance. Other hypnotic agents such as the benzodiazepines provide sedation but often interrupt REM sleep. A small dose of amitriptyline administered at night will often provide appropriate regulation of the sleep cycle. Lack of sleep is often cited as a significant factor in lowering the pain threshold so this side effect is extremely beneficial.

Antidepressants may be used as primary analgesics or as adjuvant agents in the treatment of a variety of chronic painful conditions. The choice of an appropriate agent must be predicated on experience gained with adult patients because large-scale controlled

Antidepressants used in pediatric pain management

All of these drugs, except trazodone, are tricyclic antidepressants. Trazodone belongs to a newer class of antidepressants loosely termed heterocyclics.

Agent	Daily dosage		Frequency	Side effects
	Starting (mg/kg)	*Maintenance (mg/kg/day)*		
Amitriptyline	10	1 to 3	Once at bedtime	Sedation, dry mouth
Nortriptyline	10	1 to 3	Once at bedtime	Sedation, dry mouth
Desipramine	75	1 to 2	Once at bedtime	Sedation, agitation
Doxepin	30	2 to 4	Once at bedtime	Sedation, dry mouth
Trazodone	50	1 to 2	Once at bedtime	Sedation, priapism

studies of antidepressant use in children are not available. Clinicians have used antidepressants in patients with headache, cancer, low back pain, and a variety of neuropathies. In addition, patients with such chronic disorders as rheumatoid arthritis have gained relief from trials of these agents. Children with these disorders or any other condition in which adults have been treated effectively with antidepressants should be considered candidates for trial antidepressant use. The choice of an individual agent is often made on the basis of clinician familiarity and side-effect profile. Therapy is usually administered at bedtime and low doses of medications are begun in order to minimize side effects. Because children tend to be rapid metabolizers, relatively large doses may eventually be needed. Reaching appropriate serum levels may be time-consuming as side effects such as daytime drowsiness are balanced against the need to maintain patients' ability to function. An analgesic effect may not be noted for 7 to 10 days even if appropriate serum levels have been reached. The monitoring of serum TCA levels has been suggested for patients who require high doses, are refractory to therapy, or are at high risk for cardiovascular side effects.

Side effects of antidepressants

Drowsiness is not the only side effect of the antidepressants. Dry mouth, blurred vision, and constipation are common, even at relatively low doses. These anticholinergic responses can be ameliorated by time and slow increases in dose.

Cardiovascular changes are sometimes seen in children using heterocyclic compounds, including heterocyclic antidepressants. These

Antidepressant treatment for adolescent headache

A 14-year-old female is referred to the Pain Management Center for evaluation of chronic headache. After a thorough evaluation, including psychological screening and a complete physical examination, a treatment plan is formulated, including relaxation training, physical therapy, and amitriptyline. Her baseline ECG appears normal. A single daily dose of 25 mg amitriptyline at bedtime is started, and the patient is scheduled for a follow-up visit in 2 weeks.

At that time, the patient reports dry mouth and constipation but no drowsiness. The headaches have improved but are still bothersome. Her amitriptyline dosage is increased to 50 mg at bedtime, and she is advised to increase the fiber in her diet. At the next visit, she is headache-free and reports minimal side effects from her medication. The amitriptyline is continued for 6 months, during which time she is headache-free. The dose is weaned over 6 weeks, and the patient continues headache-free after 1 year.

children are usually asymptomatic, but there is now some concern over the risk of malignant arrhythmias in patients. There are numerous case reports of deaths of children in which TCAs and other antidepressants have been implicated. Many experts now suggest a baseline ECG prior to the implementation of antidepressant therapy and further close monitoring if treatment is prolonged or if doses are above those usually recommended.

Abrupt withdrawal from antidepressants may produce alterations in mood, appetite changes, disturbances of the sleep cycle, or GI symptoms. These problems may be ameliorated by slow tapering of the drug dose. (See *Antidepressant treatment for adolescent headache.*)

Anticonvulsants

Certain pain syndromes are unresponsive to opioids and other similar analgesic compounds. Neuropathies caused by trauma, disease, or drugs produce dysesthetic pain that is extremely difficult to treat. Fortunately, certain compounds unrelated to the usual analgesics have been found effective in the treatment of these disorders. Anticonvulsants such as diphenylhydantoin (Dilantin) and carbamazepine (Tegretol) are known to suppress aberrant neurologic activity in the periphery as well as in the CNS. This action occurs without the sedation associated with opioids and is relatively dose-dependent. (See *Anticonvulsants used in pediatric pain management.*)

Anticonvulsants used in pediatric pain management

Agent	Daily dosage (mg/kg/day)	Frequency	Side effects
Phenytoin	5	Twice daily	Gingival hyperplasia, blood abnormalities, hepatic toxicity
Carbamazepine	10	Twice daily	Blood abnormalities, hepatic toxicity

Hematologic side effects of the anticonvulsants may occasionally limit their use in patients with chronic neuropathies. A baseline complete blood count as well as frequent follow-up checks will identify dose-dependent suppression of bone marrow hematopoiesis. Hepatic toxicity is also dose-dependent and can be evaluated by periodic tests of liver function and destruction. It is reasonable to assess indices of toxicity every other month in patients who are stable. (See *Anticonvulsant therapy for a child*, page 366.)

Local anesthetics

Some pain syndromes, such as reflex sympathetic dystrophy and certain neuropathies, are difficult to treat, especially if they are well established. Many drugs have failed to reduce appreciably the pain level in patients with these processes. One class of drugs, the local anesthetic agents, have been found useful in some patients. For example, intravenous infusions of lidocaine have been found to be useful in treating patients with diabetic or toxic neuropathy (see *Lidocaine for a young adult*, page 367). After confirmation of a therapeutic effect obtained via intravenous infusion, patients usually require transition to an oral medication in the same class. Though this technique is not widely reported in pediatric patients, it has been demonstrated to be safe and effective in adults. Values for serum therapeutic levels in infants and children are readily available.

Analgesic properties of the local anesthetic agents may be related to their ability to desensitize peripheral receptors. These receptors may have been damaged by metabolic processes or drugs and may fire abnormally in response to no identified stimulus. The toxicity of the local anesthetics themselves can be monitored by physical assessment of the patient and evaluation of serum drug levels. This ability to correlate serum levels with clinical effect makes the local anesthetics a drug of choice for refractory chronic pain associated with peripheral neuropathy.

📁   **PATIENT HISTORY**

Anticonvulsant therapy for a child

A 10-year-old with acute lymphocytic leukemia comes to the Pain Management Center for evaluation and treatment of pain associated with his disease. The child describes areas of numbness and tingling in both feet in the same distribution as his socks. He also complains of lancinating pain from hip to foot bilaterally. This pain is debilitating and he has been unable to attend school. His physical examination reveals decreased reflexes in his lower extremities. There is no point tenderness over his spine or in the periphery. The straight leg raise test is negative.

This child suffers from peripheral neuropathy probably caused by vincristine, a chemotherapeutic agent commonly used in children with acute lymphocytic leukemia. After a baseline complete blood count (CBC) and liver function tests, the child is started on carbamazepine 50 mg twice a day. This dose is ineffective in reducing his dysesthetic pain and the dose is increased to 75 mg after 1 month. Repeat CBC and liver function tests are done at 1 and 3 months. The child feels much better after 2 months and, because his pain has decreased, he is able to resume school and rejoin his peers.

Neuroleptic agents and alpha agonists

Certain neuroleptic agents have been used as analgesics in children, although it is difficult to separate their efficacy in pain relief from their intrinsic sedative properties. Clinicians may utilize drugs in this class after the failure of other agents in patients with chronic and severe pain. Methotrimeprazine is probably the drug most commonly used in this way. It is a phenothiazine derivative and has been reported to have an analgesic efficacy similar to morphine. In addition to its putative analgesic action, methotrimeprazine has an intrinsic antiemetic property, which is especially useful in cancer patients and others with intractable vomiting. Significant side effects, such as tardive dyskinesia, hypotension, or dysphoria, may limit the use of this drug.

Central alpha adrenergic receptor agonists, such as clonidine, have recently shown promise as analgesics for chronic and acute pain. Alpha agonists act at alpha-adrenergic receptor sites in the spinal cord and can be administered via the oral, transcutaneous, or spinal route. Hypotension may limit the use of clonidine as a primary analgesic. Data on the use of this drug in children is limited.

Capsaicin, the active ingredient in hot peppers, has been used as a local analgesic agent in patients suffering from herpes zoster and arthritis. It is thought that this compound derives its effect from depleting substance P from tissues in the area of painful lesions. Substance P is thought to be an important mediator of pain in some circumstances. A significant reduction in tissue levels may require

PATIENT HISTORY

Lidocaine for a young adult

A 20-year-old female presents for evaluation and treatment of severe diabetic neuropathy. The patient suffers dysesthetic pain in all extremities. This pain has been unresponsive to narcotics, tricyclics, and anticonvulsants. After a complete evaluation, a local anesthetic trial is suggested.

The patient is taken to the Post Anesthesia Care Unit and is monitored during I.V. infusion of lidocaine. An initial bolus of 100 mg lidocaine is given, followed by an infusion of 2 mg/minute for 2 hours. The infusion is then discontinued. The extremity pain improves during the infusion and for about 12 hours afterward.

The patient returns to the Pain Clinic 2 weeks later for follow-up. Because of the relative success of the initial infusion, the patient is once again infused with lidocaine. This infusion also reduces the pain level with no apparent side effects. The patient is started on oral procainamide with monitoring of serum levels as an outpatient. The patient's pain is reduced significantly over the next 6 weeks, and the procainamide is weaned over the ensuing 6 months.

weeks of treatment. Initial treatment with this compound is often complicated by its local toxicity.

Coanalgesia

Opioid compounds have been used as primary analgesic agents since prehistory primarily because of their potency and lack of a ceiling effect. Unfortunately, the side effects of this class of drugs sometimes severely limit their use. Nausea, constipation, sedation, and respiratory depression are common when high doses are used and are especially troublesome in patients who require chronic treatment. In addition, certain pain syndromes are not responsive to opiates. For example, posttraumatic and metabolic neuropathies, reflex sympathetic dystrophy, and migraine headache can often remain unimproved with narcotics.

For these reasons, it is often necessary to use low doses of multiple analgesic agents in order to reduce opioid side effects or enhance the total analgesic potential of the pharmacologic regimen. The use of multiple analgesic agents, referred to as *coanalgesia*, may provide additive or synergistic drug effects as well as reduce side effects.

Examples of coanalgesia are familiar to most clinicians (see *Coanalgesia for a patient with hemophilia*, page 368). Fixed-dose combinations, such as acetaminophen with codeine and buffered aspirin with caffeine, are commonly used and are more potent than the individual parent compounds. The addition of nonsteroidal com-

---

Coanalgesia for a patient with hemophilia

An HIV-positive 20-year-old with hemophilia A is referred to the Pain Management Center for treatment of leg and abdominal pain. The patient complains that he is always tired and suffers from pain in all of his extremities, his abdomen, and his back. Initial evaluation reveals an elevated amylase indicative of significant pancreatitis as well as indications of peripheral neuropathy. Because of his advanced pancreatic disease, narcotic compounds are felt to be appropriate as analgesics. A patient-controlled analgesia device is utilized with hydromorphone as the agent. Amitriptyline (25 mg at bedtime) is started to combat the neuropathy, and acetaminophen is administered around the clock. The combination of these three agents is effective in reducing his pain level and improving his sleep pattern while not producing excessive side effects. The patient is discharged on this regimen and is followed subsequently as an outpatient.

---

pounds to an analgesic regimen that includes PCA usually reduces narcotic consumption and often reduces nausea, vomiting, itching, and urine retention. Occasionally, multiple nonnarcotic analgesics can be used simultaneously in order to provide relief in either acute pain or chronic pain syndromes. Such use may be especially important in helping to avoid narcotic usage in patients with chronic non-malignant pain.

Nonpharmacologic approaches

Numerous other modalities are available for the treatment of pain in children. Hypnosis, acupuncture, acupressure, guided imagery, and massage are extremely effective in reducing the levels of narcotics or other drugs that are necessary for the treatment of acute or chronic pain. Hypnosis and guided imagery reduce stress and increase pain tolerance. Physical modalities, such as exercise, heat or cold application, massage, may act by reducing nociceptive input at the spinal cord or by increasing the production of endogenous opioids. Individual and group psychotherapy, family therapy, and patient or family education are also integral parts of successful management of chronic pain. For information, see Chapter 5, Psychological Aspects of Pain, and Chapter 6, Noninvasive Techniques for Managing Pain.

Practitioners of physical and occupational therapy are important in the treatment of children with pain, especially chronic pain. Often the patient loses significant function as a result of pain. Physical assessment prior to therapy and follow-up with exercise, stress reduction, and skill-building during the course of therapy greatly improve the chances of functional development. In adult pain management, physical and occupational therapy interact to produce "work hardening." For children, work hardening means progressive improvement in physical function so that return to school and normal social life is possible.

Managing the pain of medical procedures

The pain associated with medical procedures represents a major public health problem in the United States. Pediatric practitioners now almost routinely consider the impact of surgical incisions on infants and children but may deny the stress and pain associated with a bone marrow biopsy or a lumbar puncture. Mechanisms are available to improve the lot of children forced to undergo these procedures. Unfortunately, the knowledge base required to adequately assess and treat these children is sometimes not readily available.

The management of painful procedures in children requires knowledge of the child's history and developmental level. Children with long-standing disease may not tolerate what appear to be relatively benign diagnostic procedures without decompensating. This is often true of the 3- to 5-year old but may also occur in the adolescent. Thus, the levels of pharmacologic intervention required for pain management for these children will vary greatly, depending on individual history.

Pharmacologic management of painful procedures may include the use of local anesthetic agents for the placement of I.V. catheters, the use of potent anxiolytic agents, and the use of general anesthetic agents. For example, the Eutetic Mixture of Local Anesthetics (or EMLA) that is commonly absorbed through the skin is also available as a cream. This compound, when placed on the skin one hour prior to the procedure, allows an I.V. catheter to be placed without pain. Midazolam, a potent drug in the benzodiazepine class, provides amnesia to all but the most stressful events. Propofol , a general anesthetic agent, is as potent as the short-acting barbituate thiopental, and yet it allows early recovery with no drug hangover. Certainly, the use of these medications requires appropriate monitoring and proper attention to details of airway management. As before, the amount of drug required and thus the level of sedation produced often depend on developmental assessment and timely psychological and behavioral intervention before the procedure begins.

Behavioral management

Behavioral approaches to the management of procedural pain may be as important as pharmacologic intervention. Behavioral techniques rely heavily on knowledge of developmental psychology and the use of age-appropriate interventions. For example, a two-year-old patient may be coaxed into the treatment room through the judicious use of bubbles, talking books, and puppets. Distraction techniques along with appropriate local analgesia may allow placement of I.V. lines or other procedures while the child is otherwise engaged. Parents may be extremely helpful in this regard and can be instructed in the use of simple distraction techniques.

Of note is the child with chronic disease or the child who has had numerous diagnostic or therapeutic procedures. Many of these children regress to a lower developmental level under the stress of medical intervention and may decompensate with what appears to the clinician to be minimal pain. These patients require individual consideration. Parents can often assist greatly in devising behavioral strategies to help these children cope.

Pain treatment for infants

The management of pain in newborns and infants received public attention in the 1970s as the lay press and medical care providers began to recognize the physiologic maturity of the neonatal nervous system. Subsequent treatments of the subject by Eland and others revealed a lack of knowledge of the impact of pain on the well-being of infants (Eland and Anderson 1977). Suggestions of possible treatment protocols for infantile surgical procedures such as circumcision were met with skepticism. Unfortunately, outcome studies revealing reductions in morbidity and mortality were not and are not now available. One original report by Anand et al. appeared to demonstrate improvements in mortality in critically ill newborns after cardiac surgery. In this study, patients in which the stress response was reduced postoperatively with infusions of potent narcotics did better than those who received conventional therapy (1992). Because of methodological issues relating to the analysis of this data, the conclusions of this study have been called to question.

Pain assessment is a major issue in the management of pain in infants. Validated pain scales are available but lack of familiarity with them has minimized their use. In the late 1980s, Attia and colleagues produced a multidimensional neonatal pain scale that has served as a platform for many of the subsequent attempts to define a pain scale for infants.

Pain scales for infants rely heavily on aberrations in physiologic parameters as indicators of stress. Changes in pulse rate, blood pressure, and oxygen saturation of the blood continue to be the major diagnostic features in the management of pain in the neonate.

Procedural pain in infants

The treatment of pain is, of course predicated on diagnosis. Fortunately, much of the pain suffered by neonates and infants is related to operative procedures and can be well treated by the judicious use of local anesthetics. Penile blocks for circumcision, caudal epidurals for hernia repairs and surgical procedures on the lower extremities, as well as the careful use of other techniques of regional analgesia have revolutionized the postoperative management of the infant. The use of local anesthetics blocks the pain of surgical incisions for hours after the procedure is finished. Available evidence suggests that the routine use of local anesthesia prior to the incision may prevent pain input to the CNS from ever reaching the intensity that would obtain without it.

In considering the use of these techniques, attention must be paid to the unique characteristics of infantile pharmacokinetics. These patients bind local anesthetic poorly and have a reduced ability to metabolize drugs. Elevated levels of local anesthetics can occur rapidly with resultant cardiovascular depression and central nervous system excitation. Seizure and cardiopulmonary arrest have been reported, and strict guidelines for dosage should be followed.

The use of narcotics in neonates requires skill and attention to the details of monitoring. Narcotic compounds are cleared more slowly in newborns than in older children, probably due to hepatic immaturity. Healthy 6-month olds, however, attain near-adult clearance levels. The periods of observation required for these patients vary with age, size, acuity of illness, and ability of the liver to metabolize the drug.

Pain control for premature neonates is as important an issue as it is for full-term neonates. The ability to diagnose pain, however, is reduced by the lack of validated pain scales, lack of information concerning the development of the CNS, and fear that treatment will produce a bad outcome. Information regarding analgesic usage versus treatment outcome in premature neonates is slow in coming, but premature neonates routinely undergo procedures that would cause pain in children and adults. It seems reasonable to assume that these infants experience pain associated with medical procedures. Attention to issues of pharmacokinetics and individual toxicities of medications should be considered in the management of these patients.

Management of chronic pain in children

Headache, abdominal pain, and low back pain occur in children as they do in adults. These and other entities, when present for 6 months or longer, constitute chronic pain. Chronic pain can be considered as important a health problem of childhood as cystic fibrosis or asthma.

The impact of chronic pain in childhood

Adults with chronic pain often manifest their difficulties by job loss or inability to maintain employment. Children reveal the impact of chronic pain by behavior changes and school absences. These absences, unfortunately, are not as easily translated into economic terms as are the loss of work days by adults. That reduces the perceived impact of chronic pain, even though it does not reduce the morbidity.

Because of the impact of chronic pain on the child, parent, and family a multidisciplinary approach to management is optimal. Psychologists, social workers, nurses, and physical therapists should all participate in determining how the disease process has affected the family. Psychological assessment is extremely important in these patients. The development of depression is a well-known component of chronic pain in adults; there is little reason to believe that this should not be a problem in children also. Parental stress is often superimposed on the family because of the need for complex medical care and the lack of available health care resources. Siblings may require counseling because the presence of a child with chronic pain produces family rivalries that are deep-seated and destructive.

The pharmacologic treatment of children with chronic pain varies with the particular disease process. It is important to consider, however, the presence or absence of narcotic analgesics in the treatment regimen. Although often appropriate for acute pain, narcotics are rarely appropriate for the treatment of chronic pain disorders. The constellation of side effects renders these drugs less than effective in the management of chronic pain. In addition, the probability of the development of addiction, while not high, is documented in adults and should have a similar epidemiological distribution among chilren. The use of nonnarcotic analgesics as well as the use of nonpharmacological methods are often effective in the management of chronic pain in children.

REFERENCES

Anand, K.J., et al. "Halothane-Morphine Compared with High-Dose Sufentanil for Anesthesia and Postoperative Analgesia in Neonatal Cardiac Surgery," *New England Journal of Medicine* 326(1):1-9, January 2, 1992.

Anand, K.J., et al. "Randomized Trial of Fentanyl Anesthesia in Preterm Babies Undergoing Surgery: Effects on the Stress Response," *Lancet* 1:62-66, January 10, 1987.

Berde, C.B., et al. "Pediatric Pain Management," *Pediatric Anesthesia,* vol. 2, 2nd ed. Edited by Gregory, G.A. New York: Churchill Livingstone, 1989.

Berman, D.,et al. "The Evaluation and Management of Pain in the Infant and Young Child with Cancer," *British Journal of Cancer* 66(Suppl. 18):S84-S91, August 1992.

Beyer, J.E., et al. "Patterns of Postoperative Analgesic Use with Adults and Children Following Cardiac Surgery," *Pain* 17(1):71-81, September 1983.

Bhatt-Mehta, V., and Rosen, D.A. "Management of Acute Pain in Children," *Clinical Pharmacy* 10(9):667-85, September 1991.

Bramwell, R.G.B., et al. "Caudal Block for Postoperative Analgesia in Children," *Anaesthesia* 37(10):1024-28, October 1982.

Brill, J.E. "Control of Pain," *Critical Care Clinics* 8(1):203-18, January 1992.

Dalens, B., et al. "Lumbar Epidural Anesthesia for Operative and Postoperative Pain Relief in Infants and Young Children," *Anesthesia & Analgesia* 65(10):1069-73, October 1986.

Eland, J.M., and Anderson, J.E. "The Experience of Pain in Children," in *Pain: A Sourcebook for Nurses and Other Health Professionals.* Edited by Jacox, A.K. Boston: Little Brown & Co., 1977.

Gaukroger, P.B. "Paediatric Analgesia: Which Drug? Which Dose?" *Drugs* 41(1):52-59, January 1991.

Hertzka, R.E., et al. "Are Infants Sensitive to Respiratory Depression from Fentanyl?" *Anesthesiology* 67:A512, 1987.

Hollingworth, P. "The Use of Non-Steroidal Anti-Inflammatory Drugs in Paediatric Rheumatic Diseases," *British Journal of Rheumatology* 32(1):73-77, January 1993.

Lindsley, C.B. "Uses of Nonsteroidal Anti-Inflammatory Drugs in Pediatrics," *American Journal of Diseases of Children* 147(2):229-36, February 1993.

Lloyd-Thomas, A.R. "Pain Management in Paediatric Patients," *British Journal of Anaesthesia* 64(1):85-104, January 1990.

Lynn, A.M., and Slattery J.T. "Morphine Pharmacokinetics in Early Infancy," *Anesthesiology* 66(2): 136-39, February 1987.

Mather, L., and Mackie, J. "The Incidence of Postoperative Pain in Children," *Pain* 15(3):271-82, March 1983.

Maunuksela, E. "Nonsteroidal Anti-Inflammatory Drugs in Pediatric Pain Management," in *Pain in Infants, Children, and Adolescents.* Edited by Schechter, N.L., et al. Baltimore: Williams & Wilkins, 1993.

Maxwell, L.G., et al. "Penile Nerve Block Reduces the Physiologic Stress of Newborn Circumcision," *Anesthesiology* 63:A432, 1986.

Miser, A.W., and Miser, J.S. "The Treatment of Cancer Pain in Children," *Pediatric Clinics of North America* 36(4):979-99, August 1989.

Naito, Y., et al. "Responses of Plasma Adrenocorticotropic Hormone, Cortisol, and Cytokines during and after Upper Abdominal Surgery," *Anesthesiology* 77(3):426-31, September 1992.

Owen, M.E., and Todt, E.H. "Pain in Infancy: Neonatal Reaction to a Heel Lance," *Pain* 20(1):77, September 1984.

Pollack, M.H., and Rosenbaum, J.F. "Management of Antidepressant-Induced Side Effects: A Practical Guide for the Clinician," *Journal of Clinical Psychiatry* 48(1):3-8, January 1987.

Ptefferbaum, B., and Hagberg, C.A. "Pharmacological Management of Pain in Children," *Journal of the American Academy of Child and Adolescent Psychiatry* 32(2):235-42, March 1993.

Schechter, N.L., et al. "Status of Pediatric Pain Control: Comparison of Hospital Analgesic Use in Children and Adults," *Pediatrics* 77(1):11-15, June 1986.

Shapiro, B.S., et al. "Experience of an Interdisciplinary Pediatric Pain Service," *Pediatrics* 88(6):1226-32, December 1991.

Waldman, S.D., and Kilbride, M.J. "The Nonsteroidal Anti-inflammatory Drugs—Current Concepts," *Pain Digest* 2:289-94, 1992.

Williamson, P.S., and Williamson, M.L. "Physiologic Stress Reduction by a Local Anesthetic During Newborn Circumcision," *Pediatrics* 71(1):36-40, January 1983.

Yaster, M., and Deshpande, J.K. "Management of Pediatric Pain with Opioid Analgesics," *The Journal of Pediatrics* 113(3):421-29, September 1988.

CHAPTER 12

Care of elderly patients with pain

Betty R. Ferrell, RN, PhD, FAAN

Bruce A. Ferrell, MD, FACP

Although pain management is an integral component of geriatric care, it is a frequently undertreated problem. Pain is commonly thought to be a normal part of aging, so appropriate pain management is not viewed as an urgent geriatric care need. The elderly suffer significant pain problems associated with increased risks for functional impairment and decreased quality of life. The barriers that make pain assessment and management particularly challenging in the elderly include a high frequency of cognitive impairment, including dementia, ineffective communication, multiple medical diagnoses and pain problems, and increased sensitivity to drug side effects (Ferrell, B.A. 1991).

The risk for undertreatment of pain in elderly people is similar to that seen in pediatric patients. Although frail elderly patients are more sensitive to side effects associated with opioids and adjuvant pain management medications, they still require aggressive diagnostic evaluation and management of pain. Many pain problems can be sucessfully managed through more careful use of analgesic drugs combined with common nonpharmacologic strategies, including exercise programs and other physical therapies. Structured education in pain management and systematic, routine pain assessment of elderly patients are needed to improve the management of pain in geriatric settings. Interdisciplinary involvement in pain management is critical to address the many facets of the pain problem in the elderly.

Despite recent medical progress in diagnosis and alteration of specific biological processes, geriatric medicine remains unable to cure most chronic illnesses. Many elderly people undergo futile efforts to prolong life, while supportive care to improve quality of life is not provided. Elderly patients and their families often believe pain is expected to accompany aging and that complaining may have negative effects on to their care (Ferrell, B.A. et al. 1990). It is also important to acknowledge that the primary caregiver for an elderly patient in pain is often an elderly spouse with chronic medical problems.

Effective pain management has important implications for improving the functional status and quality of life of elderly patients and reducing the caregiving burden of family members (Ferrell, B.R., et al., *Postgraduate Medical Journal*, 1991). Unfortunately, the elderly have been largely excluded from pain research and are also an often neglected population when it comes to the design of clinical services. This chapter presents an overview of pain evaluation and management in elderly patients across a variety of settings, including nursing homes, home care, and acute care settings.

Elderly patients as a vulnerable population

Pain is a multidimensional experience, usually initiated by sensory stimuli, then modified by individual memory, expectations, emotions, and behavior. Neuroanatomic and neurochemical findings indicate an overwhelmingly complex central nervous system (CNS) for nociception and psychological responses to painful stimuli (Wall and Melzack 1990; Wall, R.T. 1990). Age-related changes in pain sensation have been proposed to occur (Wall, R.T. 1990; Harkins and Price 1992; Melding 1991). Elderly people are known to present with painless myocardial infarctions and intra-abdominal catastrophes (Bayer et al. 1986; Barsky et al. 1990; Bender 1989; Norman and Yoshikawa 1983). Whether these clinical observations result from altered pain reporting as opposed to age-related changes in pain receptors, nerve transmission, or CNS processing remains to be proven.

Studies using a variety of methods to induce pain experimentally in volunteers have shown mixed results (Ferrell, B.A. 1991; Harkins et al. 1984). Moreover, the clinical relevance of these studies remains questionable because experimentally induced pain may not be analogous to the experience of disease-associated pain. In the final analysis, the widespread belief of many clinicians that aging results in decreased pain sensitivity or increased pain tolerance lacks scientific support.

The Agency for Health Care Policy and Research identified elderly patients as a population at risk for undertreatment of acute pain, postoperative pain, and cancer-related pain. (Acute Pain Management Guideline Panel, 1992). These guidelines point out that most pain management research has systematically excluded elderly subjects and that relatively little attention has been paid to the topic of pain management in elderly populations in medical and nursing textbooks or in medical and nursing school curricula. Thus, substantial research and education are needed to manage this special population more successfully.

Epidemiology of geriatric pain

Clinical experience suggests that pain is common in elderly people. Population-based studies have estimated 25% to 50% of community-dwelling elderly people suffer significant pain problems (Ferrell, B.A. 1991; Crook et al. 1984). A 1984 Canadian study reported that 16% of people from a randomly selected sample of Ontario households had significant pain problems. In this study, the morbidity of pain was twofold higher in those over age 60 (250 per 1,000) compared with those younger (125 per 1,000) (Crook et al. 1984).

The overall prevalence of pain has been reported to be as high as 45% to 80% in the nursing home setting (Ferrell, B.A. et al. 1990; Roy and Michael 1986; Lau-Ting and Phoon 1988). A sample of 92 residents from a single multilevel care facility found that almost 25% complained of constant or continuous pain, and 47% reported intermittent pain, over half of whom reported pain on a daily basis. The sources of pain observed included low back pain (40%), previous fracture sites (14%), neuropathies (11%), leg cramps (9%), and claudication (8%). Of these patients, 36% described more than one source of pain, with a median of five medical problems (Ferrell, B.A. et al. 1990). The majority of pain complaints in the nursing home are probably related to arthritis and musculoskeletal problems, particularly degenerative arthritis and low back pain (Ferrell, B.A. et al. 1990; Lau-Ting and Phoon 1988; Davis 1988).

Cancer is also a source of severe pain in the elderly population. Most forms of cancer are more common in elderly people. In all cancer patients, one-third to one-half of those undergoing active treatment have pain, and among those with advanced disease, two-thirds have severe pain (Foley 1985).

A number of other specific pain syndromes are known to affect this population disproportionately, including peripheral vascular disease, herpes zoster, temporal arteritis, and polymyalgia rheumatica (National Institutes of Health 1979). Other common pain problems in the elderly include leg cramps, headaches, and diabetic neuropathies (Ferrell, B.A. et al. 1990; Parmelee et al. 1991).

Consequences of geriatric pain

The consequences of pain are, of course, also widespread among the elderly. Depression, decreased socialization, sleep disturbance, impaired ambulation, and increased health care utilization and costs have all been associated with the presence of pain (Ferrell, B.A. et al. 1990; Parmelee et al. 1991; Lavsky-Shulan et al. 1985). Deconditioning, gait disturbances, falls, slow rehabilitation, polypharmacy, cognitive dysfunction, and malnutrition are among the many geriatric conditions potentially worsened by the presence of pain (Ferrell, B.A. 1991). These facts highlight the need to recognize pain as a complication with substantial potential to disrupt treatment goals and overall quality of life for the elderly.

Assessment of pain in elderly patients

One of the challenges of pain management in the elderly is adequate assessment. Accurate pain assessment begins with asking about pain, believing patients' responses, and taking pain complaints seriously. Multiple concurrent illnesses, underreporting of pain, and the prevalence of cognitive impairment make pain evaluation much more difficult among the elderly than among other adult populations. Moreover, the absence of diagnostic facilities in settings such as nursing homes often complicates comprehensive evaluation of pain (Ouslander 1989).

Assessment of any pain complaint should begin with a thorough history and physical examination. Because pain management often relies on management of underlying disease, the importance of establishing a medical diagnosis cannot be overemphasized. For frail elderly patients, any history of trauma should be thoroughly evaluated because of the increased likelihood of occult fractures and other injuries (Ferrell, B.A. and Ferrell, B.R. 1989).

Elderly patients may present special problems in obtaining an accurate pain history. Many elderly patients don't complain despite having severe pain that affects their mood and functional status. They may think pain is to be expected with aging, or they may fear the meaning of pain. For cancer patients, pain is a metaphor for advancing disease and approaching death (Ferrell, B.R. et al., *Oncology Nursing Forum*, 1991). Patients often believe that their pain cannot be relieved or that they may avoid being labeled a "complainer" because of potential negative effects on their overall care (Ferrell, B.A. et al. 1990). In developing pain histories of elderly patients, it is essential to consult the nursing staff and family caregivers, for the observations and comments of those familiar with patients provide invaluable information.

Cognitive impairment

It has been estimated that more than 3% to 15% of community-dwelling elderly people and 50% of nursing home residents have substantial cognitive impairment or dementia (Kane et al. 1989; Ouslander et al. 1991). Pain-assessment instruments such as visual analog scales, word descriptor scales, and numerical scales, while helpful among younger patients, have not been validated in elderly populations. The high prevalence of cognitive, visual, hearing, and motor impairments may impede the direct adaptation of many of these instruments to the elderly. Behavioral scales based on facial grimace and posturing have been investigated in preverbal children, but have not been well established for clinical use in elderly patients who cannot provide a verbal report of pain.

Clinical observations and ongoing research indicate that most nursing home residents with mild to moderate cognitive impairment can report present pain intensity. Recent tests have been made of five unidimensional pain-intensity scales (word descriptor scales, a visual analog scale, and a graphic rating scale) in 134 cognitively impaired nursing home residents who were in pain (Ferrell, B.A. et al. 1995). The scales had been previously established as valid for younger patients. The nursing home residents demonstrated moderate to severe cognitive impairment as evidenced by an average score of 12.1 on the Folstein Mini–Mental Status (normal score being greater than 24 out of a possible 30 points). The Folstein Mini–Mental Status Examination is a multidimensional mental status scale widely used in the geriatric population to screen and evaluate the severity of dementia or delirium.

Results of the tests suggest that even though only one-third of the patients in pain could complete all of the pain-intensity scales, 83% of subjects could complete at least one of the scales. This research does indicate limitations in the ability of cognitively impaired patients to recall, integrate, and report pain intensity over preceding days or weeks. These observations may indicate the need for a systematic approach that involves frequent monitoring of pain rather than relying on patients' recall of pain.

Psychological evaluation

Psychological evaluation should be conducted in elderly patients because of the psychological sequelae that often accompany chronic pain (Parmelee et al. 1991). Most patients with chronic pain will have substantial depressive symptoms at some time and may benefit dramatically from psychological or psychiatric intervention. Likewise, anxiety may be an important psychological factor in the management of chronic pain. However, care must be taken to avoid attributing pain to depression or psychogenic causes.

Clinical experience suggests that psychogenic pain (pain for which no pathologic process can be identified other than psychological origins) is unusual in elderly patients. More often, such patients have multiple potential sources of pain, and care must be taken to avoid attributing pain only to preexisting illness. Making this problem worse is the fact that chronic pain is not usually constant. Its character and intensity fluctuate with time. Pain associated with trauma as well as with acute disease, such as gout and calcium pyrophosphate crystal diseases, are easily overlooked. Only astute questioning and comprehensive evaluation can avoid these pitfalls.

Physical findings and functional status

Physical examinations should include focus on the musculoskeletal and nervous systems, with special attention given to palpating for trigger points and inflammation. Trigger points may result from tendinitis, muscle strain, or nerve irritation, any of which may be treated with local injections of steroids or local anesthetics or through specific physical therapy. Maneuvers that reproduce pain, such as straight leg raising and joint motion, may be useful in diagnosis as well as in functional assessment. A thorough neurologic examination should also be conducted, including attention to signs of autonomic, sensory, and motor deficits suggestive of neuropathic conditions and nerve injuries which may require specific treatments (Ferrell, B.A. and Ferrell, B.R. 1989; Kane et al. 1989).

Evaluation of functional status is important as an outcome measure for pain management so that mobility and independence are maximized. Functional assessment may include information from histories and physical examinations as well as from several available functional assessment scales. Scales frequently used in routine geriatric evaluation include the Katz Activities of Daily Living scale or the Lawton Instrumental Activities of Daily Living scale (Rubenstein 1987). These scales have been very helpful in the care of elderly people because they have been shown to have high predictive value for dependency needs, placement in alternative care settings, and overall survival. For ambulatory patients, quality of life and engagement in advanced activities of daily living or "elective" activities, such as ambulation and psychosocial function, may be better proxy measures for evaluating the presence and severity of pain (Ferrell, B.A. 1991).

State-of-the-art diagnostic procedures and expertise may be difficult to obtain for frail elderly patients. Laboratories and other diagnostic facilities are often not accessible to those confined to home care or nursing homes. Many physicians and consultants do not make house calls or visit nursing homes because they are not sufficiently reimbursed for the time necessary for assessment and development of treatment plans for complex problems among patients confined to home or nursing homes. Physicians tending patients in these settings are sometimes tempted to send patients to emergency departments or to distant facilities for examinations and procedures. Transportation to other facilities often results in missed meals and medications, making the trip for most frail elderly people not only physically exhausting and emotionally disruptive, but also fraught with potential for iatrogenic illness. For some patients, however, short hospitalization may be appropriate for risky or highly technical procedures related to severe pain problems for the above reasons or because some home care agencies and nursing homes are just not equipped to manage acute illnesses (Ouslander 1989).

Pain-education program

Increasingly, cancer is managed on an outpatient basis, with the responsibility for pain management being assumed by the family at home. Recent research evaluated a structured pain-education program that included three components: basic pain-management principles and assessment, pharmacologic interventions, and nondrug treatments (Ferrell, B.R. et al. 1993). The pain education intervention was implemented across three home visits with two points of follow-up evaluations. Sixty-six elderly patients with cancer completed the education program that included measures of patients' quality of life, measures of knowledge and attitudes regarding pain, and use of self-care logs to document drug and nonpharmacologic interventions and their effectiveness. Results indicated improved patient understanding of the causes and effects of pain, more positive attitudes regarding the ability to self-manage pain, and better understanding of how to use both drug and nonpharmacologic interventions to control pain.

Outcomes of the quality-of-life instrument suggest that pain has significant effects on all aspects of quality of life, including physical well-being, psychological well-being, social concerns, and spiritual well-being (Ferrell, B.R. et al. 1994). The pain-education program and materials such as the self-care log are also applicable to populations other than the elderly. (See *Self-care pain-management log*, page 382, and *Pain-education program*, page 383.)

Geriatric pain management

That pain management in the elderly has received little attention is exemplified by the dirth of research and literature available in medical textbooks. Fewer than 1% of the more than 4,000 papers on the subject of pain published each year focus on pain in elderly people, and few studies have been published to describe the effectiveness of available pain management strategies in the elderly population (Melding

Self-care pain-management log

Name _____

Please use this pain assessment scale to fill out your self-care log.

NO PAIN   0   1   2   3   4   5   6   7   8   9   10   WORST PAIN

Date	Time	How severe is the pain?	How distressing is the pain?	Describe action or medicine taken	How severe is pain after 1 hour?	Comment

1991). For the most part, pharmacologic research has been limited to single-dose studies in young or middle-aged adults, and data on the actual frequencies of complications associated with most analgesic drugs in the elderly are not available (Acute Pain Management Guideline Panel 1992). Most reports from rehabilitation programs or specialized pain centers have excluded elderly subjects or have included only selected subjects such as the more mobile elderly with resources for transportation and substantial support systems (Crook et al. 1989; Sorkin et al. 1990).

Pharmacologic treatments

The control of most acute and postoperative pain relies initially on diagnosis and treatment of the underlying condition and short-term administration of analgesic drugs. Chronic pain, on the other hand,

PAIN MANAGEMENT PRINCIPLES

Pain-education program

A structured pain-education program involves the following components.

General overview of pain
- Defining pain
- Understanding the causes of pain
- Assessing pain and using pain-rating scales to communicate pain
- Using a preventive approach to controlling pain
- Involving the family in pain management

Pharmacologic management of pain
- Overview of drug management of pain
- Overcoming fears of addiction
- Fear of drug dependence

- Understanding drug tolerance
- Understanding respiratory depression
- Talking to the doctor about pain
- Controlling other symptoms, such as nausea and constipation

Nonpharmacologic management of pain
- Importance of nonpharmacologic interventions
- Use of nonpharmacologic modalities as an adjunct to medications
- Review of previous experiences with nonpharmacologic methods
- Demonstration of use of heat, cold, massage, relaxation, distraction, and imagery

may often require a multidimensional approach using a combination of nonpharmacologic interventions as well as analgesic and adjuvant drug therapies (Foley 1990). Patients with malignant pain usually respond well to constant administration of opioids (Foley 1985). However, long-term use of narcotic analgesics for chronic nonmalignant pain remains more controversial (Portenoy 1991). Neuropathic pains, such as herpes zoster and post-CVA thalamic pain, may respond initially to traditional analgesic drugs but in the long run may require adjuvant drug strategies, such as tricyclic antidepressants (TCAs), anticonvulsant therapy, or the more recently described cardiac antiarrhythmic drugs (Portenoy 1987).

In general, using a combination of both pharmacologic and non-pharmacologic techniques may result in more effective pain control with less reliance on medications that have major side effects in the elderly (Melzack 1990). Multiple trials with various combinations of drug and nondrug strategies may still be required in some cases.

The traditional approach to pain management is the use of oral analgesic medications, either opioids or nonsteroidal anti-inflammatory drugs (NSAIDs). Acetaminophen is in a separate category with analgesic and antipyretic properties but little anti-inflammatory activity and with a site of action different from most NSAIDs. A variety of other drugs, such as TCAs and anticonvulsants have been found useful for specific pain problems, such as trigeminal neuralgia, herpes zoster neuralgia, and diabetic neuralgia. These drugs have been referred to as adjuvant analgesic drugs because they have no inherent analgesic properties of their own. For the most part, they are only partially effective when used alone but are very effective as adjuncts to other pharmacologic or nonpharmacologic pain-management strategies (Ferrell, B.A. 1991).

Pain management with NSAIDs

NSAIDs act peripherally in the CNS, affecting pain receptors, nerve conduction, and inflammatory conditions that may stimulate pain (Kantor 1984). Individual drugs in this class vary widely in their analgesic properties, metabolism, excretion, and side-effect profiles. A recent study by Rochon et al. has pointed out that older people have generally been omitted from clinical trials of NSAIDs. Between 1987 and 1990, 83 randomized controlled trials consisting of over 9,600 subjects, were found to include no patients over age 85 and only 2.3% over age 65 (1993).

The analgesic activity of NSAIDs is limited by a low ceiling effect. A ceiling effect is occurrence of a certain level of analgesia at a given dosage of drug; analgesia does not increase beyond this point, even after increasing dosage. Bradley et al. have shown that in patients with chronic osteoarthritis of the knee, 4,000 mg/day of acetaminophen results in analgesia similar to that provided by ibuprofen, regardless of whether the ibuprofen is administered in an analgesic dose (1,200 mg/day) or an anti-inflammatory dose (2,400 mg/day) (1991). This study demonstrates that acetaminophen may be a better analgesic choice because of its lower side-effect profile. The study also highlighted the ceiling analgesic effect above 1,200 mg/day often seen with ibuprofen.

NSAIDs often work well when given alone or in combination with narcotic analgesics for metastatic bone pain and inflammatory conditions. However, NSAIDs have been associated with a variety of side effects in the elderly, including peptic ulcer disease, renal insufficiency, and bleeding diathesis. Among frail elderly, NSAIDs have also been reported to cause constipation, cognitive impairment, and headaches (Roth 1989). (See *Prescribing NSAIDs for elderly patients.*)

Pain management with opioids

Opioids act on the brain and spinal cord to decrease the perception of pain. Some of these drugs, including morphine, may also act as local anesthetics and have recently found widespread use in epidural administration (Morgan 1989). Opioids have no ceiling to their effects and have been shown to relieve multiple types of pain. Short-term studies have shown that elderly patients are more sensitive to the

Prescribing NSAIDs for elderly patients

Drug	Potential advantages	Potential problems	Potential solutions
Aspirin	Standard to which others are compared.	Gastric bleeding; abnormal platelet function.	Avoid high dose for prolonged periods.*
Acetaminophen	Analgesia simillar to aspirin; no gastric or platelet toxicity.	Hepatotoxic at high dose; little anti-inflammatory activity.	Keep dose to < 4 g/24 hr
Diflunisal (Dolobid)	May provide better analgesia than aspirin.	Weak anti-inflammatory activity; side-effect profile similar to other NSAIDs; requires loading dose.	Give continuously for maximum effectiveness.
Ibuprofen (Motrin)	May be superior to aspirin.	Gastric, renal, and platelet toxicity may be dose- and time-dependent; constipation, confusion, and headaches may be more common in elderly patients.	Avoid high dose for prolonged periods.*
Naproxen (Naprosyn)	Is similar to ibuprofen.	May require a loading dose; similar toxicity to ibuprofen.	Avoid high dose for prolonged periods.*
Sulindac (Clinoril)	Is similar to ibuprofen.	Similar toxicity to ibuprofen.	Avoid high dose for prolonged periods.*
Salsalate (Disalcid)	May have less gastric toxicity.	Prolonged half-life of 8 to 12 hr; similar toxicity to ibuprofen; may develop classic salicylate toxicity at high dose.	Salicylate levels may be necessary occasionally to avoid toxicity.*
Trisalicylate (Trilisate)	Has lowest side-effect profile for gastric, renal, and platelet activity; prolonged half-life (12 to 24 hours).	May have less analgesic and anti-inflammatory activity.	Avoid drug accumulation with q 24-hour dosing.
Indomethacin (Indocin)	Has more anti-inflammatory activity.	Highest incidence of gastric and other toxic effects.	Avoid entirely in elderly patients, or give minimum doses for short periods.*
Ketorolac (Toradol)	Is the only NSAID approved for parenteral use.	Has side-effect profile similar to other NSAIDs, including gastric and renal toxicity as well as antiplatelet activity.	Avoid prolonged use (longer than 2 weeks).*

* Gastric toxicity may be at least partially prevented by the concomitant use of misoprostol (Cytotec).

Adapted from Ferrell, B.A., "Pain," in *Ambulatory Geriatric Care*. Edited by Yoshikawa, T.T., et al. St. Louis: Mosby—Year Book, Inc. 1993. Used with permission.

pain-relieving properties of these drugs than are younger patients (Kaiko 1980; Bellville et al. 1971; Kaiko et al. 1982). Advanced age is associated with a prolonged drug half-life and enhanced sensitivity to opioids. Thus, elderly patients may achieve pain relief from smaller doses of opioids than do younger patients.

Opiate drugs have an increased potential to cause cognitive disturbances, constipation, and respiratory depression among elderly persons. Clinical experience suggests that opioids, like other psychoactive drugs, may produce paradoxical excitement and agitation more commonly in elderly than in younger patients. Morphine remains the standard by which all other opioids drugs are judged because its effects are the best understood and most predictable.

Thus, morphine is the opioid of choice for severe pain in elderly people (Acute Pain Management Guideline Panel, 1992; Melzack 1990). Among patients taking morphine for both malignant and nonmalignant disease, recent studies have shown that:

• Drug tolerance is usually related to worsening disease.
• Drug addiction is exceedingly rare.
• When drug dependency does occur, it is surprisingly easy to manage (Melzack 1990).

This does not imply that morphine and other opioids can be used indiscriminately, only that dependency and other side effects do not justify withholding effective therapy from most elderly patients.

Tolerance occurs to some of the side effects of opioids. This may have the beneficial result of reducing the risk for respiratory depression and drowsiness. Thus, opioids as well as other analgesic drugs should be administered around the clock as opposed to on an as-needed basis whenever possible. This policy results in reduced overall drug consumption, continuous analgesia, and improved tolerance to drowsiness and respiratory depression (Melzack 1990). On the other hand, some side effects of opioids, such as constipation, do not diminish with time. Because these side effects make overall pain management more difficult, it is important to begin a bowel protocol early, when opiates are first started. Increased fluids, bulk agents, lubricating agents, and bowel stimulants may be required while opioids are administered (Ferrell, B.A. 1991).

Nausea results from direct stimulation of a chemoreceptor trigger zone in the brain. Antiemetic drugs, such as antihistamine, phenothiazine and others, have been the mainstay for preventing opioid-related nausea and vomiting. It is important to remember that elderly patients are especially sensitive to the anticholinergic side effects from these drugs, including bowel or bladder dysfunction, delirium, and movement disorders.

Prescribing opioid analgesics in elderly patients

Drug	Potential advantages	Potential problems	Potential solutions
Morphine sulfate	Standard to which others are compared; opioid of choice for severe pain.	Short half life; elderly patients are more sensitive to side effects compared with younger patients.	Start low and titrate to comfort. Give continuously (q 3 to 4 hr); avoid PRN use. Anticipate and prevent opioid side effects.
Sustained-release morphine (MS Contin)	Appears to be well tolerated in majority of elderly patients; no ceiling dose.	Potential for drug accumulation; potency and toxicity similar to plain morphine sulfate; requires short-acting drugs for breakthrough pain.	Use q 12 hr doses (q 8 hr rarely required); escalate dose slowly to avoid accumulation (daily or every other day).
Codeine (including combinations) (Tylenol #3; Empirin #3)	Weak opioid for mild to moderate pain.	NSAID or acetaminophen combinations limit maximum dose; constipation a major issue.	Avoid high doses; anticipate and prevent NSAID side effects; begin bowel program early.
Oxycodone (Percodan [oxycodone/aspirin]; Tylox [oxycodone/acetaminophen])	More potent than plain codeine; side-effect profile may be milder than codeine or other codeine derivatives.	NSAID or acetaminophen combinations limit maximum dose.	Now available uncompounded (Roxicodone); anticipate and prevent NSAID side effects; begin bowel program early.
Hydrocodone (Vicodin [hydrocodone/acetaminophen]; Lortab [hydrocodone/aspirin])	Potency similar to oxycodone.	NSAID or acetaminophen combinations limit maximum dose; toxicity similar to codeine.	Avoid high doses; anticipate and prevent NSAID side effects; begin bowel program early.
Hydromorphone (Dilaudid)	More potent than morphine.	Short half-life (3 to 4 hr). Toxicity similar to morphine.	Similar to morphine; start low and titrate to comfort; give continuously (q 3 to 4 hr); avoid PRN use. Anticipate and prevent side effects.

Source: Ferrell, B.A., "Pain," in *Ambulatory Geriatric Care*, Yoshikawa, T.T. et al., eds. St. Louis: Mosby–Year Book, 1993. Adapted with permission.

Precautions for opioid use

A variety of opioids are available and they differ widely with respect to analgesic potency and side effects among the elderly. *Prescribing opioid analgesics in elderly patients* lists precautions and recommenda-

Analgesics to avoid in elderly patients

Drug	Precautions	Potential solutions
Meperidine (Demerol)	Extremely low oral potency and short duration of analgesia compared to morphine. Metabolite, normeperidine, may accumulate and cause confusion, agitation, and seizure activity, especially among renal-impaired patients.	Choose a drug with higher oral potency. There are no advantages of either oral or parenteral meperidine over other opioids.
Pentazocine (Talwin)	Mixed opioid agonist-antagonist activity often leads to CNS excitement, confusion, and agitation.	Avoid all use in frail elderly patients.
Propoxyphene (Darvon)	Potency no better than aspirin or acetaminophen. Significant potential for dependency and renal injury.	Choose an NSAID, acetaminophen, or a more effective opioid.
Methadone (Dolophine)	Plasma half-life may be extremely prolonged in elderly people. Analgesic half-life relatively short.	Sustained-release morphine appears to be a better alternative.
Transderm fentanyl (Duragesic)	Extremely potent; tissue reservoir results in prolonged half-life; may be expensive when high dosage is required.	Avoid in opioid-naive patients.

Adapted from Ferrell, B.A. "Pain," in *Ambulatory Geriatric Care*. Edited by Yoshikawa, T.T., et al. St. Louis: Mosby–Year Book, Inc., 1993. Reprinted with permission.

tions for prescribing opioids for frail elderly patients. Because of particular problems in older persons, certain opioids should probably be avoided in the elderly (see *Analgesics to avoid in elderly patients*). Propoxyphene (Darvon) is a controversial drug that is probably overprescribed for the elderly. Reports suggest that its efficacy is no better than aspirin or acetaminophen and it has significant potential for renal injury (Beaver 1988). Pentazocine (Talwin) should be avoided because it frequently causes delirium and agitation in the elderly. This effect seems to be related to the drug's mixed agonist-antagonist opioid receptor activity (Hanks 1987).

Meperidine (Demerol) is also particularly hazardous in the elderly because of its unique toxicity in patients with renal impairment or those receiving antidepressants of the monoamine oxidase inhibitor class. The active metabolite, normeperidine, is particularly prone to accumulation and is often associated with delirium and seizure activity (Acute Pain Management Guideline Panel 1992; Kaiko et al. 1983). Methadone should also be used with caution because of its propensity to accumulate. More importantly, methadone may be a poor choice because its analgesic effect may be short compared with its serum half-life, increasing its potential for accumulation or overdosage in elderly people (Foley and Inturrisi 1987). Finally, transdermal fentanyl is an extremely potent drug (perhaps 50 times as potent as morphine) with a potential for complications (Steinberg et al. 1992). The transdermal delivery system relies on a tissue reservoir of fentanyl to produce analgesia, resulting in a serum half-life of 36 hours (Payne 1992). Because of the extreme potency and potential for overdosage, this drug should not be used in opioid-naive elderly patients or those unaccustomed to the respiratory depression of opioids.

Pain management with adjuvant analgesics

Adjuvant analgesic drugs may be helpful for some types of recalcitrant pain syndromes. It is important to remember that in most cases, these drugs are only partially successful and work best when used along with other opioids and other pharmacologic and nonpharmacologic pain management strategies. TCAs such as amitriptyline (Elavil and Enovil), may be helpful in the management of diabetic neuralgia and other neuropathic pain syndromes (Portenoy 1987). Recently, desipramine, a TCA from a different chemical class, was found to be as effective as amitriptyline for the management of diabetic neuralgia, thus offering an alternative for patients unable to tolerate the high side-effect profile of amitriptyline (Max et al. 1992). In the same study, it was noted that fluoxetine, a bicyclic antidepressant, (Prozac) was no more effective than a placebo.

As early as 1942 it was demonstrated that the antileptic drug phenytoin (Dilantin) could relive the pain of trigeminal neuralgia. Subsequently diabetic neuralgia and other neuropathies were also found to respond occasionally to other antileptic drugs, including carbamazepine, sodium valproate, and clonazepam. I.V. administered local anesthetics such as lidocaine and procaine also possess antileptic activity and are now known to have analgesic effects independent of nerve conduction blockade (Swerdlow 1988). Randomized trials have found both oral tocainide and mexiletine (lidocaine analogues used as antiarrhythmics) to be effective in trigeminal neuralgia and diabetic neuralgia respectively (Lindstrom and Lindstrom 1987; Stracke et al. 1992). Although these drugs may have serious side-effect profiles, the dosage for mexiletine may be one-half the dose traditionally used for cardiac indications (Swerdlow 1988; Stracke et al. 1992). Thus, a variety of adjuvant drugs are potentially useful for neuropathic pain syndromes recalcitrant to other forms of therapy.

Finally, capsaicin, a drug applied topically, has been shown to deplete free nerve endings of substance P by blocking its reuptake. The drug may be useful as a topical anesthetic for herpes zoster neuralgia, diabetic neuropathy, and postoperate neuropathies (Watson et al. 1988; Tandan et al. 1992; AMA Drug Evaluations Annual 1992). Although now available without a prescription, its overall efficacy for arthritis and other painful syndromes remains more controversial. A burning sensation normally caused by the drug may be intolerable to some patients and has led to speculation that a gate-control mechanism may also contribute to its action.

Guidelines for geriatric analgesia

A number of generalizations should be considered when prescribing analgesic drugs for elderly patients. Pain management for frail elderly patients must be based on a plan of care that is reasonable for the given resources and skills available. Short-acting analgesics should be prescribed for breakthrough pain or incident pain associated with physical therapy, bathing, or other potentially painful activities. Medication regimens should be as simple as possible. Long-acting analgesics provide greater duration of comfort and require fewer administrations of drugs. It is best to prevent pain by routine analgesia and avoid giving medications on an as-needed basis when possible. Treatments should be simplified so that nighttime monitoring requirements are minimized. Remember that pharmacy and formulary restrictions may result in delays in obtaining prescriptions. Develop contingency plans for pain management so that delays do not occur during medication changes or dosage adjustments. Finally, the regulations governing prescriptions for analgesic medications, such as requirements for triplicate prescriptions and limited refills, may represent substantial barriers to effective pain management for which careful planning is the only solution (Zullich et al. 1992).

Nonpharmacologic treatments

Clinical experience suggests many nonpharmacologic techniques are quite effective in individual cases. Physical methods including heat, cold, and massage should not be underestimated. These measures relax tense muscles and are soothing for a variety of complaints. Some of these techniques can be applied by patients themselves, thus providing a sense of personal control over symptoms and treatment. Precautions should be taken to avoid thermal burns from the use of either heat or ice among patients with cognitive impairment. Physical therapy directed at stretching and strengthening specific muscles and joints as well as maintenance exercise programs, available in most nursing homes, are useful in improving muscle strength, reducing muscle spasm, and fostering enhanced functional activity. Consultation and therapy with a skilled therapist, available in many nursing homes, is appropriate for safe and effective rehabilitation from many painful conditions.

Transcutaneous nerve stimulation (TENS) has been used successfully in a variety of chronic pain conditions in elderly patients (Thorsteinsson 1987). Painful diabetic neuropathies, shoulder pain or bursitis, and fractured ribs have been shown to respond to TENS therapy. Although some patients have been relieved for years, the effectiveness of TENS usually diminishes with time. Strong placebo effects have been associated with its use (Deyo et al. 1990). An important issue in the success of TENS therapy is the appropriate placement of the electrodes and the current adjustment. This involves meticulous searching, with the help of a trained physical therapist, for the best settings for each individual's optimum comfort. Also, care must be taken to avoid skin irritation and possible burns from the electrodes.

Some psychological maneuvers may be quite effective in controlling pain. Biofeedback, relaxation, and hypnosis may be helpful for some patients. These methods usually require high levels of cognitive function and therefore may not lend themselves to patients with significant impairment. A trained psychologist or therapist should be consulted for these techniques.

Finally, a variety of distractions may be effective in decreasing the perception of pain. Many patients find comfort in prayer, meditation, or music. Involvement in activities, exercise, and recreation should be encouraged to the greatest degree tolerable. Inactivity and immobility may contribute extensively to depression and increased pain.

High-technology pain management in elderly patients

Recent developments in pain management have focused on a variety of highly technical drug-delivery systems for the management of pain. Available are both external and implantable infusion pumps that can supply continuous or intermittent analgesic drug infusions via S.C., I.V., or intraspinal routes. Some pumps are fully programmable, a feature that allows patients to titrate medication within limits programmed by the physician. With appropriate supervision and education, this technology has become feasible for selected patients (Kerr et al. 1989; Hecker and Albert 1988; Morgan1989; Waldman and Coomb 1989; Sjogren and Banning 1989). A randomized trial found that patient-controlled analgesia (PCA) using morphine infusions is safe and effective for postoperative pain management among selected elderly men (Egbert et al. 1990). However, continuous morphine infusions are expensive and may cost several thousand dollars a month.

Although these procedures have been effective in selected cases, more research is needed to define expanded roles of these technologies among elderly patients. The usual approach, because of cost and potential side effects, is to consider high-tech strategies only after failure of oral medications and all other treatments. Whether these technologies have risk-benefit ratios sufficient to justify their routine use for nonmalignant pain or less intense pain syndromes needs further study. Although most of these techniques are expensive, they are often partially reimbursable by Medicare and other insurers. Unfortunately, simpler modalities such as oral medications are not reimbursable under Medicare for patients outside the acute hospital setting.

Summary and future directions

Pain is a common problem that has considerable potential to influence the physical function and quality of life of the elderly. Unfortunately, little geriatric research and education has focused on this important topic. Pain management involves the careful use of appropriate pharmacologic and nonpharmacologic pain management strategies. The incorporation of pain management into geriatric and medical education at all levels will result in long-term-care professionals who are skilled in pain management and in comforting those with chronic pain. All geriatric pain management should incorporate the standards of care given. (See *Principles of pain management in elderly patients*.)

Substantial research is needed to further the understanding of pain and its management among elderly people. Valid and reliable pain measures, such as pain-intensity scales, functional scales, and behavioral observations, need to be established for cognitively impaired people. New drugs with milder side-effect profiles are urgently needed. Nonpharmacologic pain-management strategies, such as exercise and other physical methods, should be investigated. Indications for high-tech pain management strategies, such as morphine pumps and chronic spinal infusions, need to be clarified in this population. And finally, comparative studies of the long-term outcomes of pain- management strategies are needed.

As the elderly population grows, more and more people will require effective pain management to maintain their dignity and quality of life. It is the obligation of all health care providers to do everything possible to provide comfort and effective pain management for these people during their remaining years.

PAIN MANAGEMENT PRINCIPLES

Principles of pain management in elderly patients

- Always ask elderly patients about pain. Many expect to have pain and avoid complaining.
- Accept patients' reports of pain and its intensity.
- Remember that pain is not normal with aging.
- Don't underestimate the impact of pain on quality of life in elderly people.
- Determine the underlying cause of the pain. Optimum treatment depends on accurate diagnosis.
- Treat pain before diagnostic procedures. Unrelieved pain reduces patients' tolerance for diagnostic tests.
- Use a combination of drug and nondrug interventions.
- Involve patients in pain management.

- Remember that physical and psychosocial mobility are important in treatment.
- Use analgesic drugs appropriately. Start low and go slowly with elderly patients.
- Achieve adequate doses of analgesics and anticipate side effects.
- Treat anxiety and depression as common symptoms that influence pain in elderly patients.
- Evaluate patients' response to treatment and continue assessment.
- Address elderly patients' frequent fears of addiction, tolerance, and respiratory depression.
- Involve family caregivers in the treatment plan for elderly patients.

REFERENCES

Acute Pain Management Guideline Panel. *Acute Pain Management: Operative or Medical Procedures and Trauma. Clinical Practice Guideline.* AHCPR Pub. No. 92-0032. Rockville, Md.: Agency for Health Care Policy and Research, Public Health Service, U.S. Department of Health and Human Services, February 1992.

American Medical Association. *AMA Drug Evaluations Annual.* Chicago: American Medical Association, 1995.

Barsky, A.J., et al. "Silent Myocardial Ischemia: Is the Person or the Event Silent?" *JAMA* 264(9):1132-35, September 5, 1990.

Bayer, A.J., et al. "Changing Presentations of Myocardial Infarctions with Increasing Old Age," *Journal of the American Geriatrics Society* 34(4):263-66, August 1986.

Beaver, W.T. "Impact of Nonnarcotic Oral Analgesics on Pain Management," *American Journal of Medicine* 84(5A):3-15, May 20, 1988.

Bellville, J.W., et al. "Influence of Age on Pain Relief from Analgesics," *JAMA* 217(13):1835-41, September 27, 1971.

Bender, J.S. "Approach to the Acute Abdomen," *Medical Clinics of North America* 73(6):1413-22, November 1989.

Bradley, J.D., et al. "Comparison of an Anti-Inflammatory Dose of Ibuprofen, an Analgesic Dose of Ibuprofen, and Acetaminophen in the Treatment of Patients of Osteoarthritis of the Knee," *New England Journal of Medicine* 325(2):87-91, July 11, 1991.

Crook, J., et al. "An epidemiological Follow-up Survey of Persistent Pain Sufferers in a Group Family Practice and Specialty Pain Clinic," *Pain* 36(1):49-61, January 1989.

Crook, J., et al. "The Prevalence of Pain Complaints in a General Population," *Pain* 18(3):299-314, March 1984.

Davis, M.A. "Epidemiology of Osteoarthritis," *Clinics in Geriatric Medicine* 4(2):241-55, May 1988.

Deyo, R.A., et al. "A Controlled Trial of Transcutaneous Electrical Nerve Stimulation (TENS) and Exercise for Chronic Low Back Pain," *New England Journal of Medicine* 322(23):1627-34, June 7, 1990.

Egbert, A.M., et al. "Randomized Trial of Post-operative Patient-Controlled Analgesia vs Intramuscular Narcotics in Frail Elderly Men," *Archives of Internal Medicine* 150(9):1897-1903, September 1990.

Ferrell, B.A. "Pain Management in Elderly People," *Journal of the American Geriatrics Society* 39(1):64-73, January 1991.

Ferrell, B.A., and Ferrell, B.R. "Assessment of Chronic Pain in the Elderly," *Geriatric Medicine Today* 8(5):123-34, 1989.

Ferrell, B.A., et al. "Pain in the Nursing Home," *Journal of the American Geriatrics Society* 38(4):409-14, April 1990.

Ferrell, B.A., et al. "Pain in Cognitively Impaired Nursing Home Residents," *Journal of Pain and Symptom Management* 10(8):591-98, 1995.

Ferrell, B.R., et al. "Development and Implementation of a Pain Education Program," *Cancer* 72(suppl. 11):3426-32, 1993.

Ferrell, B.R., et al. "Family Factors Influencing Cancer Pain Management," *Postgraduate Medical Journal* 67(suppl. 2):S64-S69, 1991.

Ferrell, B.R., et al. "Pain as a Metaphor for Illness. Part I: Impact of Cancer Pain on Family Caregivers," *Oncology Nursing Forum* 18(8):1303-09, November-December 1991.

Ferrell, B.R., et al. "Pain Management for Elderly Patients with Cancer at Home," *Cancer* 74(suppl. 7):2139-46, 1994.

Foley, K., and Inturrisi, C. "Analgesic Drug Therapy in Cancer Pain: Principles and Practice," *Medical Clinics of North America* 71(2):207-32, March 1987.

Foley, K.M. "Pain Management in the Elderly," in *Principles of Geriatric Medicine.* Edited by Andres, R., et al. New York: McGraw-Hill, 1985.

Foley, K.M. "The Treatment of Cancer Pain," *New England Journal of Medicine* 113(2):84-95, July 11, 1985.

Hanks, G.W. "The Clinical Usefulness of Agonist-Antagonistic Opioid Analgesics in Chronic Pain," *Drug and Alcohol Dependence* 20(4):339-46, December 1987.

Harkins, S.W., and Price, D.D. "Assessment of Pain in the Elderly," in *Handbook of Pain Assessment.* Edited by Turk, D.C., and Melzack, R. New York: The Guilford Press, 1992.

Harkins, S.W., et al. "Pain in the Elderly," in *Advances in Pain Research and Therapy,* vol. 7. Edited by Benedetti, C. New York: Raven Press, 1984.

Hecker, B.R., and Albert, L. "Patient-Controlled Analgesia: A Randomized, Prospective Comparison between Two Commercially Available PCA Pumps and Conventional Analgesic Therapy for Postoperative Pain," *Pain* 35(1):115-20, October 1988.

Kaiko, R.F. "Age and Morphine Analgesia in Cancer Patients with Postoperative Pain," *Clinical Pharmacology and Therapeutics* 28(6):823-26, December 1980.

Kaiko, R.F., et al. "Central Nervous System Excitatory Effects of Meperidine in Cancer Patients," *Annals of Neurology* 13(2):180-85, February 1983.

Kaiko, R.F., et al. "Narcotics in the Elderly," *Medical Clinics of North America* 66(5):1079-89, 1982.

Kane, R.L., et al., eds. *Essentials of Clinical Geriatrics,* 3rd ed. New York: McGraw Hill, 1994.

Kantor, T.G. "Peripherally-acting Analgesics," in *Analgesics: Neurochemical, Behavioral and Clinical Perspectives.* Edited by Kuhar, M., and Pasternak, G. New York: Raven Press, 1984.

Kerr, I.G., et al. "Continuous Narcotic Infusion with Patient-Controlled Analgesia for Chronic Cancer Pain in Outpatients," *Annals of Internal Medicine* 108(4):554-57, April 1988.

Lau-Ting, C., and Phoon, W.O. "Aches and Pains among Singapore Elderly," *Singapore Medical Journal* 29(2):164-67, April 1988.

Lavsky-Shulan, M., et al. "Prevalence and Functional Correlates of Low Back Pain in the Elderly: The Iowa 65+ Rural Health Survey," *Journal of the American Geriatrics Society* 33(1):23-28, January 1985.

Lindstrom, P., and Lindblom, U. "The Analgesic Effect of Tocainide in Trigeminal Neuralgia," *Pain* 28(1):45-50, January 1987.

Max, M.B., et al. "Effects of Desipramine, Amitriptyline, and Fluoxetine on Pain in Diabetic Neuropathy," *New England Journal of Medicine* 326(19):1250-56, May 7, 1992.

Melding, P.S. "Is There Such a Thing as Geriatric Pain?" *Pain* 46(2):119-21, August 1991

Melzack, R. "The Tragedy of Needless Pain," *Scientific American* 262(2):27-33, February 1990.

Morgan, M. "The Rational Use of Intrathecal and Extradural Opioids," *British Journal of Anaesthesia* 63(2):165-88, August 1989.

National Institutes of Health. "Pain in the Elderly: Patterns Change with Age," *JAMA* 241(23):2491-92, June 8, 1979.

Norman, D.C., and Yoshikawa, T.T. "Intra-abdominal Infections in the Elderly," *Journal of the American Geriatrics Society* 31(11):677-84, November 1983.

Ouslander, J.G. "Medical Care in the Nursing Home," *JAMA* 262(18):2582-90, November 10, 1989.

Ouslander, J.G., et al. *Medical Care in the Nursing Home.* New York: McGraw-Hill, 1991.

Parmelee, P.A., et al. "The Relation of Pain to Depression among Institutionalized Aged," *Journal of Gerontology* 46(1):15-21, January 1991.

Payne, R. "Transdermal Fentanyl: Suggested Recommendations for Clinical Use," *Journal of Pain and Symptom Management* 7(suppl. 3):S40-S44, April 1992.

Portenoy, R.K. "Chronic Opioid Therapy for Persistent Noncancer Pain: Can We Get Past the Bias?" *APS Bulletin* 1(2):1, 1991.

Portenoy, R.K. "Drug Treatment of Pain Syndromes," *Seminars in Neurology* 7(2):139-49, June 1987.

Portenoy, R.K. "Opioid Therapy for Chronic Noncancer Pain: The Issue Revisited," *APS Bulletin* 1(4):4-7, 1991.

Rochon, P.A., et al. "Reporting of Age Data in Clinical Trials of Arthritis," *Archives of Internal Medicine* 153(2):243-48, January 25, 1993.

Roth, S.H. "Merits and Liabilities of NSAID Therapy," *Rheumatic Diseases Clinics of North America* 15(3):479-98, August 1989.

Roy, R., and Michael, T. "A Survey of Chronic Pain in an Elderly Population," *Canadian Family Physician* 32:513-16, 1986.

Rubenstein, L.Z., ed. "Geriatric Assessment: An Overview of Its Impacts," *Clinics in Geriatric Medicine* 3(1):1-15, February 1987.

Sjogren, P., and Banning, A. "Pain, Sedation and Reaction Time during Long-Term Treatment of Cancer Patients with Oral and Epidural Opioids," *Pain* 39(1):5-11, October 1989.

Sorkin, B.A., et al. "Chronic Pain in Old and Young Patients: Differences Appear Less Important than Similarities," *Journal of Gerontology* 45(2):P64- P68, March 1990.

Steinberg, R.B., et al. "Acute Toxic Delirium in a Patient Using Transdermal Fentanyl," *Anesthesia and Analgesia* 75(6):1014-16, December 1992.

Stracke, H., et al. "Mexiletine in the Treatment of Diabetic Neuropathy," *Diabetes Care* 15(11):1550-55, November 1992.

Swerdlow, M. "The Use of Local Anaesthetics for Relief of Chronic Pain," *The Pain Clinic* 2(1):3-6, 1988.

Tandan, R., et al. "Topical Capsaicin in Painful Diabetic Neuropathy," *Diabetes Care* 15(1):15-18, January 1992.

Thorsteinsson, G. "Chronic Pain: Use of TENS in the Elderly," *Geriatrics* 42(12):75-77, 81-82, December 1987.

Waldman, S.D., and Coombs, D.W. "Selection of Implantable Narcotic Delivery Systems," *Anesthesia & Analgesia* 68(3):377-84, March 1989.

Wall, P.D., and Melzack, R., eds. *Textbook of Pain*, 3rd ed. London: Churchill Livingstone, 1994.

Wall, R.T. "Use of Analgesics in the Elderly," *Clinics in Geriatric Medicine* 6(2):345-64, May 1990.

Watson, C.P.N., et al. "Post-Herpetic Neuralgia and Topical Capsaicin," *Pain* 33(3):333-40, June 1988.

Zullich, S.G., et al. "Impact of Triplicate Prescription Program on Psychotropic Prescribing Patterns in Long-Term Care Facilities," *Annals of Pharmacotherapy* 26(4):539-46, April 1992.

Index

i refers to an illustration; t refers to a table.

i refers to an illustration; t refers to a table.

i refers to an illustration; t refers to a table.